# Making Babies

# Making Babies

## A PROVEN 3-MONTH PROGRAM FOR MAXIMUM FERTILITY

**Sami S. David, MD,** AND **Jill Blakeway, LAc**

**Little, Brown and Company**
NEW YORK   BOSTON   LONDON

Little, Brown and Company
Hachette Book Group
237 Park Avenue, New York, NY 10017
www.HachetteBookGroup.com

The publisher is not responsible for websites (or their content) that are not owned by the publisher.

First Edition: August 2009

The information herein is not intended to replace the services of a trained health care professional. You are advised to consult with a health care professional with regard to matters relating to your health, and in particular regarding matters that may require diagnosis or medical attention.

A complete list of references is available at www.makingbabiesprogram.com.

Little, Brown and Company is a division of Hachette Book Group, Inc. The Little, Brown name and logo are trademarks of Hachette Book Group, Inc.

Illustrations and Basal Body Temperature charts by J. Gregory Barton
Massage techniques courtesy of Rosita Arvigo, DN, and Nicole Kruck, LMT

Library of Congress Cataloging-in-Publication Data
David, Sami S.
     Making babies : a proven 3-month program for maximum fertility / Sami S. David and
Jill Blakeway. — 1st ed.
          p. cm.
     Includes index.
     ISBN 978-0-316-02450-1
     1. Conception.   2. Fertility, Human.   3. Infertility — Alternative treatment.
I. Blakeway, Jill.   II. Title.
     RG133.D38 2009
     618.1'78 — dc22                                                    2008054935

10   9   8   7   6   5

RRD-IN

Book design by Fearn Cutler de Vicq

Printed in the United States of America

To my beloved wife, Rena, who awakened and inspired my interest in the integration of Western and Eastern medicine; to my family, who encouraged me to pursue medicine as a profession; and to my mentor, the late Dr. Luigi Mastroianni, who kindled my passion for the practice of making babies.

—S.D.

To my daughter, Emma, who has been such a source of joy that I am inspired to help other women to become mothers.

—J.B.

# Contents

## Part IV: Common Fertility Problems and Solutions

## Part V: Pre-mester: The 3-Month Making Babies Program

## Part VI: Getting Pregnant with a Little Help

# Introduction

One in eight couples in the United States has trouble getting or staying pregnant — one in three couples in which the woman is over 35 and one in two in which the woman is over 40. And these figures have been on the rise for decades. Right now, more than nine million American women seek treatment for fertility issues every year, and their partners need treatment, too.

If you are reading this book, you are likely one of them. Or maybe you're just planning to get pregnant and want to be as well prepared as you can be. In any case, you are certainly not alone, and you are facing an amazing frontier. Western medicine is standing by, eager to assist you with every technological tool available, spare no expense. Just about everyone else in the world, from your grandmother and your neighbor to your yoga teacher and the celebrity you read about in *People,* has "helpful" advice for you: Do it every day. Do it every other day. Douche. Don't douche. Drink chaste tree berry tea. Drink Mountain Dew. And, the classic, "Just relax!" (Right, no problem.)

You want to do everything you can, but you want to be smart about it. You don't want to rush into expensive treatments with their inherent risks and side effects. You don't want to waste your time any more than you want to waste your money. You don't want to be guided by unproven old wives' tales, but you don't want to dismiss something that just might work either. Truth be told, you'd try just about anything if it meant having a baby.

This is just the position our patients are in. No matter whether they've sought out a reproductive endocrinologist and microsurgeon (Sami) or a Chinese medicine practitioner and integrative medicine expert (Jill), they need both optimistic messages (there are simple and effective strategies you can use) and word-to-the-wise advice (don't get drawn into in vitro fertilization, or IVF, too quickly). And whether a patient is 32 (or under) or 42 (or over), together we *can* help her get pregnant.

Our joint approach is uniquely complementary. We draw on the best of both Eastern and Western medicine, and the lessons learned from forty years of collective experience in guiding our patients (and their approximately four thousand pregnancies). This book brings what we do face-to-face in our offices in New York to women everywhere, who can now benefit from the same careful, individualized attention and personally tailored action plans. Making Babies is a three-month program designed to help any woman get pregnant *as naturally as possible*.

Infertility medicine today is all about aggressive surgical, pharmacological, and technological intervention. It's a high-stakes, high-pressure world. But making babies is still best as a natural process. So we aim to support a woman's ability to bear a child with just enough help to get nature to do its thing. What constitutes "just enough" varies from person to person, from a simple douche, a course of antibiotics, or the shedding of five or six pounds, to a few months of Chinese herbs, precisely *de*creased doses of fertility drugs, or acupuncture in conjunction with IVF. What's always the same is the fact that minimizing harsh intervention is better for the mother, better for the baby, and better for the couple. There are hundreds of thousands of families out there that exist thanks to intensive and aggressive medical intervention — and here's to them! — but for many women, there *is* a better way.

The Making Babies program is valuable for all would-be parents in their 20s, 30s, or 40s. It has all the answers you need (as well as all the questions you need to ask), whether you are only beginning to wonder what is taking so long, are just stepping into the whirlwind that is fertility medicine, or are already battle-scarred veterans — or even if you have been turned away from advanced treatments, having been told that you'll likely never bear children.

If you are trying to get pregnant — or are thinking about trying to get pregnant — you will benefit from the Making Babies program. If you have been having unprotected sex for six months but still aren't pregnant, you *need* it. If you are a woman over 35 trying to get pregnant, or if you are trying to get pregnant with a man over 40, you need it, too. Making Babies provides you with a clear path to getting pregnant with as little medical intervention as possible. We estimate that as many as half of the women who use IVF could get pregnant without it—if they receive carefully individualized care. We have absolutely nothing against using every trick of technology available to help you get pregnant. We're just against using reproductive technology unnecessarily and unwisely.

## THE PROGRAM

So before you make the huge investment (financial and otherwise) in IVF and other assisted reproductive technologies (ARTs), invest three months in the Making Babies program. We know that, like a lot of our patients, you probably feel pressured to make this thing happen. So it is our solemn promise that taking these few months will be well worthwhile.

The Making Babies program is designed to prepare your body for healthy, natural conception. Using strategies that are best for you, you can prime your body to do what comes naturally and identify and overcome common roadblocks that may be getting in the way. Detailed but easy-to-follow instructions show you how to implement lifestyle changes and early-intervention strategies. For many women, this may be all it takes: within ninety days, they'll be pregnant.

Some couples will need to continue with professional help for more intensive intervention. The program will still be a boon, optimally preparing the body for any further fertility treatment, increasing the chances of success as well as the ease with which it is achieved. These couples will enter (or reenter) the technological path to conception with their bodies physically prepared to be most receptive to the appropriate medical intervention(s), their minds open to letting nature and medicine work together without undue stress, and a step-by-step plan to pinpoint precisely—then safely, efficiently, and effectively solve—any problems blocking their way to biological parenthood. The Making Babies program expands to support the various ARTs, ensuring the best chances of success.

The Making Babies program closely follows what we do with our patients in our offices. Both innovative and time-tested, it pulls together the best of both our worlds into one comprehensive program that you can follow on your own or with your doctor or other health care practitioner.

You will learn from our patients who got pregnant after pursuing one or more of the following strategies:

- Taking antibiotics to clear up a common, asymptomatic infection in the man's sperm
- Gaining a few pounds and using herbs and acupuncture to rebalance hormones
- Thickening the endometrium with herbs and acupuncture
- Thinning cervical mucus with an over-the-counter cold remedy
- Lowering the temperature of the man's daily bath by four degrees
- Taking progesterone to stop extremely early miscarriages
- Restoring regular cycles and ovulation in a case of polycystic ovarian syndrome with a very low-carb diet and the elimination of coffee and alcohol
- Decreasing the intensity of daily workouts to limit endorphin rushes contributing to repeated extremely early miscarriages
- Douching with baking soda
- Improving sperm motility and morphology from poor to perfect by cutting out alcohol and overhauling dietary choices
- Having sex *more* often
- Having sex *less* often
- Taking steroids to block an allergic reaction to sperm
- Dramatically lowering the dose of fertility drugs used for IVF
- Using herbs and acupuncture to prepare for IVF—only to conceive naturally before the day of the IVF appointment even arrived

And of course much more. But you get the idea.

We start by giving you a look at the way fertility medicine is practiced today—and why that can be a big problem. Then we go back to basics to review how the male and female reproductive systems work—and how they work *together*—as well as everything you need to know about how, exactly, to get pregnant. (You might *think* you know everything you need to know, but we bet you'll be surprised at least in part.) The next chapter is devoted to the many lifestyle choices you make every day that have a big impact on your fertility—the type of exercise you choose, for example, your weight, the environment, and even your cell phone habits. Managing stress is the topic of the next chapter, followed by two chapters on nutrition—both what you eat and what supplements you need (and don't need).

Then comes the heart of the book: a guide to determining your specific fertility type. These types distill the complexities of Chinese medicine to the most salient factors for fertility. Simple checklists help you determine whether you are Tired, Dry, Stuck, Pale, or Waterlogged. Knowing your type lets you focus on just the issues and advice most relevant to you and your situation throughout the rest of the book and the Making Babies program. By identifying and understanding the subtle signs your body is providing, you'll be able to save yourself time, energy, money, and heartache by homing in on what you most need to be concerned about and addressing it as efficiently and effectively as possible.

The chapters that follow explain all the common (and some not-so-common) fertility problems our patients run into, the "who, how, and why" of what tests you should be having to pinpoint your issue(s), and the available (but not always necessary) ARTs you'll want to know about. We cover just about everything, but you'll have to bone up on only a handful of conditions, dictated by your type.

After all that, you'll be more than ready for the Making Babies program. The program provides both specific lifestyle advice geared toward enhancing fertility and guidance on necessary testing in one detailed plan of action, so that you can put everything into play over the course of just three months. You'll follow the version of the program specific to your fertility type. For women, there's a second layer to the program that breaks it down a bit further according to what's going on in the menstrual cycle. Tired types don't need to do the same things as Stuck types, for example. Stuck types may need to do one thing during their periods and something slightly different during ovulation to maximize the benefits of the program.

By the end of this book, you'll know:

- How to tell if you have a fertility problem (and what exactly is behind it)
- Simple yet often overlooked medical treatments that can restore fertility immediately

- Key lifestyle choices that enhance or impede fertility
- Which problems can be tackled naturally and which need to be addressed with pharmaceuticals, surgery, or advanced laboratory techniques
- When to move to the next level of treatment
- How to combine Eastern and Western approaches in a systematic and beneficial way
- How to find the likeliest path to success for you and why what works will likely be different from what worked for your neighbor, sister, or friend
- How to determine your fertility type and how your type should guide all your choices about conception
- The potential hazards of the infertility industry (which all concerned tend to choose to downplay) and the alternatives that provide a better way
- How to understand, evaluate, and prepare for the complicated problems, processes, techniques, and emotions you face when coping with a fertility issue
- A host of surprisingly simple solutions most doctors will probably never mention
- Why many women using assisted reproduction could conceive much more naturally and how you could be one of them

## TRULY COMPLEMENTARY

Within our respective fields of expertise, we have each helped countless women conceive and bear the children they've been dreaming of. But working together, we've witnessed the extraordinary benefits of a middle way. We make a great team! Taking full advantage of both approaches, we cherry-pick the best techniques according to highly individualized diagnostic procedures. Then we press them into service so that each strategy best supports all the others. Benefits begin with (but are certainly not limited to) effectiveness. To put it plainly, *more women get pregnant more easily using our combined approach than they would strictly using one or the other*. This is truly complementary medicine.

When it comes to infertility, Western medicine now routinely creates what once would have seemed like miracles. There's been a huge proliferation of options for women who are having trouble conceiving.

But these don't come without costs — of many kinds. With the wisdom of thousands of years behind it, Chinese medicine can also create what seem like miracles, but it too has its limits. Both fields tend to create more ideologues than practitioners who are open-minded enough to embrace a totally different paradigm. The Making Babies program bridges the gap between the two worlds.

Three-quarters of infertility patients seeking conventional treatments already use "alternative" approaches as well. If you are one of them, you know how hard it is to get these approaches coordinated in any meaningful way. Perhaps you've tried to discuss what else you are doing with your health care practitioner (of any stripe), only to get not much more than a polite nod in response. The Making Babies program pulls together all the best practices for you, so instead of one from column A and one from column B, you can integrate both styles so that they work together, while avoiding any counterproductive conflict.

To harness the power of both Eastern and Western traditions, you need to know how to apply them so they support and enhance each other, rather than hinder progress or even work against each other. As a layperson, you can't really do that on your own, and few and far between are the practitioners who can help you do it. Our patients seek us out for the truly integrative approach we've put down in this book. They want a comprehensive plan that takes the best of alternative medicine and combines it with the best of conventional medicine. They want help in weighing the risks and benefits of all their choices. They want to try the most natural options first. But they also need advice they can trust about when to consider ARTs. We've written *Making Babies* to do all that for everyone who can't come in to our offices.

We are proud of our reputations for helping people find their way through the complicated maze of fertility medicine with compassion and good humor, as well as careful detective work, and we've tried hard to retain all that on the written page. We hope that you, too, will appreciate what's so funny about the detailed analysis of cervical mucus, discussions of choices in scented "personal lubricants," and the mad dash home from the office for a quickie when your fertility chart tells you IT IS TIME. What we're really all about, though, is taking each and every patient seriously and recognizing him or her as an individual with his or her own particular issues that can never be adequately addressed by cookbook medicine or factory-like clinics. There's no reason for the joyous work of helping people have babies to be dreadfully dull. After all, isn't it about bringing more love into the world?

Every day, separately and together, we work through complicated cases with women from all over the country and even from around the world. And always, it is our mission to leave no stone unturned until we figure out exactly what's going on. Once we've shined a light on whatever is standing in the way of a healthy pregnancy, we do whatever it takes to get rid of the barrier, always with a focus on what's closest to how the body does it naturally.

Simply put, we have essentially one job, and one job only: to get women pregnant, often when all other methods have failed. Sometimes we even get first crack at it, as soon as it looks as if there may be a problem. Then not only do we get the deeply satisfying pleasure of helping people become parents, but we also get to save them a lot of time, effort, anxiety, risk, and heartbreak—exactly as we aim to do with *Making Babies*.

# PART ONE

# Making Babies

# CHAPTER ONE

# Modern Fertility Medicine:
# The Risks and Overuse of
# (Sometimes) Terrific Technologies

Pamela had been through ten cycles of in vitro fertilization (IVF) at three different centers but had never been pregnant. Some of the best fertility doctors in New York had told her she was too old (39) and probably had "bad eggs."

Over the course of ten years of trying to have a baby, Evelyn's doctors had pumped her up with a total of fifty cycles of fertility drugs, really strong ones. She'd made hundreds of eggs, but still she wasn't pregnant. Not one of the four doctors she'd seen had ever stopped to ask *why* she wasn't getting pregnant.

Stephanie took high doses of fertility drugs in preparation for her first IVF cycle at the best clinic in the city. The doctors harvested lots of eggs, made nine embryos, and discovered on testing that every single embryo was genetically abnormal. Although they'd been willing to give IVF a try with her, they now told her there was nothing more they could do because of her age (41).

The good news is that, in the end, all these women got pregnant and had babies. The bad news is that they underwent difficult, unnecessary, and futile treatments before anyone figured out why they weren't getting pregnant and what to do about it. The worse news is that these women are not exceptions to the rule. The way fertility medicine is practiced today routinely generates stories like these.

Reproductive technologies also create a lot of expanded families, and we never want to discount the blessing that can be. What we long for is a new era in which technological successes will be *unadulterated* blessings, because the technology will be offered and used only when it is necessary. Everyone else will be able to get the appropriate help they need to conceive and bear children as naturally as possible — because that's what's gentlest, safest, and often most effective, even in the face of some serious fertility issues.

One in 100 babies born in the United States today was conceived with the help of assisted reproductive technologies (ARTs), according to the American Society for Reproductive Medicine (ASRM). Worldwide, more than 3 million babies have been born who were conceived through IVF — more than 400,000 of them in the United States. Each year in this country, 250,000 families consider IVF, and about half of those give it a try. They do so at their pick of 461 clinics nationwide.

The numbers have skyrocketed since IVF technology was introduced three decades ago. The number of ART births more than doubled between 1996 and 2002. A Centers for Disease Control (CDC) report from 2004 counted almost 50,000 babies born after ART interventions in this country that year. Just six years earlier, the figure was 28,000 — and that was announced as evidence of the rapid growth in the use of these technologies. Over time, the nature of the industry itself has changed as dramatically as the number of babies born as a result of it, with ART morphing from an option of last resort, available to only a few, to the first choice for every player in the game.

We both celebrate regularly with patients who bring home babies thanks to amazing technological interventions, and we are always glad to do so. And we are both grateful, professionally speaking, to have something to refer patients to when our areas of expertise can't address their needs. But the sad truth underlying the good news is that ARTs, and in particular IVF, are frequently misused, grossly overprescribed, and too aggressively administered. We've arrived at this place because of a culture, both in society at large and in reproductive medicine in particular, that always goes for the quick fix regardless of other options or possible consequences, emphasizes personal gain, and values technology for its own sake. Added to that grim picture are the risks and side effects of the procedures themselves.

Based on our experience with thousands of patients coming to us in various phases of fertility treatment, as well as on what we hear from our colleagues, we estimate that as many as half of all women who receive IVF could conceive naturally or with minimal medical intervention. This is not just a theoretical best-practices argument. The consequences of fertility treatment for women, couples, and families are immense—even when they succeed. When they don't succeed, that failure adds another layer of heartbreak to an experience that is already extremely stressful physically, emotionally, and financially. Proud parents of babies born thanks to ARTs will say that it was worth everything they went through. But the more important point is not whether it is ultimately worth it, but whether it was *necessary*.

These technologies can be miracle makers, but they must be used wisely to be used well. As a society, we are not yet applying that wisdom. There is a better way, modeled by the Making Babies program. This is it in a nutshell: use all options available *in their proper place and time,* with a preference always for what's closest to the way nature intended and what's best (and most likely to work) for the patient. The truth is, with careful diagnosis, basic fertility education, and simple but detailed diet and lifestyle advice, many women using ARTs could conceive much more naturally. If any drugs or other interventions turn out to be necessary, minimal doses and least invasive procedures can be used, minimizing risks as well as unpleasant side effects—all while increasing success rates.

The stories that opened this chapter ultimately illustrate the possibilities.

Pamela, who'd had ten IVF attempts and a diagnosis of "bad eggs," also had scar tissue from having fibroids removed, which was effectively keeping her eggs from getting into her fallopian tubes. She'd started IVF to get around the scar tissue—a common approach. But clearly something about the IVF wasn't working for her, even if it was circumventing the obvious roadblock. When she came to see me (Sami), I couldn't find any other issues to explain her problem, so I recommended surgery to clear away the scar tissue. (The same laparoscopic procedure can diagnose and correct this problem all at the same time.) Two months after I performed the surgery, Pamela was pregnant, with no drugs and no IVF.

Evelyn, who'd been treated with fertility drugs since before her 30th birthday, finally became pregnant at age 40 after a single course of antibiotics cleared up a mycoplasma infection in her cervical mucus. Two years after her daughter was born, she went on to have a son with no treatment and no delay.

Stephanie, all of whose embryos had tested genetically abnormal, fit into a pattern we have seen all too often: high doses of injectable fertility drugs predisposing eggs in older women to develop chromosomal irregularities. Stephanie had been given too many fertility drugs for a woman of 41. My (Sami's) approach was to recommend a much lower dose of essentially the same drugs. This time, her eggs and embryos were perfectly normal — and so is her young son.

It is not our intention to set anyone's mind against IVF or any other ART. But we do want anyone who goes that route to do so with eyes wide open — and to know, before he or she heads down that road, that there are many other ways through the forest that are easier, safer, quicker, and cheaper. They all end up in the same place, so the difference between what exists now and the world you envision is understanding that you have a choice, including, but not limited to, ART. So before we get into the details of how to do this right, let's take a bit of time to look at what's wrong with the way it's done now.

## PATIENTS WITHOUT PATIENCE

We're about to pin a lot of this on doctors and the infertility industry, but consumers of these services need to take a look at their own behavior as well. Most couples, their hearts set on having a baby and with an acute sense that time is of the essence, want the fastest solution possible. Many feel that technology is their only choice. People struggling with infertility may feel vulnerable and desperate enough to try anything that promises they'll have a child, without doing any of the due diligence and critical thinking they'd apply to making a decision in any other area of their lives. Their doctors bear much of the responsibility, of course, but lots of couples accept IVF without examining other (and usually far better) options.

There are also plenty of people treating IVF more or less as a lifestyle choice, or as just another modern convenience. No room in the schedule for well-timed sex? Let the lab take care of the details! Long-distance relationship? Ship sperm overnight! In certain populations, the culture downplays or ignores the reality of fertility diminishing with age, with an unspoken and maybe even unconscious reliance on technology to bail out those who simply wait until it is too late to conceive naturally. There are plenty of good reasons to delay childbearing. But doing so is not without risks — the risk of never being able to conceive and/or the risks you expose yourself and your baby to in the use of technology. The plain fact is that many people who do wait (and wait, and wait) before trying to get pregnant don't really do so for hard-and-fast reasons. For too many people, when they are faced with the reality of infertility, in hindsight their reasons for waiting no longer seem compelling.

Although it is true that fertility is not an area where you want to drag your feet in finding a solution, that does not mean that everyone should jump immediately to the most drastic measures. No one should do so without knowing his or her diagnosis and options, with the pros and cons of each. Some people have more time to work with than others, but everyone can confidently take three months to explore the possibility of conceiving as naturally as possible with the Making Babies program. We've devised the program to be as efficient as it is effective. And even if the program itself is not sufficient in your case, it will thoroughly prepare you for the next steps, physically and mentally, giving you the very best odds of success as you move forward.

## DOCTORS WITHOUT PATIENCE

Lest anyone think we are blaming the victim, we now want to give the medical profession its due. We've watched from inside the industry as it has experienced explosive growth over the past three decades. And we are sad to report that too often the culture of modern fertility medicine harms more than it helps.

Because infertility patients are so often vulnerable and desperate, they are also easy to persuade — and some doctors take advantage of this dynamic. Driven by patient pressure for a quick fix, financial pressures, overenthusiasm, greed, or just plain thoughtlessness, they are steering women immediately toward drastic medical interventions and unnecessarily exposing patients to the expense, stress, and risks of IVF. Doctors often fail to produce a working diagnosis for their patients and often consider even an established diagnosis as irrelevant in the face of technology. Many fail to identify, explain, explore, and evaluate all options available to couples.

Money has corrupted health care across the board, and nowhere is that plainer than in fertility medicine. It's become an industry more than a field of medicine, and a highly commercialized one at that. Highly profitable tests and procedures are performed at ridiculously high rates, at times with no proven benefit to the patient (though the financial benefit to the doctor is high). As one patient who is an advertising executive remarked to us, "Fertility doctors are masters of marketing." That's definitely not the area of expertise you most want from your health care professional.

Some fertility doctors overmedicate patients, fail to tell patients about the downsides of fertility treatments, neglect to offer other (less profitable) treatments that may work just as well and/or be less invasive, turn away candidates they perceive as more difficult cases (because they rely on their success rates as a marketing tool), and, in the rare extreme case, perpetrate outright fraud, such as the swapping of embryos.

There are plenty of talented, well-intentioned practitioners out there, of course. Yet even they reap enormous profits from the aggressive use of technology, and it's the rare one who stands against the current. Furthermore, the irresponsible practitioners among them smear the whole profession. Even if all infertility doctors were good ones, the industry itself is woefully underregulated. Indeed, the way infertility treatment is carried out today is problematic in many ways.

## WHAT'S WRONG WITH YOU?

Most of the patients who come to see us have already seen at least one fertility doctor. When we ask new patients, "What's your diagnosis?" eight out of ten of them say they don't know. But what is truly appalling is, *neither do their doctors.* The way fertility medicine runs these days, the diagnosis is seen as almost inconsequential. *Why figure out why she's not getting pregnant,* the thinking goes; *we're just going to give her drugs anyway.* Or, *I don't need to know if he's making healthy sperm in normal amounts; we'll get enough to combine with the eggs for IVF.* The general attitude is that doctors are more powerful than nature and can simply force a woman's body to become pregnant.

This is not good medicine, and we find it offensive. Even if we could put those things aside, however, this approach simply makes no sense. If the sperm count is low, why not try one of the easy fixes that may be possible rather than jumping straight to serious intervention? And if the sperm aren't healthy, do you really want to use them to fertilize hard-won eggs for IVF? The only function of fertility drugs is to make more eggs release. They won't help a bit if the problem is bad sperm, an infection, or something toxic in the environment. You can pump out as many eggs as you like, but if the sperm can't get to them or penetrate them, or the body can't implant them or keep them once they're implanted, it's not going to get you any closer to having a baby. Fertility drugs can get more eggs released, but they can't make a woman more fertile.

The first order of business must always be to find out why someone is not getting pregnant. Roughly 10 percent of all infertile couples will not be able to find out why they cannot conceive. The medical profession is left to shrug its collective shoulders and explain to these people that they are something of a mystery. They are offered ARTs, but without there being a clear idea of what is being fixed, the outcome remains uncertain. It is impossible to determine the best course of treatment without the crucial insight of just what is wrong. What works for someone with blocked fallopian tubes is not going to work for someone with a bacterial infection that's preventing implantation, and what works for that person is not going to help someone who simply doesn't know when she is ovulating or how best to time intercourse.

## THE MISUSE AND OVERUSE OF IVF

The culture among both doctors and patients has led fertility medicine in general astray, but the effect is most glaring when it comes to IVF. We'd argue that even in the best practices, IVF is used too often, is insufficiently considered, and is too harshly pursued.

As in all areas of medicine, fertility practices are getting more and more specialized, and so we have plenty of clinics devoted solely to IVF. Psychologist Abraham Maslow famously wrote, "If the only tool you have is a hammer, you tend to see every problem as a nail." These days, IVF doctors are pounding nails just as fast and as hard as they can.

Often women are run through IVF clinics like cattle. Doctors know their treatment strategy before they even meet a particular patient. Doctors make themselves too busy, then don't have enough time to spend with each patient. Many doctors are more concerned with their own success rates than they are with their individual patients. Most IVF doctors go all out to convince a woman that they can make her pregnant. Then, if it turns out they can't, they blame it on her, telling her that her eggs are "bad." The big guns are always drawn first; there's almost never an effort to try every basic thing that makes sense for a particular patient before proceeding to more drastic measures. It's the rare woman who walks into one of these practices and isn't told she needs IVF (at thousands of dollars per cycle). That's like everyone who consults a cardiologist being told that he or she needs heart surgery.

On the flip side, many women are turned away from IVF treatment but never presented with any other options, with the possible exception of donor eggs. The system has mostly given up on women with high levels of follicle-stimulating hormone (FSH) — levels that generally increase with age — on the theory that they probably won't respond well to the standard treatments. Imagine oncologists refusing to treat patients who "probably" won't respond to cancer treatments, picking and choosing whom they will treat based on the likelihood of quick success. Yet many fertility practices seem to have no qualms about turning away less likely prospects. They always have one eye on how they'll look on paper, focusing on the stats they have to report each year to the government, for publication. If you've already started the process of ART yourself, you know just what we're talking about. What was the first thing you did when choosing a doctor? Bet you anything it was look up the relevant batting averages.

All this despite the fact that FSH on its own is not a good indicator of fertility prospects (see page 216), although it may predict possible IVF failure. There are many other options for women with high FSH that might allow them to conceive naturally or prepare their bodies so that IVF may indeed work for them. It's become a familiar story: a woman walks into one of our offices frantic over what other doctors have said to her, panicked that she'll never have a child (often because she's been told she'll never have a child), and within months she needs to go back to her ob-gyn — for prenatal care.

## PLAYING GOD

In the early 1980s, I (Sami) was the first doctor to successfully perform IVF in New York. I was working as part of a team, but I was the one who actually extracted the eggs and then implanted them once they were fertilized. I placed the cell cluster that was to become the first baby born in the city conceived outside the womb.

And I didn't like it.

I felt like I was playing God, and that just wasn't right for me. I didn't like holding life literally in my hands. It was a kind of surreal experience, still vivid in my memory: the embryologist over my left shoulder, handing me a syringe with three air bubbles in the fluid, telling me that there were four embryos between the bubbles. I just kept thinking, *These are babies inside this little syringe*.

I can't think of anything more satisfying than helping people who want babies to have babies, but I knew that day that this wasn't going to be the way for me to do it. I understood that I was in the middle of a major revolution for medicine — for humanity — but I also understood that I couldn't be part of it any longer. Not that way.

My professional peers by and large saw it differently. Although our training was fundamentally the same, almost all of them made a full conversion into IVF-oriented practices. And for that, I'm often grateful: they're there when I need to refer a patient, and there are a whole lot of children in the world thanks to them.

But the shift in the field of reproductive medicine to focus so intensely on IVF is a decidedly mixed blessing. It has reached an extreme of specialized practices run like fertility factories with one-size-fits-all treatment strategies, where doctors decide on treatments without knowing what they are actually treating. It's like treating a symptom without looking to discover the disease that's causing it. In the process of this upheaval, we've forgotten a lot of what we once knew, and we've been blind to better solutions, old and new.

In my practice today, I focus on medical and surgical treatment of infertility in women of all ages, specializing in recurrent pregnancy losses and women over the age of 39. I consider myself a traditional doctor. Some might say "old-fashioned" — I've made house calls — but I've got a number of cutting-edge techniques in my repertoire as well. I'm a surgeon, but I approach infertility first medically, then surgically if necessary. I take only about 10 percent of my patients into the operating room. The way I see it, the less invasive a treatment is, the better (of course, it still has to work). I don't put anybody on fertility drugs unless I have to, which turns out to be less than half the time. And when I do prescribe fertility drugs, I use only one-quarter of the dose most IVF docs do. Some couples I see need drugs, but not fertility drugs — they need antibiotics or steroids. Some benefit from simply taking over-the-counter cough medicine or plain old aspirin. Some of my patients simply need to douche with baking soda before intercourse.

I'll do whatever works best for the patient, even referring for IVF — but only for people who really need it. My preference is always for the gentlest option that will be effective. When the more natural ways don't work, I'm all for making use of more aggressive interventions. Almost always, good medical detective work will uncover the cause of a patient's infertility and so reveal the appropriate solution. And despite what you'd think if you walked into just about any IVF clinic in this country, the solutions don't often involve major invasive interventions.

## WHAT'S THE PROBLEM?

IVF is just the most widely used — and the most widely overused — ART. Other techniques are overused as well — and patients are charged even more for them — including genetic screening and intracytoplasmic sperm injection (ICSI), both of which are discussed in chapter 25. ARTs in general have a significant physical, financial, and emotional impact on any couple. The drugs and techniques used pose short- and long-term health risks for the mother and the baby, on top of producing unpleasant (if transient) side effects. Many are not covered by health insurance. Even if they are covered, patients may bear a high proportion of the costs out of pocket. Psychological stress and emotional problems are common — even when the procedures are successful, and even more so when they aren't. That's in addition to the plain old physical stress of going through the procedures. Among other things, treatment disrupts people's personal and professional lives. Appointments (and there are a lot of them) may be made for the convenience of the doctors and staff rather than the patients. In any case, they have to be squeezed into already very full lives. If you go to a fertility clinic at six in the morning, you're likely to see women lined up there already, waiting to get their blood taken or have a sonogram. All in pursuit of a goal that's anything but a sure thing.

Even if IVF were always carefully considered and judiciously recommended, it would still be a mistake to rely on it as completely as mainstream fertility medicine does, simply because the odds are so great that it won't work. Success rates have greatly improved since the dawn of the IVF era and are inching up each year, but, even so, the chances of having a healthy full-term baby after one cycle of IVF hovers at around 30 to 40 percent (and generally varies between roughly 10 and 50 percent, depending on the age of the mother). One of the best IVF programs in the country, for example, sends about 47 percent of patients under the age of 35 home with a baby in any given IVF cycle. The best program and the most-likely-to-succeed patients — and still patients get what they came for less than half the time.

## WHY RISK IT?

The possible health risks of many fertility treatments are often glossed over — and not just by doctors who don't want to emphasize them, but also by patients who don't really want to think about them. The risks are an important part of the big picture, however. *They are small but real.* Negative effects on both mothers and babies are seen more frequently in children of ARTs than in naturally conceived babies. If you've already tried any of these techniques, we want you to keep these risks in perspective. In fact, everyone should keep them in perspective, because there may come a time when these *are* the right strategies for you. These may be risks you are ready to assume. What we wish for all couples trying to conceive is that any risks are *necessary* risks. What breaks our hearts is people opening themselves up to potential problems when safer options are available.

Our aim is not to scare women but rather to underscore why they must view ARTs as options of last resort. The risks are worth it when there is no other way to have a baby, but they are unnecessary if you can get pregnant in a more natural way. Following the Making Babies program will allow you to avoid the potential problems associated with fertility drugs, IVF, and other ARTs, including an increased risk of ovarian cancer in the mother; a tubal pregnancy; eggs or embryos with genetic defects; fetal abnormalities; perinatal complications; pregnancy with two or more babies at once (and all the potential health problems that go along with that); premature birth (and all the potential health problems that go along with that); neurological and physical handicaps, developmental delays, learning disabilities, and mental and behavioral disorders later in life; and possible infertility (for the baby) later in life.

There are potential immediate health risks for the mother from ARTs as well, including allergic reactions to fertility drugs, infection, injury during retrieval of eggs, bleeding, blood clots, and damage to organs or blood vessels. Poor lab work, including mix-ups of samples and/or results as well as basic quality issues, introduces another kind of risk in pursuing technological solutions to fertility problems.

### The Risks of Fertility Drugs

Most of the risks to the mother come from fertility drugs, and we'll look at the potential problems in more detail in chapter 25. On their own, fertility drugs are the most common approach to infertility issues, and each cycle of IVF begins with fertility drugs. In both cases, the drugs are used to stimulate the ovaries to release more eggs. The usual strategy boils down to using more and more of the drugs, in an attempt to get more and more eggs. But some women receive doses that are too high. Others are given too many courses of the drugs. And some are given drugs when they don't really need them or have a fertility problem the drugs can't solve.

High-dose fertility drugs put women at risk in both the short and long term and increase the risks for babies as well. At the most basic level, many women experience headaches, hot flashes, and mood swings, among other familiar unpleasant signs of hormones at work. These effects may not be dangerous, but they can make a woman quite miserable, and they place even more physical and emotional stress on women and couples already pushed to the edge by fertility issues.

Over the long term, the repercussions are more serious. Some studies show an increase in cancer risk from fertility drugs, which aligns with what we've seen in some patients with a history of extreme fertility drug use. The most common serious side effect of fertility drugs is ovarian hyperstimulation syndrome (OHSS; see page 323). The most severe cases require hospitalization and sometimes termination of pregnancy. Even with careful monitoring by their doctors, up to 10 percent of women using these drugs for IVF experience OHSS, with up to 2 percent having severe cases. OHSS is widely considered to be an overreaction to the drugs. We might do better to see it as a sign that we are overreacting in our use of such high doses of these extremely powerful drugs.

Once women go to all this trouble to get more eggs, it isn't exactly smooth sailing from there. Many eggs harvested this way are abnormal, increasingly so as a woman gets older, and are more likely to produce embryos with genetic defects than those from a natural cycle. These defects can cause fertility treatment to fail. Experts worry, too, that the drugs may be causing problems that have yet to be pinpointed in children born as a result of fertility drug pregnancies.

### The Risks of Multiples

The goal of using large doses of fertility drugs is to get lots of eggs. Not surprisingly, this raises the risk of pregnancy with more than one baby at a time. Only about 2 percent of naturally conceived children are twins. Fertility drugs alone increase the chances of multiples between 6 and 20 percent, depending on the medication. With IVF the number of multiples goes up even further — about a third of IVF pregnancies are twins — thanks to the standard American approach of transferring multiple embryos in each cycle to increase the chances of conception.

Multiples pregnancies are high-risk pregnancies. Essentially, a system designed to grow one new human being is strained to the limit by larger demands. Multiples pregnancies are more likely to end in miscarriage. They are more likely to involve cesarean delivery, premature birth (more than half of twins are born prematurely), and/or low birth weight. (The number of babies born prematurely has increased drastically over the past two decades, right alongside the number of babies conceived with technological assistance.) Babies born early or small have more health problems at birth and over the long term, as well as a higher risk of death in infancy, than full-term infants. Consider, too, the high economic costs of the neonatal intensive care premature babies require.

Even the "solution" to the problem of multiples pregnancies created by IVF is problematic. "Reduction" — the euphemism used for selective abortion of one or more fetuses to lower the risks of the pregnancy — is a horrible situation to have to contemplate. And now evidence is showing that single infants born after selective (or spontaneous) reduction have many of the same risks and problems as twins.

### The Risks of IVF

Research shows that babies conceived through IVF are at greater risk, even when they are in single pregnancies. If you've used any ART, or if you think you might, it is important to remember that the risks of serious, long-term problems in children born through ARTs are small. For couples with no other viable options for getting pregnant, these are acceptable risks. But for the many couples for whom these are *avoidable* risks, it is unnecessary to run them.

Less than 2 percent of naturally conceived children have birth defects, and although that figure certainly provokes some anxiety in would-be parents, it rightly doesn't dissuade anyone from conceiving that way. In babies born through ARTs, the risks are 50 percent higher: 3 percent. If you could lower the risks for your child even 1 percent, wouldn't you?

IVF babies also are two and a half times more likely than spontaneously conceived babies to have low birth weight, and that brings with it a raft of health risks, just as multiple and premature births do. Scientists do not yet agree on what to blame for the increased risks with ARTs. What is clear is that the more involved or intense the fertility intervention, the more likely it is that some problems will emerge over the long term.

### The Risks of Not Knowing

Of all the risks faced by people struggling with fertility issues, the biggest one is not having a child. That's what makes all the other risks acceptable — *when they are necessary*. But the way the infertility industry operates in America today, these very real risks are too easily dismissed, never really considered, or taken for granted. If nothing else, they should give you pause, even if they don't change your decision in the end.

Modern infertility medicine poses subtler risks as well, and these receive even less consideration. There's the risk of receiving a diagnosis and being told there's nothing to be done about it (and so you'll never have a baby). There's also the risk of receiving the vague diagnosis of "unexplained infertility," meaning, really, that Western medicine can't find anything that needs fixing and so, again, there's nothing to be done.

So many patients come to us having failed IVF, or having been turned down as candidates for IVF, and their doctors don't have anything else to offer them, with the possible exception of donor eggs. They've been told that they'll never have a baby, perhaps because they are too old or their FSH is too high. For these women, that's a terrifying position to be in.

These are the risks of not knowing — not knowing what is preventing pregnancy and/or not knowing what to do about it — which the one-size-fits-all approach of fertility medicine today not only deems acceptable but also implicitly encourages. But you don't have to accept them if you follow the Making Babies path.

## A BETTER WAY

The program laid out in this book will guide you through the process of conceiving as naturally as you can given your own particular situation. This decreases the risks of ARTs and comes as close as is humanly possible to eliminating the risk of not having a child. It's the paralyzing fear of that worst risk coming true that drives the whole crazy way the infertility industry works today. The latest and greatest technologies are sold as the one true path to salvation, the only things keeping patients away from the abyss. But fear is a terrible place to proceed from.

What a couple being pushed that way really needs is basic information, good advice, judicious use of conventional and adjunctive treatments, and a certain amount of clearheaded patience. What they often *don't* need is IVF. They don't need the physical strain of extreme hormone doses and repeated invasive procedures. They don't need the long-term increased health risks to mother and baby. They don't need the emotional strains the IVF roller coaster puts couples on. (In psychological testing measuring stress levels, infertility patients score higher than cancer patients.) They don't need the tremendous expense — in the New York metropolitan area, we're talking an average of $12,000 to $14,000 *per cycle* — and they don't need the additional stress that comes with that expense.

All these patients really need is a baby. When that goal proves difficult to achieve, they need careful detective work to uncover what's really going on and to so reveal how best to address it. Then they need a wise guide to help them navigate through their choices — *all* their choices — until their primary need is fulfilled. Sometimes the solution is indeed IVF, but most times something far less drastic will do the trick.

High-tech medicine produces all kinds of miracles for all kinds of people, not the least of which are people desperately wanting to be parents. It isn't that we shouldn't use the technology available to us. It's just that we should use it wisely and well. The widespread availability of IVF and all ARTs is undeniably a good thing. The overreliance on them is not. In this book, we aim to help you walk the fine line of what is best for *you*. Let technology work wonders for those who need it. Let nature work *its* wonders for those who don't.

## Making Babies Action Plan

❏ Try to get pregnant as close to the way nature intended as possible by following the Making Babies program.

❏ Understand the basics of how to get pregnant, including how your body works, how your partner's body works, and how they work together.

❏ Be patient (within reason).

❏ Consult with health care practitioners dedicated to treating you as a whole person and to considering all your options with you.

❏ Know your diagnosis.

❏ Weigh the negative aspects of IVF and other ARTs against the potential benefits.

❏ Use ARTs when and as appropriate.

# PART TWO

# Getting Pregnant Naturally

# CHAPTER TWO

# How to Get Pregnant: The Basics

We are going to assume that by this point in your life, you have a reasonable grasp of the birds and the bees. But we are not going to assume that you know everything you need to know to get pregnant. Most of us spend our early reproductive years focusing on how *not* to get pregnant. What you need to know now can be subtly but significantly different. Or at least there are crucial details that may never have been important to you before that are now pretty much key to the whole thing.

We are on occasion astonished at how little many of our clients know about how to conceive a baby — even those who have been obsessing on the subject for a year or more. Even more amazing is how often some basic education is all they need to remove whatever roadblock they've been stumbling over. We've both celebrated the birth of many babies where our main contribution has been just a guided tour of the female and male reproductive systems, specific instructions on establishing when a couple is most fertile, or advice on when (and how) to have sex when a couple wants to make a baby. So it is exactly those topics we are going to cover in this chapter.

## IT ALL STARTS WITH THE MOTHER

The conception of a baby really begins with the conception of that baby's mother. Female fetuses have oocytes in their ovaries well before birth — the oocytes that will eventually mature into eggs. At birth, a baby girl has roughly 1 to 2 million of them, though they'll be pared back to "only" about 300,000 by the time she has her first period. Those immature eggs just hang out in the ovaries until puberty, at which point they take turns "ripening," then bursting out of their follicles to be released through ovulation as part of the menstrual cycle. A trip down the fallopian tubes is only for the lucky few, however, as hundreds of eggs are reabsorbed into the body each month and never released. Just one makes an official debut through ovulation (with, on occasion, a little company—IVF isn't the only way to have twins, you know!). This process keeps going until all the eggs are gone: menopause.

By contrast, sperm are more about the short term. From first formation to ejaculation, any given sperm has been in a man's body for about three months at most. And whereas an egg is essentially a solo act, sperm show more of a mob mentality. At puberty, sperm begin to be produced by the testicles—many millions every single day, roughly 5,000 every single minute! It takes only about forty-eight hours to form a sperm and another two weeks for the sperm to mature, during which it gains the ability to "swim" (*motility*). The testicles store the millions of tiny sperm cells until they are called for in ejaculation, at which point they take off, roughly 40 million to 200 million at a time, mixed in with fluid to create semen. The final bit of development doesn't occur until the sperm are in the female reproductive tract and the membrane around each one changes in ways that will allow it to penetrate and merge with the egg.

Which brings us to the fun part: having sex. Specifically, vaginal intercourse, but we're guessing we don't have to tell you that. Sperm are ejaculated into the vagina. Right off the bat, the semen coagulates, and only about a tenth of the sperm survive to swim on. Perhaps 10 minutes later, the semen liquefies again, which lets the sperm get through the cervix. The sperm move along tiny tracks formed by proteins in fertile cervical mucus. As they progress, they shed their protective coating, a process called *capacitation,* which leaves them able to penetrate an egg (should they get the chance).

If the timing is right and an egg is on its way down a fallopian tube while the sperm are swimming up it, whichever sperm wins the race and has all the required skills gets to fertilize the egg. This will happen within a few hours of ovulation, if it happens at all, somewhere along the fallopian tube, closer to the ovary than to the uterus. The first sperm in sets off a reaction in the egg that makes it impermeable to any other sperm, although the minions will keep on trying as long as they have any swim left in them.

The union of the egg and the sperm creates what is technically known as a *zygote*. The zygote finishes the journey into the uterus, swept along by tiny hairs (*cilia*) lining the fallopian tubes. The trip takes about five days. Upon arrival, the zygote nestles into the endometrium, which will nourish its development. The cells multiply and begin to specialize. After eight weeks, it is an *embryo*, with about thirty-two more weeks to go before its official debut.

All through this process, the egg, the sperm, and the zygote they create are dancing to a tune called by a cascade of hormones orchestrated by the pituitary gland, operating under the influence, chemically and physically, of their environment. It's an intricate web, and success depends on everything working as it should, when it should.

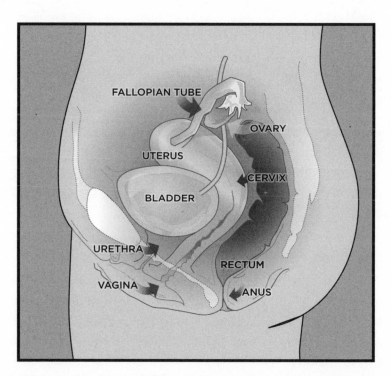

**Fig. 1:** Oocytes develop in follicles in the ovaries until one takes the lead, bursting from its follicle and becoming a mature egg. The egg is drawn into and through one of the fallopian tubes into the uterus. If fertilized on its journey, the egg, now a zygote, attaches to the uterine lining (endometrium). If not, the egg disintegrates by the time it reaches the uterus. Then the endometrium is sloughed off and moves out of the uterus through the cervix and into the vagina as menstrual flow.

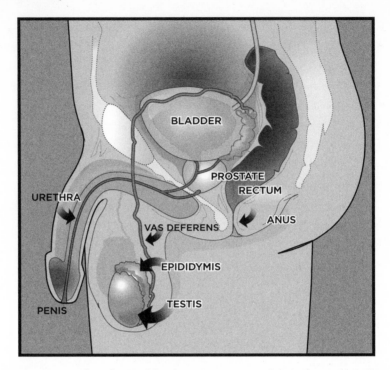

**Fig. 2:** Sperm are first formed in the testes, or testicles, then move into the epididymis to mature further and be stored. At ejaculation, sperm move into and through the vas deferens, mix with fluid from the prostate and the seminal vessels to create semen, and then move through the urethra and leave the body.

## THE CYCLE

Now we want to back up for a minute and break down the female reproductive cycle in a bit more detail. A woman's menstrual cycle is typically divided into two phases—follicular and luteal. For our purposes, however, there are four significant phases to the cycle, and as you get into the Making Babies program, you'll find that in many instances our advice changes for each phase. We're going to tell you a bit about each phase here—first from a Western and then from an Eastern perspective—so that you'll have a basic understanding of the mechanics underlying the practical applications to come.

### Phase 1: Menstruation

In the hours before you get your period, blood vessels in the endometrium lining the uterus tighten up, restricting blood flow to the endometrium. This causes it to start to die. Then the blood vessels relax again, which triggers the gradual shedding of the endometrium: you get your period. This goes on for between four and seven days on average, with the majority of the shedding happening in the first twenty-four hours, and so the heaviest bleeding occurs on the first or second day.

The endometrium wastes no time in starting to regenerate itself so it will be ready to accommodate an embryo later in the cycle. Regrowth begins within two days of when you start to bleed. By day 3, estrogen and progesterone receptors form in the endometrium, and your hormones take control of endometrium building. By day 6, the endometrium is about 1 to 2 mm thick.

While all this is going on, the ripening process starts in the follicles on your ovaries that house your eggs, one egg to a follicle, beginning on about day 4. The follicles are less than 4 mm across at this point, but they will quintuple in size, to about 20 mm.

The whole shebang — endometrium shedding, endometrium regenerating, follicles growing — is orchestrated by the interplay of hormones. Estrogen and progesterone kick it off; their falling levels signal the release of gonadotropin-releasing hormone (GnRH), which triggers menstrual bleeding. GnRH in turn signals the release of follicle-stimulating hormone (FSH), which, appropriately enough, stimulates the growth of follicles.

### Phase 2: Pre-ovulation

During menstruation, a signal from the pituitary gland at the base of the brain causes FSH levels to start to rise. The FSH stimulates the ovaries, causing fifteen to twenty follicles on them to begin ripening in preparation for release of the egg each one holds. In this phase, FSH continues to rise, still signaling to the follicles. Each follicle produces estrogen — the estrogen that will determine when you ovulate — so estrogen rises gradually through this phase.

Full follicle development usually takes about two weeks, from day 4 or so of your period up to ovulation, though a normal follicular phase may last anywhere from ten to twenty days. Typically, by day 6 or 7 of your cycle, one follicle has become dominant, and the rest simply shrink away.

Rising estrogen tells your body to reduce FSH, so no more follicles are produced. Estrogen levels peak on about day 12 or 13, signaling the pituitary gland for the release of luteinizing hormone (LH), which in turn triggers the release of an egg. (In men's bodies, sperm production also proceeds under the influence of FSH and LH.)

As estrogen levels rise, you may notice that your vagina feels more moist and your cervical mucus shifts from being sticky or rubbery to being opaque, whitish, and creamy, like hand lotion. This is not yet fertile cervical mucus. As estrogen rises even higher, it will thin out and become transparent and stretchy, like egg whites.

All the while, the endometrium has been regenerating. It thickens further as estrogen rises, and by ovulation a healthy endometrium will be about 7 to 10 mm thick.

### Phase 3: Ovulation

Ovulation typically occurs on day 14 of an average cycle, although it could be as early as day 10 or as late as day 20, and as long as the cycle is regular, it's nothing to worry about. It usually occurs within twenty-four hours of the surge in LH. Occasionally, a cycle produces no egg, which is normal. From time to time, two eggs are released, always within twenty-four hours of each other. This is how we get fraternal twins. Twenty-four hours after ovulation, progesterone levels rise to the point at which any further release of eggs is impossible. Contrary to popular belief, ovulation doesn't necessarily alternate from one ovary to the other from month to month.

Whichever side it comes from, the egg is about the size of the period at the end of this sentence. Upon its release from the lead follicle, the egg is quickly drawn into the fallopian tube, a process that takes only about twenty seconds.

The egg remains alive for twelve to twenty-four hours, traveling toward the uterus. When its time is up, if the egg has not been fertilized by the sperm, it disintegrates and is eventually reabsorbed into the body. If an egg is going to be fertilized, it happens within a matter of hours of ovulation, probably by a sperm that's been waiting there for it. Sperm need fertile cervical mucus to swim through to reach the egg—mucus in which they can survive for up to three or four days—and that mucus is produced thanks to increasing estrogen levels in the later days of the follicular phase.

Within eighteen to twenty-four hours of ovulation, progesterone thickens the mucus, and it once again becomes opaque and no longer conducive to sperm survival or movement. Once an egg is fertilized, it continues on its way toward the uterus, a journey of about six days.

## Phase 4: Potential Implantation

Progesterone is the dominant hormone in the second, post-ovulation half of your cycle, known as the luteal phase. Progesterone switches off production of FSH and LH, thereby preventing the release of any more eggs. It thickens the endometrium and helps it secrete nutrients so that it will be ready to nourish an embryo if called upon to do so. And it causes your basal body temperature (BBT) to rise (which is favorable to implantation), closes the cervix, and thickens cervical mucus, forming a plug that is meant to prevent more sperm from entering the cervix after fertilization. All this progesterone is released by the corpus luteum, which is formed from the collapse of the empty follicle that released the egg.

The length of the luteal phase is determined by how long the corpus luteum lasts, generally between twelve and sixteen days. The luteal phase needs to last at least eleven to twelve days, or there won't be enough time for an embryo to implant, and even if an egg has been fertilized, no pregnancy will result or an early miscarriage may take place.

The embryo arrives in the uterus by the fifth or sixth day of the journey, cells busily dividing all the way. Generally it implants — attaches to the endometrium — within a day after that. The uterus itself assists with implantation by actually pressing its front and back walls together, holding the embryo in place. To achieve this, the body removes fluid from the endometrium in a process called pinocytosis.

Once the fertilized egg has nestled into the endometrium, it gives off the pregnancy hormone human chorionic gonadotropin (HCG), the signal your standard pregnancy test "pee stick" is looking for. That HCG also tells the corpus luteum back in the ovarian wall to continue releasing progesterone to sustain the endometrium, instead of shutting the uterine lining down after the usual twelve to sixteen days. (Five to six weeks later, the placenta will take over the task of producing progesterone and maintaining the endometrium.) At this point, the menstrual cycle is effectively finished (for the next nine months, anyway), and pregnancy has begun. After eight weeks of pregnancy, the little ball of cells has developed and differentiated enough to officially be known as a *fetus*.

If there is no fertilization or no implantation, the corpus luteum begins to degenerate, ultimately stopping the flow of progesterone, and the blood vessels leading to the endometrium begin closing down, in preparation for endometrial shedding. Estrogen levels begin to fall as well, and the drop in estrogen and progesterone trigger the release of GnRH and FSH, bringing the process full circle: the next period begins. The drop in progesterone is what may cause the symptoms we know as premenstrual syndrome (PMS).

## THE CHINESE VIEW

Chinese medicine considers menstruation to be essentially yin. The period—the shedding of the endometrium—requires the movement of blood. Follicle building also requires yin. And endometrium building requires blood and yin.

Nourishing yin governs phase 2 as well. The estrogen predominating is considered to be a yin hormone. Yin promotes growth (of follicles) and building (of the endometrium). The production of fertile cervical mucus also requires yin. Developing follicles require good blood flow as well as yin. The quality of yin affects the quality of the egg itself, as well as the growth of the follicle around it. Preparing the uterine lining also requires blood and yin, as well as jing.

At mid-cycle, yin cedes its dominance to the yang energy required by the hormonal transformation necessary for ovulation. This shift is

### TALK THE TALK

The vocabulary of Chinese medicine can be daunting, so we've limited our use of specialized terms. But there are a handful of immensely useful words that can't be fully translated. Here are their basic definitions.

**Blood**—blood, with emphasis on its moving and nourishing functions.

**Jing**—reproductive essence; also, prenatal inheritance (genetic makeup).

**Qi**—life force; energy; activating spark.

**Yang**—the body's functions related to movement, transformation, and heating; the complementary opposite of yin.

**Yin**—the body's functions related to nourishment, moistening, and cooling; the complementary opposite of yang.

reflected in the changing of the dominant hormone from estrogen to progesterone. This hormonal changing of the guard requires an even flow of qi and blood to occur smoothly and in a timely fashion. Qi also guides the release of the egg and its progress down the fallopian tube.

In Chinese medicine, the luteal phase (our phase 4) is dominated by yang energy, which is warming and energizing. The body needs yang energy to sustain progesterone levels. If you are deficient in yang (or progesterone), your BBT may climb too slowly in the luteal phase, or drop too soon, making implantation less likely. Generally, women's bodies are warmer in the luteal phase, and for thousands of years doctors of Chinese medicine have stressed the importance of a warm uterus for implantation. Implantation also relies on a good flow of blood to the uterus to create a strong endometrium.

If you are not pregnant, your progesterone level drops in this phase. To negotiate this transformation smoothly, your body needs qi and blood to flow smoothly. When they don't, the result is PMS symptoms, including mood swings, breast tenderness, bloating, food cravings, fatigue, and headaches.

Yang energy flows once again into yin on the first day of your period, a significant transformation in the Chinese medicine view of things.

## HOW TO HAVE SEX

Here again, we're going to presume you pretty much have a handle on this. But there are a few things you need to know to enhance fertility.

First, don't forget the foreplay. Just because you have a job to do now doesn't mean that you should make this too much like work. For one thing, you want to try to keep sex from becoming a stressor. For another, sexual stimulation improves cervical mucus and increases the flow of hormones, which in turn increases fertility. In addition, one study found that men who were turned on by a partner had higher sperm counts than those who masturbated by themselves. It's in your best interest not to give sex short shrift by letting it become too goal oriented.

Second, the missionary position is the best one to use when you are trying to conceive. Any other time, you should of course use whatever position(s) you enjoy. But right now, you need to be a little more task oriented, and your immediate task is to get those sperm just as far along their journey as you can. The missionary position allows for penetration closest to the cervix.

---

### Case Study: Cherie

Cherie had been trying to get pregnant for six years when she finally came to Manhattan to see me (Sami). During the part of the intake interview where I ask about sexual positions, she looked as if she thought I was getting a bit too personal, but she told me that when she and her husband had sex, she was always on top. I ran a postcoital test (see page 197) that very day, and it showed no sperm swimming around. I didn't find any other red flags, so I sent Cherie home with the recommendation that she and her husband switch to the missionary position for the time being. They did, and when Cherie came back for another postcoital test, sure enough, there were sperm. Within a couple of months, Cherie was pregnant, with no other intervention.

---

In addition, this may not be the best time for anal penetration. Obviously, that's not going to lead to conception, but until you are pregnant, you might want to abstain even during the times in your cycle when you know you're not likely to get pregnant. That's because you could be facilitating the transfer of bacteria into the vagina and/or the urethra, which might lead to an infection that could threaten fertility. (See chapter 16 for more about infections.)

---

### Case Study: Thea and Bob

I (Sami) once saw a couple who both tested positive for *Streptococcus fecalis* in their reproductive tracts, though the only symptom it was causing was the inability to get pregnant. Both Thea and Bob took antibiotics, and their infections cleared up. But still no pregnancy occured.

So I retested them, only to discover that the strep was back. This went on through three rounds of antibiotics, until it finally occurred to me to ask them if they ever had anal intercourse. They told me they did. I explained that I thought that was the source of the recurring strep, prescribed antibiotics one more time, and never heard from them again. Months later, a new patient called to schedule an appointment, saying that Thea had referred her to me. "Oh, and how is she?" I asked. "Pregnant!" the woman reported. And, I presumed, strep-free.

---

After sex, stay put for ten to twenty minutes — especially if you're the woman. (Though wouldn't this be a nice time to cuddle for both of you?) I (Jill) once had a patient, a yoga devotee, who used to stand on her head after intercourse to maximize the effects of gravity. This is not necessary. Just don't make the sperm fight gravity along with everything else. You may also have heard that the woman should lie with her legs up a wall. That's certainly not going to hurt anything, but it isn't necessary either. Just stay lying down. If you're one of those women just dying for a pee after you've had sex, please don't withhold urine so long that you give yourself a urinary tract infection. But you'll be fine for fifteen minutes, if you can manage to hold it.

### "Intimate Moisturizers"

Sexual lubricants (especially scented varieties) can interfere with conception. They are, in general, too acidic for the sperm to survive and swim well in. In addition, the concentration of salts in the lubricants can cause sperm to either shrink or swell beyond their capacity to perform normally.

If you need a little extra moisture — and many couples do at ovulation or under the stress of trying to conceive — you don't have to do without. Look for Pre-Seed lubricant, which is specially designed for couples trying to conceive. It does not contain any glycerin or propylene glycol, the mischief makers in most lubricants. Its pH is the same as fertile cervical mucus, and it contains roughly the same amount of salts. It also has striations in it, little channels that ease the sperm's movement, just as fertile cervical mucus does (though it lacks the nutrients that mucus also provides). A new Cleveland Clinic study of lubricants published in the journal *Fertility and Sterility* found that Pre-Seed was the only commercially available vaginal lubricant that didn't decrease sperm motility or compromise sperm DNA.

Beware of some of the other common suggestions for lubrication, such as using a little warm water. Don't! Water can kill sperm on contact. Or how about trying a little saliva? Wrong! Saliva contains digestive enzymes that stop sperm from swimming. Maybe you've heard that egg whites are a good lubricant. We don't recommend them because of the risk of salmonella in raw eggs. (In addition, many patients who have tried it tell us it made them feel rather like an omelet!) Some doctors recommend mineral oil (sexual lubricants may contain it), but studies show that it may limit the ability of sperm to penetrate the egg. None of these effects is powerful enough to rely on as a birth control method, mind you, but when the idea is to get the sperm up to the egg, you do not want to make things any more difficult for them than they already are.

---

### Case Study: Stella

Stella, age 39, flew all the way to New York from Peru to consult with me (Sami) because she'd been trying for almost three years to get pregnant. A little detective work revealed a whole lot of nothing suspicious—except that she and her husband liked to use a particular fragrant lubricant. I told her to skip it for a while. No sooner had she stopped using it than she got pregnant.

---

### Frequency

Here's one good way to get pregnant: have lots of sex.

Forgive us if it seems we are stating the obvious, but we think it bears repeating. We've both had plenty of patients focused like lasers on the exact day of the woman's cycle when they should have sex to conceive, having sex on that day and maybe one day just before that as well, and then not having sex for the rest of the month. And we've had lots of patients who'd read on the Internet all about letting sperm build back up between ejaculations and were limiting sex in some kind of rationing effort.

Unless the male partner has been diagnosed with a low sperm count or low semen volume, you can pretty much feel free to have all the sex you want. (It is a good idea to keep it to once a day.) Not only won't it hurt anything, but it will greatly increase your chances of conceiving. (It could reduce stress levels a bit, too, if you do it right.) Of course, it's fine if you're not inclined to have sex every day, but every other day around ovulation is important. And if a postcoital test (see page 197), done twelve to eighteen hours after intercourse, shows dead sperm, you do need to have sex every day at mid-cycle to maximize your chances of conceiving.

Research has shown that couples who have sex about once a week have a 15 percent chance of conceiving in any given cycle, while those having sex every day kick up their chances to 50 percent. One study found that only 12 percent of couples reported having intercourse five times a week or more, but for those who did, there was no negative impact on fertility.

Another study, looking to advise couples in which the fertility issue had been traced back to the man on how long to abstain before collecting semen for ARTs, found that sperm and semen quality peaked between one and three days of abstinence, with significant decreases in quality as the period of abstinence stretched on. Although the sperm count went up, the older sperm started to deteriorate. Note that this was in men with a diagnosed fertility problem. But the study found that the official guideline most commonly followed, to go two to seven days without ejaculating before collecting sperm, did not serve the couples' best interests. Men with no reason to maximize their sperm counts surely have even less reason to limit the amount of sex they have.

If you are working with a sperm count that's low or low normal, you might want to keep ejaculation to every other day to give the count a chance to build up a bit, at least around the time of the woman's peak fertility. But there's no need to limit it any more than that, and in fact there seems to be a benefit to *not* abstaining any longer.

---

### Case Study: Donna

For some people, it *is* possible to overdo it on sex. That's what happened to Donna, who had consulted with a feng shui expert about her trouble getting pregnant some months before she met me (Jill). The feng shui expert advised placing a plant beside the bed and a bowl of water under the bed. Each time Donna and her husband had intercourse, they were to pour the water on the plant. If the plant thrived, they would conceive. Well, it wasn't long before the plant was all but dead—from overwatering! And Donna still wasn't pregnant. That's when she came to see me.

I found that in their eagerness to conceive, Donna and her husband were having too much sex, given his low-normal sperm count. With some good fertility counseling, focusing especially on how best to time intercourse, Donna was soon pregnant. (No word on the health of the plant!)

---

### It's All in the Timing

If you and your partner are healthy and have no particular fertility challenges, the single most important thing you can do to help this process along is to know when to have sex. Which is to say, you need to know when you ovulate and to time the swimming of the sperm accordingly.

We'll get to the particulars of how to predict ovulation in a minute. But once you know when you ovulate, the key is to have sex ahead of time. Once they're in your body, the sperm will hang out for a bit, just swimming around, looking for something to do — just waiting for an egg to debut. The egg will not lollygag, so if you wait until you think it's on the move, you have a very short window of time for the sperm to catch up to it. Having sex on the day ovulation is about to occur may be ideal, but better the day before than the day after, when it will be too late. Think of boarding a cruise ship. Sometimes you can board a couple of days before launch, but once it pulls away from the dock, you are out of luck. That ship has sailed, and you're just going to have to wait for the next one.

Researchers at the National Institute of Environmental Health Sciences studied more than two hundred healthy women planning to get pregnant. They tracked their estimated ovulation and the days on which they had intercourse. Conception took place only when intercourse occurred in the six days leading up to ovulation, and the likelihood of conception increased dramatically the closer sex was to the actual day of ovulation. Only a small number of pregnancies were due to sperm that were three or more days old, and none occurred with sex after the day of ovulation.

## Case Study: Lee Anne

Lee Anne, age 41, had been trying to get pregnant with a second child for a year. She'd had no trouble conceiving the first one. (This "secondary infertility" seems particularly baffling to doctors.) She and her husband had been diligently following her doctor's advice to have sex on the eleventh, thirteenth, and fifteenth days of her cycle. What the doctor hadn't taken into account, however, was that although Lee Anne, like many women as they get older, had a regular menstrual cycle, it had become shorter than average, only about twenty-four days. So by the time she was at day 11, she had already ovulated. By having sex on the days recommended, she and her husband were sure *not* to conceive. They were actually practicing the "rhythm method" form of birth control.

My (Sami's) advice to Lee Anne was simple: have sex fourteen days before you expect your period to start. Counting backward from your next period is a more reliable indicator of when ovulation will occur than counting forward from your last period. The number of days from ovulation to the start of the next period varies from woman to woman, but it is generally the same from month to month for an individual woman. It is also likely to stay near the average fourteen-day length, or at least in the eleven- to fourteen-day range. By contrast, the number of days from the start of your period to ovulation is more likely to shift from cycle to cycle. It's that first part of the cycle that accounts for longer or shorter than average cycles, as well as for irregular cycles.

Once Lee Anne and her husband more productively timed when they had intercourse, she conceived promptly and had a lovely baby girl.

Sperm generally live for seventy-two hours—that's three whole days—as long as they have good, alkaline cervical mucus to sustain them, and they can sometimes make it for up to seven days. An egg, meanwhile, is fertilizable for only twenty-four hours, and that time frame may squeeze down to just twelve hours as women get older. So your best bet is to have the sperm ready and waiting for the egg when it is released, and that means the best time to have sex is on days 12 through 14 of a standard twenty-eight-day cycle, where ovulation is on day 14. You'll have to get to know your own cycle to get the timing exactly right, and just how to do that is coming up next.

## HOW TO KNOW WHEN YOU ARE MOST FERTILE

To know most accurately when you ovulate, the following three strategies will serve you well: charting your BBT (see page 40), monitoring your cervical mucus, and feeling for changes in the position of your cervix.

Your temperature alone is not enough to tell you when you are most fertile. It will tell you whether or not you are ovulating at all—good to know!—and will give you some other helpful information, including patterns that can help determine your fertility type or your fertility diagnosis. But the fact remains that your temperature rises *after* ovulation. Since the name of the game is knowing when you *will* ovulate, just charting your temperature won't tell you what you most need to know. This is why we begin with a section on getting to know your cervical mucus. If you use only one of these three strategies, this should be it. And though all of these approaches are pretty simple, this is the easiest one of all.

Although we give you an overview of these fertility signs and how to track and interpret them, the acknowledged master in this area is Toni Weschler, author of the classic *Taking Charge of Your Fertility*. If you want more detailed guidance in this regard, we enthusiastically recommend her book.

### Cervical Mucus

Paying attention to the cyclical changes in your cervical mucus (your vaginal discharge) is your single best guide to ovulation. Yet cervical mucus is rarely discussed. Your doctor is no more likely to mention it than is your best girlfriend (despite the details you might get about her period). And so most women know next to nothing about it and the messages it carries about their fertility. The normal ebbs and flows in this mucus are open to misinterpretation for the same reason, and more than one woman has become convinced that she has a yeast infection when what she's really experiencing is an increase in cervical mucus at ovulation.

Learning how to hear what your body is telling you is really quite simple. What you're looking for is fertile cervical mucus—fluid that will be the most hospitable to sperm, helping them along their journey toward the egg. This section is about how to recognize it when you see (and feel) it, how to know when to expect it, and how best to take advantage of the opportunity it signals. As you are getting to know your body's rhythms in more detail, you may want to jot down your observations in a log or diary for a few months to help you pinpoint your personal pattern. If you keep a BBT chart (see page 40), that's a great place to record any notes on cervical mucus as well.

### *Getting Started*

First a few ground rules. You need to check your cervical mucus at a time when you are not sexually aroused, or you won't be able to sort out whether you are observing lubrication or regular fluids. Artificial lubricants, spermicides, and semen will all cloud the results as well, so choose a time when none of those will be running interference. Vaginal infections can also confuse matters. If you have one, don't begin your monitoring until after it is cleared up. Antihistamines can dry up cervical mucus, so you won't be able to learn much if you take them regularly. (And because of this, you're going to want to avoid them while trying to get pregnant.) If you are dehydrated, the mucus may be quite scanty, so keep drinking that water!

Anytime you are checking your cervical mucus, tune in to vaginal sensations as well. Do you feel dry? Wet? Slippery? One easy way to see what's going on is to wipe yourself with a tissue, from front to back, and note how easily the tissue slides.

### *Early Days*

You'll begin to attend to your cervical mucus on the first day after your period ends. Your vagina will feel dry or very slightly moist. After a few days — and about a week before ovulation, so around day 7, 8, or 9 of your cycle — you'll begin to have some mucus discharge, which will be thick, a bit sticky, or rubbery and springy. It may be white or yellowish. How long this lasts varies from woman to woman, but once you start paying attention, you'll quickly be able to identify your body's pattern.

Then for a few days, your vagina will feel wet, and your mucus will become opaque and quite creamy, like hand lotion. It will still be white or yellow. There will be enough to make a mark on your underwear. There's not a lot of water in the mucus at this point, so the mark it makes will be rather square or oblong.

### Fertile Days

Next comes the fertile cervical mucus you've been waiting for, thinner and transparent. It will be slippery and very stretchy; many people say it looks like raw egg white. Usually it is clear, but it can be pink or blood-tinged. It may also be watery. Your vagina will feel very wet and lubricated. The discharge will now form a round, moist patch on your underwear (there's more water in it); it will show up more clearly on dark underwear. Fertile cervical mucus won't dissolve in water like the other secretions; it'll form little balls, like opaque marbles, in the toilet bowl. You're most likely to see it after a bowel movement, when you've been straining a little.

You are at your most fertile during this time. Fertile cervical mucus lasts three days on average. Young women have up to five days of it; older women may have only two days, or even just one. (This is one reason young women get pregnant more easily.) Higher estrogen levels create the fertile mucus. When estrogen levels drop and progesterone appears, the fertile mucus dries up within a day. *Your peak fertility is the last day of this egg-white mucus.* Most women are pretty consistent from month to month as to how many days of fertile mucus they have, so once you're familiar with your pattern, you'll be able to target the very best day to have intercourse. For example, if you usually have three days of fertile mucus, on the first day you can make a date for the day after tomorrow. Feel free to throw in the rest of the days, too, of course; it can only help (so long as your partner's sperm count is normal). If you don't experience egg-white mucus as we've described it, try having sex on the last day of the wettest cervical mucus you do observe.

We call the egg-white stuff fertile mucus because besides marking for you when ovulation will occur, it is in and of itself a great boost to fertility. Cervical mucus is the equivalent of semen in men. Men are fertile all the time, so they produce seminal fluid all the time. Women are fertile only once a month, so they produce fertile cervical mucus only once a month.

Sperm can live longer in fertile cervical mucus—up to five days—than in regular cervical mucus. It has nutrients for the sperm, and little striations, sort of like channels, for the sperm to swim in. All this means that there can be a reservoir of sperm waiting for an egg to be released, headed toward it, so timing intercourse doesn't have to be so precise. The mucus also capacitates sperm—that is, it prepares the sperm to fertilize the egg. Without the chemical changes the mucus makes possible, the sperm could not attach to or penetrate an egg. Mucus also helps filter out bacteria and prevents bacteria from taking hold in the uterus. The pH of fertile mucus matches that of semen, and this alkalinity protects sperm from an environment in the vagina that is generally acidic, which is detrimental to sperm.

So in addition to cracking the code of your cervical mucus to help you know when you're ovulating, you'll also want to make sure you have healthy mucus for its own sake. If you have to put a finger inside your vagina to get any fertile mucus, you probably don't have enough. If, however, your underwear is wet with it, you have quite a lot. If you have too little mucus, you need to double-check that you aren't taking any medications that could be drying it up. (The most common culprits are diuretics, antihistamines, decongestants, and high-dose vitamin C.) If your mucus is too thick or is otherwise "hostile" to sperm, you may want to use the over-the-counter decongestant guaifenesin (Mucinex or Humibid) or a natural alternative to liquefy thick mucus or otherwise balance it out (see chapter 18).

After ovulation takes place, progesterone makes the mucus very thick, thereby preventing sperm from swimming into the uterus. It will get cloudy again, compared to the transparency of the fertile stuff. It will likely be so thick that it more or less stays in place, and you may not see it at all during this phase. In most cases, women have essentially no discharge until their periods start again, eleven to fourteen days after ovulation. Thanks to the drop in progesterone, some women get a wet, watery sensation just before their periods.

## Cervical Position

While tracking your cervical mucus, you should also track your cervix itself. The lower part of the uterus, the "neck" where the uterus and the vagina come together, moves up and down a bit and changes texture under the influence of shifting hormones through the menstrual cycle.

### *Getting Started*

If you want to know where your cervix is, what it's up to, and what it can tell you about your fertility, you're going to have to stick a finger up into your vagina to find out. For some of you, that's no big deal. But if you have a less relaxed relationship with the unseen portions of your anatomy, promise us you'll give it a try. We think you'll find it *is* no big deal, and you'll soon get the hang of it, even if it is a bit awkward at first.

To get useful information from your cervix, you'll have to check it regularly. Every day, in fact, except while menstruating, for at least for a few cycles. You're looking for changes than can be subtle and signs that are relative. You'll need a clear idea of what it was like yesterday to understand what you are observing today.

Here again, you may want to jot down what you observe, at least at first while you are becoming familiar with your own pattern. You can do that on a BBT chart if you are keeping one, on your calendar, or in a notebook or diary.

### *How to Check It*

So once your period is done, here's what you do. First, wash your hands. (Do *not* check your cervix if you have vaginal sores, a herpes outbreak, or a yeast infection.) Choose a time to check when you do not have a full bowel, which can make the cervix feel as if it is positioned lower than it really is. Figure out a comfortable and accessible way to position your body — we recommend squatting or standing with one leg up on the toilet lid. Find what works for you, then stick with it. You need to use the same position consistently.

Slide a finger into your vagina until you touch your cervix. Use your finger to gauge how far up it is (low, midway, or high in the vaginal canal). Press gently to see how the cervix feels (firm, soft, or medium). Feel for the opening to get an idea of its size (open, partially open, or closed). If you haven't already, note the quality of the mucus you feel (wet or dry; sticky, creamy, or slippery). That's it! You're done.

### *Are You Ready to Ovulate?*

Right after your period ends, your cervix will be hard, like the tip of your nose, and low. The opening will be closed and feel something like a dimple. (There will be little or no cervical mucus.) In the one to three days before ovulation, the cervix will move higher in the vaginal canal, as estrogen tightens the ligaments that hold it in place. It will start to feel soft, almost like your lips. By ovulation, the cervix will be open, to allow the sperm to swim into the uterus on their way to the fallopian tubes, and with practice you'll be able to feel that, too. And of course the texture of the mucus you feel will be changing during this time frame, as described in the previous section. At ovulation, you should experience wetness coming from the cervix.

After ovulation, in the luteal phase, the cervix will again be low, hard, and closed.

Toni Weschler provides a handy acronym in her book to help you remember what to look for at ovulation: SHOW, for soft, high, open, and wet. If you let it, your cervix will SHOW you when you are most likely to conceive.

## Basal Body Temperature

Your body temperature shifts subtly throughout your menstrual cycle, and tracking its changes is a great way to understand your body's rhythm and to help figure out when you are most fertile. Over time, focusing on the day-to-day differences will give you insight into how your body works, and this information will be very useful when you're trying to conceive. It can also give you insight into what is going wrong if you have trouble conceiving.

To track these differences, you'll need to take your temperature first thing every morning — that's when you get your basal, or baseline, body temperature (BBT) — and record it on a special chart so that you can interpret the significant details of the pattern revealed. You may also note your observations about your cervical mucus and the position of your cervix on the chart.

Body temperature alone can't tell you when you ought to be having sex, because the significant change in temperature happens right at ovulation, and by the time you detect it, you'll have missed your fertile phase for that cycle. A BBT chart *can* tell you for sure that you are ovulating, a key piece of information to have if you want to conceive a baby. And it can help you determine whether your luteal phase is long enough to allow for implantation. (More about that is coming up.) The true power of the BBT chart comes in conjunction with tracking changes in cervical position and mucus, as we've been discussing. Taken all together, these signs will point you toward your peak fertility.

We have two pieces of advice before we get into the nitty-gritty of how to track your temperature. The first is a basic recommendation to bring your chart with you to any and all appointments with your health care practitioner, as he or she may want to adjust treatment accordingly. This is true for any practitioner who knows how to read a BBT chart, but especially so in Chinese medicine, where herbal formulas and acupuncture approaches will vary throughout your cycle. In addition, a professional can interpret the chart for you if you haven't mastered that yourself yet.

Which brings us to our second piece of advice: don't get bogged down in the details of tracking your fertility this way. Anyone can learn to do this quickly and easily, and most women enjoy the process of tuning in to their bodies more acutely than they ever have before. Like pregnancy itself, this can give you a fresh appreciation for and awe at the wonders of the human body. As this book goes on, you'll find that information from a BBT chart can help you identify your fertility type and sometimes help diagnose a fertility problem or suggest a treatment. It also can provide a wealth of insight for a Chinese medicine diagnosis.

If maintaining a BBT chart just seems to you like another item on your already oppressive "to do" list rather than a helpful tool, it may not be for you. Or you may need to find some happy medium, such as letting your doctor interpret your chart for you, or keeping track of your cervix but not your temperature. Find what works best for you, with an eye to decreasing, not increasing, your stress. If you don't want to keep a chart, don't. If keeping a chart is stressing you out, stop. If your doctor or practitioner thinks that keeping a chart would provide important information, you can always chart later if you decide not to now.

In any case, you need only about three months of BBT charts to detect your personal pattern. If things are changing and you or your doctor needs more information on how they are changing, you may want to continue charting beyond three months. Or if you simply like watching your rhythms unfold, by all means go ahead and keep charting.

### How to Chart

The basic idea is to take your temperature every morning and note it on your chart. After you've recorded a bunch of temperatures, you're going to look for certain trends in how your body changes through your menstrual cycle. Your temperature will be lower before you ovulate and higher afterward, normally varying by at least 0.4°F.

We recommend using a special digital BBT thermometer, which will be more accurate at measuring smaller increments of temperature than a regular thermometer. You can buy one at any drugstore for around $10. It will give you a readout in only about one minute.

Before you go to bed at night, place the thermometer within easy reach so that you will not need to move much to get it in the morning. When we say you need to take your temperature first thing in the morning, we are not fooling around. We mean *first thing:* before you cuddle, before you drink coffee, before you pee, before you even speak. Any activity will change your temperature, and you want to get a reading when you are as close to inactive as possible. (If you are one of the holdouts using a glass thermometer and we can't convince you to upgrade to a faster digital model, be sure to shake it down before you go to bed so that you don't have to in the morning.)

You should take your temperature after a minimum of five hours of sleep if at all possible. Any reading you get after less sleep won't be accurate — your body temperature won't have had enough time to settle down.

Take your temperature orally, and do it exactly the same way every time, right down to putting the thermometer in the same place in your mouth. Take your temperature at as close to the same time each day as possible. (But no alarm setting on weekends! Sleep in when you want to or can.) If you have a regular wake-up time during the week, that will be enough to establish the trend. Take 0.1°F off your temperature for each half hour you sleep beyond your usual temperature-taking time. Likewise, if you wake up earlier than usual, add 0.1°F for each half hour of sleep you have missed. And don't worry if you miss a day here or there. As long as you have enough data points to show a trend, you'll have what you need.

Start a new chart on day 1 of your cycle — the day you get your period. Mark down your temperature every day, then play "connect the dots" to join them together into one line. There's space on the chart for you to note any unusual events in your life — things that might stress you out or otherwise affect your cycle. Big presentation at work? Fight with your partner? Moving day? Jot it down. This may help you make sense of irregularities in your cycle that might otherwise cause concern. You should also record your observations about your cervical mucus and position. You may want to use the chart to record details about your period — color, amount, length, pain, clots, stops and starts — as well.

You can find a blank chart to photocopy in the appendix (page 341). You also can print out copies of the chart at http://www.making babiesprogram.com.

### Draw a Cover Line

To give you a clear visual of your temperature shift and ovulation, you'll need to draw a "cover line" on your chart. This is very simple, but until you do it once, it may sound a bit confusing. Refer to the sample chart showing the cover line to help you visualize how this works.

As you enter your daily temperature, keep an eye out for the day your temperature rises at least 0.2°F above the previous day. (You should expect this to be roughly two weeks into your cycle, although part of what a BBT chart will reveal is where your cycle differs from the average.) Count back six days from that day, marking the temperatures on those days with a highlighter or a colored pen. Pick the highest of those six temperatures and make a mark on the chart 0.1°F above it. Now draw a line all the way across the chart at the level of that mark. That's your cover line.

With the cover line in place, you'll be able to see clearly that the follicular phase temperatures fall in a cluster below that line and the luteal phase temperatures fall above it. The sample chart on the next page shows a typical twenty-eight-day cycle.

# THE MAKING BABIES
# BASAL BODY TEMPERATURE CHART

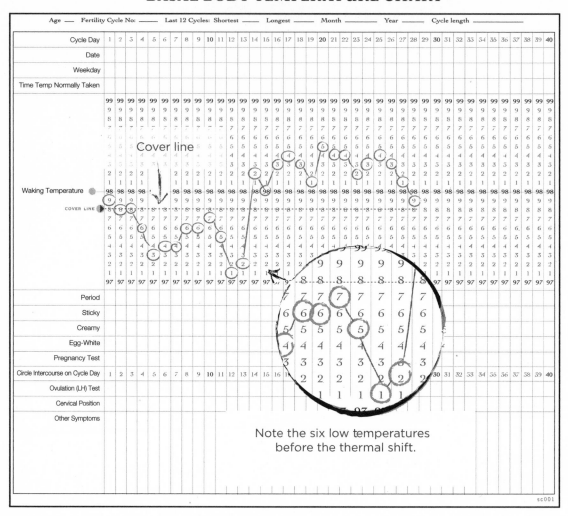

**Fig. 3:** A standard chart with the cover line drawn.

## Understanding Your Chart

The first thing to remember when interpreting your chart is to focus on the overall trend and not get hung up on individual temperature variations. This is one reason the cover line is useful, putting emphasis on the two phases rather than the little ups and downs you might see from day to day. When drawing your cover line, if you have one temperature in the first half of your cycle that is much higher than all the others (more than the 0.2°F rise you're looking for), consider it a fluke and ignore it when working out where to draw the cover line and when you ovulate. We call this the "rule of thumb"—put your thumb over the temperature that's way out of line as a way of disregarding it when you interpret your chart. Over time, you'll know more about how your chart usually looks, and it will be easier to know for sure if an off number really is a fluke. Noting anything out of the ordinary going on in your life can also help you explain a fluke high temperature (see the box on page 50). The sample chart below shows a fluke high temperature to be ignored for the purposes of the cover line.

## THE MAKING BABIES
## BASAL BODY TEMPERATURE CHART

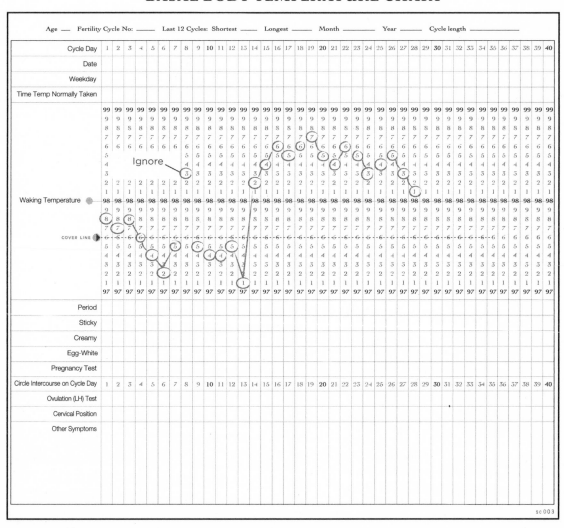

**Fig. 4:** A chart ignoring an unusually high temperature.

Looking at a chart filled in through one entire cycle, here's what you can expect to see. Estrogen predominates among your hormones during the first part of your cycle, and it turns down the thermostat a bit when it is in charge. In this follicular phase, BBT is generally between 97°F and 97.5°F and should be pretty stable. In the average twenty-eight-day cycle, this first phase—from when your period starts until you ovulate—usually lasts fourteen days, but it can last as few as twelve or as many as fifteen days.

## THE MAKING BABIES
## BASAL BODY TEMPERATURE CHART

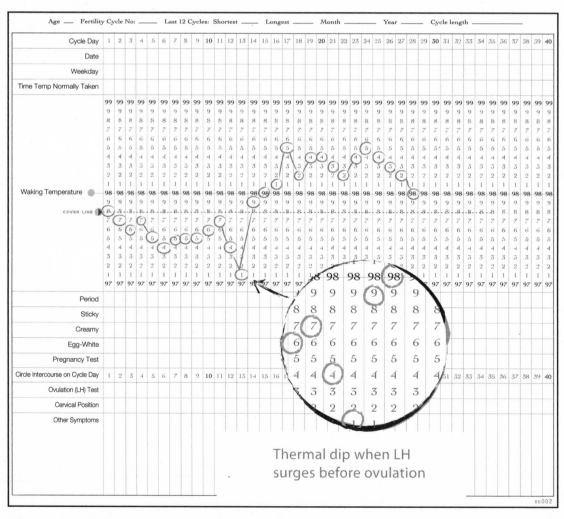

Thermal dip when LH
surges before ovulation

**Fig. 5:** A chart highlighting the temperature dip when there is a surge in LH.

Then progesterone takes the wheel, and it warms things up a bit. When you ovulate, your temperature will go up within twenty-four hours to at least 0.4°F higher than the highest temperature over the previous six days. Your temperature will generally stay up for twelve to sixteen days—the average luteal phase BBT is between 97.6°F and 98.6°F—until your period begins again. If you get pregnant, your temperature will remain elevated for more than eighteen days, as progesterone stays on as boss during implantation and gestation.

Some women get a temperature drop when LH surges just before they ovulate. If you are one of them, you can watch for this drop in your chart and take it as a sign to have sex if trying to conceive. Not everyone gets this dip, but women who do usually get it every month, and it will be obvious on your chart (see the sample chart showing this dip).

Other than that, you want to watch for the upward temperature shift so that you can be sure you are ovulating. Also pay attention to the length of the luteal phase. If it is too short, you may conceive but then have problems with implantation. (See page 200 for more on luteal phase defect, or LPD.) And, of course, once you are familiar with your body's patterns, the chart can help you predict when you will ovulate, and you can time intercourse accordingly. Just keep in mind that the chart alone won't tell you for sure that you are ovulating until it is too late to conceive in that cycle.

### What to Watch For on Your Chart
A few common BBT chart patterns can indicate fertility trouble. If you spot one of these on your chart, bring it to your doctor's attention.

**PHASE 1 (MENSTRUATION)**
- BBT that stays high for one or two days after the start of your period

**PHASE 2 (PRE-OVULATION)**
- BBT that doesn't stay steady around 97°F to 97.5°F
- BBT above 97.8°F (spikes in temperature can impair egg development and make you ovulate early)
- Consistently low BBT
- Follicular phase less than ten days/early ovulation (the uterine lining may not be thick enough for implantation)
- Follicular phase longer than twenty days (estrogen is building up too slowly; the resulting deterioration in egg

quality means an increased risk of chromosomal abnormalities, which increase the risk of miscarriage)

PHASE 3 (OVULATION)

- No spike in BBT to herald ovulation

PHASE 4 (POTENTIAL IMPLANTATION)

- BBT climbs, then sinks, then climbs again, making a saddle shape pattern (low progesterone)
- BBT drops erratically, or drops three to five days before period begins (possible luteal phase defect [LPD])

### *Am I Pregnant?*

A BBT chart can help you tell when you are pregnant. This might not be necessary in this age of easy at-home pregnancy tests, but it's cheaper than buying a large supply of those pee sticks, handy though they may be. And it's just cool to understand your body's rhythms enough to interpret them this way.

Here's what to look for:

- Eighteen days of high temperatures in the luteal phase (after ovulation)
- Luteal phase temperature that remains high three days longer than the longest luteal phase you have previously recorded
- A triphasic chart (see sample on next page) with temperature increasing from the follicular to the luteal phase, then again from the luteal phase to pregnancy (the chart looks like stair steps; the second shift in the luteal phase happens after implantation, about five to eight days after ovulation, and is a really good sign)

Spot one of these signs, and you'll know you need to make an appointment with your ob-gyn as soon as possible.

You'll find more ways to use information from your BBT chart in several upcoming chapters, including how BBT patterns can help identify your fertility type and how your chart can help you detect specific fertility problems.

# THE MAKING BABIES
# BASAL BODY TEMPERATURE CHART

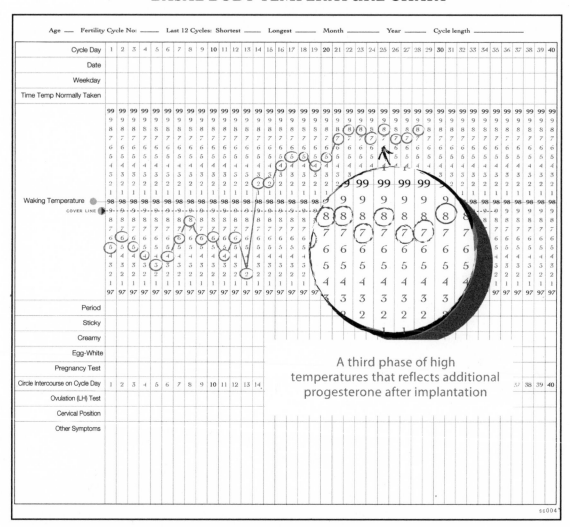

**Fig. 6:** A chart showing a triphasic pattern that indicates pregnancy.

## WHY IS MY BBT OFF?

Several common occurrences or practices can throw off your BBT. To get the most accurate chart, avoid the ones you can (no electric blankets) or make a note on the chart so you'll have a clue about why an unusual temperature might have occurred. The first three are the most common things that affect BBT.

- Having a fever
- Drinking alcohol
- Getting less than three hours of sleep or having disturbed sleep
- Taking your temperature at a different time
- Using a hot pack or electric blanket
- Breathing through your mouth while asleep or being congested (causing mouth breathing)
- Traveling to a different time zone
- Taking an anti-inflammatory or a sleep aid
- Stress

## Case Study: Joanne

Joanne didn't really know when she ovulated. Her periods were always irregular, she didn't get the cramping that some women do, and she'd never thought much about her cervical mucus, much less the position of her cervix or her BBT. She always knew when her period was coming, she told me (Jill), because she experienced PMS symptoms such as breast tenderness, fatigue, and irritability, but those signals weren't very helpful in trying to get pregnant. For months, she'd been squeezing appointments for unprotected sex with her husband into her hectic schedule, to no avail.

I explained how to keep a BBT chart, which she agreed to do. At her next appointment, one thing jumped off the chart for me: her temperature dipped just before she ovulated (when her LH surged). But it did not rise again for several days, when it should have shot up right at ovulation. She was ovulating, but it was taking longer than usual. This slow transition revealed that her body couldn't make hormonal shifts smoothly. At ovulation, her body was not responding efficiently to the rise in progesterone. She could blame the same problem for those PMS symptoms, though they were occurring as her progesterone fell.

I prescribed herbs meant to ease these hormonal transitions and persuaded her to fit acupuncture into her busy schedule. We knew we were getting somewhere as her PMS symptoms eased and her cycle got more regular. Her BBT chart kept showing the temperature drop at the LH surge, but now it was promptly followed by an appropriate rise, signaling ovulation. After six months of treatment, Joanne conceived and went on to have a baby girl.

### Other Signs That You Are Ovulating

The most reliable signals of ovulation that you can observe on your own are fertile cervical mucus, cervical position, and BBT, as described in this chapter. But lots of women experience other physical symptoms that let them know they are ovulating. If you tune in, you may notice some in yourself. We recommend letting that knowledge just confirm what the Big Three are telling you; don't count on any of them to guide your attempts at conception.

It's perfectly normal to have — or not have — any of these symptoms when you are ovulating, and the pattern will be different for every woman.

- Water retention
- Breast sensitivity or tenderness
- Heightened senses
- Increased libido (some of my [Jill's] patients have noticed that they are more desirable to the opposite sex at this time, too; one woman told me that she could always tell she was ovulating because men would approach her in the street and on the subway)
- "Mittelschmerz" — a dull pain as the follicle swells or a sharp one as the egg bursts out (felt on the same side of the abdomen as whichever ovary is releasing the egg); may be very mild, more or less like "gas pain," or more emphatic; may feel like a cramp as the follicle bursts
- Mid-cycle bleeding, caused by the sudden drop in estrogen when there's not enough progesterone to sustain the endometrium (occurs in about 10 percent of women)
- Abdominal bloating
- Swollen vulva
- Increased energy; feeling of being more dynamic and outgoing; feeling more attractive (or even thinner!)
- Increased sense of well-being and optimism
- Swollen lymph gland in groin (on whichever side ovulation is occurring)

### Ovulation Predictor Kits

There is a less hands-on way of knowing when you ovulate: an ovulation predictor kit, available in any drugstore. These kits work pretty much like a home pregnancy test, but they are looking for a different hormone: LH, which triggers the release of the mature egg from the follicle. So you pee on the stick (or "hold it in your urine stream") for a few seconds, wait a few minutes, and watch for an indicator line to appear (or not). You do one a day leading up to when you expect to ovulate. When it detects a rise in LH, you'll ovulate in the next twenty-four to forty-eight hours. Start having sex every day, or every other day, as soon as you see the faintest indication of LH.

Tracking ovulation this way costs a lot more than tracking cervical mucus changes or BBT. Each kit typically contains five tests and costs about $15. That's enough to get you through one cycle, unless you have irregular cycles, in which case you could easily need more than one box to hit the target. Regardless, you may find the convenience worth the cost.

Ovulation predictor kits have one clear advantage over charting BBT: as the name promises, they *predict* ovulation, whereas tracking your temperature will tell you only when you have ovulated. But the results can sometimes be misleading.

- Just because LH is detected does not mean you will ovulate. In some cases, LH spikes but the follicle doesn't heed the call to rupture, and no egg is released. (See the section on luteinized unruptured follicle syndrome, or LUFS, on page 212.)
- Some women have false LH surges several days before ovulation. This is especially common in women with polycystic ovarian syndrome (PCOS; see page 202). If you get a result that seems too early, keep testing to see if you get another, more realistic spike a bit further down the road.
- Women over 40 sometimes have elevated levels of LH in general, so when they use these kits, there may be several days when it looks as though they're ovulating, and they can't tell which one is the real deal.

### Ferning

Time was, if you needed to know whether you were ovulating, your doctor would take a sample of cervical mucus during an internal exam performed near the expected time of ovulation, place a drop of it on a slide, allow it to dry for a few minutes, and then pop it under the microscope to look for telltale "ferning." Near ovulation, high levels of estrogen increase the level of electrolytes (salts) in body fluids, including cervical mucus. When viewed under a microscope, those salts form a distinctive crystalline pattern resembling the leaves of a fern or frost on a window. The pattern is there only on the three or four days before ovulation. (Outside your fertile time, dried mucus looks like random dots.) So if the doctor saw the pattern, he or she knew you were in your most fertile period, just before ovulation. (The doctor would simultaneously check the mucus for spinnbarkeit, or stretchiness, to confirm the conclusion.)

With all the sensitive hormone tests available today, not many doctors are spending much time peering through a microscope looking for ferns. But if you are so inclined, you can do it yourself, using a microscope the size of a tube of lipstick and a sample of your saliva (or your cervical mucus, but the saliva is that much easier to get on the slide). You can buy a personal ovulation microscope, which magnifies things about fifty times, as part of a kit available at any drugstore or online. Expect it to set you back between $20 and $50. The slide and microscope are reusable, so this is a one-time investment and may be cheaper than an adequate supply of the pee sticks, if not quite as precise. For the best results, have sex on the day you first see the ferning and every day or every other day until the ferning disappears.

### Ultrasound

For the sake of covering all the bases, we want to mention that ovulation can also be detected by sonogram. You're not going to use this for most conception planning, but when the precise day of ovulation is key to a fertility treatment such as intrauterine insemination (IUI) or in vitro fertilization (IVF), both of which are discussed in chapter 25, this is how your doctor will tell. If that level of precision is not required, the doctor will most likely rely on hormone blood tests.

### Which Way Is Best?

What is the best way for you to figure out when you are ovulating? We recommend that you pick whichever approach seems simplest, easiest, most appealing, or niftiest to you. I (Sami) generally recommend ovulation predictor kits to my patients who want to keep closer tabs on the situation themselves. I (Jill) prefer BBT charting with cervical mucus tracking because the process of documenting ovulation also provides me with other useful information.

You may find other ovulation-related products on the market, some of which combine a few of the strategies discussed here. Sometimes we hear from patients about positive experiences with a fertility monitor or some other gadget, and who knows what will be developed next. Although we certainly haven't provided a comprehensive listing here, we have covered the simplest and most straightforward, useful, and effective methods commonly in use today.

If this all seems like more than you want to manage, we hope you'll focus on at least one message: if you see egg-white mucus, have sex! I (Jill) had a patient who had been peeing on ovulation predictor sticks for several months but still wasn't pregnant. She'd been getting erratic results with the tests because her LH was elevated across the board (not unusual for a woman of 43), so it was hard to know if she was timing intercourse correctly. Recently, she called me to report, "I remembered what you said about watching for egg whites, so when I saw it, I went right home and met my husband. And now we're pregnant!" Sometimes it's just that simple.

## WHAT ARE THE ODDS?

For the average, healthy couple, the odds of conceiving in any given cycle are about 20 to 25 percent, and they don't get any better just because you've tried before. So it can take a while to get pregnant, even when everything is normal and it's well planned out. Still, six in ten couples actively trying to conceive, having sex two or three times a week, will get pregnant within the first six months of trying, eight out of ten will succeed within the first year, and nine out of ten will succeed within eighteen months.

So the final tool you need for getting pregnant is a modicum of patience. If it doesn't happen the first month or two or three, there is absolutely no need for concern. If you get worked up about it, you're only going to make it that much harder. That's not to say everyone should go on being patient indefinitely. At some point, couples do need to seek medical assistance. Chapter 25 has more about how to know whether that time has arrived for you. But for starters, learn what you need to know from this chapter, make time in your life for sex, check out the next chapters for tips on how to make sure your overall health and well-being are most conducive to fertility, and let nature take its course.

And who knows, you may find that a little tweaking to match the guidelines in this chapter are all you will need to get pregnant. We've helped hundreds of patients conceive just by teaching them to understand when they are most fertile so they can time intercourse perfectly. Give it a chance, and maybe this will work for you, too.

## Making Babies Action Plan

- ❏ Have vaginal intercourse in the missionary position, and don't skip the foreplay.
- ❏ Stay in bed for ten to twenty minutes after sex around the time of ovulation.
- ❏ Avoid lubricants, especially scented products. Use Pre-Seed, sparingly, if you need some extra moisture. Don't use water, saliva, or mineral oil.
- ❏ Abstain from having sex during your period. According to Chinese medicine, it can interfere with proper blood flow.
- ❏ Have sex every day or every other day during your most fertile times. If your partner's sperm count is low or low normal, keep it to every other day.
- ❏ Have sex just ahead of ovulation, days twelve through fourteen of a standard twenty-eight-day cycle with ovulation on day 14.
- ❏ Track your body's cycle so you know exactly when you ovulate.
- ❏ Look for egg-white fertile cervical mucus.
- ❏ Track cervical position, looking for SHOW (soft, high, open, and wet).
- ❏ Tune in to other signs your body gives you when you are ovulating.
- ❏ Keep a BBT chart and look for the temperature shift that shows you have ovulated.

❑   Try an ovulation predictor kit, or use a personal ovulation microscope to check for ferning.

❑   Consider forgoing perfume or any other strongly scented products during phase 3 of your cycle (ovulation). At that time, your body gives off specific chemical cues (pheromones) in the form of subtle odors that signal both you and your partner that it's a good time to mate. You don't want to drown out that message. Let nature take its course.

# Lifestyles of the Naturally Fertile

The process of maturing an oocyte into an egg ready to be released at ovulation goes on for at least three months. It also takes at least three months for sperm cells to develop fully. What happens in your body during this time affects your eggs or sperm. If you want them to be healthy and active, *you* need to be healthy and active. Consider this time a three-month "pre-mester" during which you can help your body prepare to conceive. Take the same careful care of your body as you would if you were already pregnant. Do it for the same reason you do it during pregnancy (providing the best health for your baby), and you'll get a bonus: a smoother, surer path to conception. Men, follow your partner's lead and take care of your body with the same care. You'll reap the same rewards.

For the most part, the things that keep your body healthy also support fertility. So the basic principles in this chapter will probably come as no surprise. But many of the reasons behind our recommendations may shed new light on familiar ground. We'll look at the specific links to improving fertility in order to reinforce your motivation to implement any necessary changes in your life.

Wanting to have a healthy baby is a primal urge, and most women are therefore capable of being really well behaved while pregnant. What's not always as clear to our patients is that cleaning up their acts in similar ways will help them get pregnant in the first place. This is a news flash for some would-be dads, too: your health affects the likelihood and health of a pregnancy, especially before that pregnancy is ever conceived.

So on the one hand, we take a firm stand: everyone who wants to conceive will benefit by getting himself or herself in good shape before he or she even starts trying. We recommend taking a full three months to do so. On the other hand, this is not a rigid program. We won't be telling you never to let coffee cross your lips, or to exercise every day (or drop exercise altogether), or to swear off all junk food, or to quit your job so you will never experience stress (as if that would work anyway). We advocate moderation in all things. We lay out our advice clearly, but we don't want to cause anxiety by making you feel that you have to heed every last piece of it if you ever want to get pregnant. As long as you are making choices for general good health and following our guidelines whenever possible, in ways that make sense in your life, you'll be doing the right thing.

And you'll be rewarded for your efforts. British researchers surveyed more than two thousand pregnant women to assess how much lifestyle factors influenced time to pregnancy. They wanted to know if drinking, smoking, being overweight, being over age 35 for a woman or over age 45 for a man, or drinking caffeinated beverages as if you owned a Starbucks really made an impact on how long it took couples to conceive once they started trying.

They found that couples with, between them, more than four strikes against them in these areas took more than seven times longer to conceive than couples with none of these bad habits, and they were more than seven times as likely to take more than a year to get pregnant. The chances that they would conceive at all fell by 60 percent; less than 40 percent of them were able to conceive within a year. The more they smoked or drank or caffeinated themselves, the greater the impact on their fertility. Even couples with just two bad habits between them — maybe he's overweight and she's over 35, or she's into espresso and he's a beer connoisseur — took two and a half times longer to get pregnant than those without any bad habits.

Despite these findings, we see this as a good-news study. At bottom, what these scientists found was that 83 percent of the couples with fertility-friendly lifestyles got pregnant within one year. They estimated that if couples planning a pregnancy led fertility-friendly lives, they'd cut their chances of fertility problems in half. This research is backed up by findings from a study at the University of Surrey which showed that couples diagnosed with infertility who made lifestyle changes, especially in their diets, and followed a program of nutritional supplements had an 80 percent pregnancy rate. (In couples without infertility diagnoses, pregnancy rates normally range from 44 to 96 percent within a year of trying, depending on age.) Other research indicates that cleaning up your act can also help increase your chances of success with ARTs.

This chapter covers many of the most important lifestyle choices for conceiving naturally. (The next two chapters discuss two other major lifestyle factors, stress and diet.) The advice is simple: be realistic about your age, control your weight, get good exercise, get sufficient sleep, avoid environmental toxins, don't smoke, be careful with medications, don't use recreational drugs, and don't overheat your reproductive organs. Our purpose here, though, isn't just to give you commonsense advice. We mean to convince you that each of these things is crucial for fertility, not just for general good health or even the health of a future baby. Whether or not there will *be* a future baby may hang in the balance.

In upcoming chapters, you will learn how to determine your personal fertility type and get a lifestyle program to optimize fertility for your specific type. These programs are built on the foundation this chapter provides. To increase the chances of conceiving naturally, everyone, of every fertility type, should begin by following these basic recommendations.

## BE AWARE OF YOUR AGE

If we had to pin fertility on just one factor, the most important would be age. The older you are, male or female, the more likely you and your partner are to have problems conceiving and carrying a pregnancy. That's true for conceiving naturally, and it's true for conceiving with technology. As a society, our view of IVF and other high-tech fertility interventions as one giant Plan B is deeply flawed.

And so we've put age at the top of this list of lifestyle factors that influence fertility. Age might seem like a fertility factor you have no control over, at least if you are already in your 30s. But you can control a number of other factors that offset the effects of aging.

Speaking strictly from the "how easy or hard it will be to get pregnant" point of view, the best advice is to have children sooner rather than later (though of course that isn't always feasible, for so many reasons). As men and women get older, both sperm and eggs decline in quantity and quality, which leads to higher rates of birth defects, miscarriages, and pregnancy risks.

The older you get, the more the lifestyle choices matter. The strategies laid out in the Making Babies program will benefit everyone, in a variety of ways, but several will specifically combat the effects of aging on fertility. When you're 23, it will probably be a simple enough thing to get pregnant even if you party every weekend and don't eat right or get any exercise. When you're 38, it's quite a different story.

*Peak* reproductive capacity is a benefit of youth. But peak reproductive capacity is not necessary for conceiving and bearing a child. Women under age 25 have a 96 percent chance of conceiving within a year. That figure drops to 86 percent between ages 25 and 34. The odds decrease again for women at age 35, with further drop-offs at 38 and again at about 42. However, if you group all women ages 35 to 44, statistically about 78 percent of them will be able to get pregnant within a year (weighted more toward 35 than 44, of course).

But age alone cannot account for the dramatic increases in infertility rates over the past several decades. Other aspects of people's lifestyles and environments are contributing to this finding, and these need to be addressed. Our society often assumes that infertility is increasing because so many people are choosing to become parents at ever older ages, but research shows that this development is not sufficient to explain the fertility changes we're seeing—and the way we're seeing them. Even within specific age groups, the number of couples facing infertility has been increasing for years. In fact, the biggest increases in rates of infertility have occurred in the youngest women.

When age *is* the problem, it's not just the woman's age that matters. It is true that women age 35 and older do have a harder time getting pregnant (and have higher-risk pregnancies). According to figures from the American Society for Reproductive Medicine (ASRM), a woman's chances of getting pregnant in any given cycle are 20 percent for women under 30 but just 5 percent for women over 40. Pregnancy rates fall and miscarriage rates rise with a woman's age. The same is true for couples with a man age 40 or older, even if his partner is younger than 35. A couple in which the man is five or more years older than his partner, no matter what her age, can have a harder time, too.

A new study from France confirms this. It is the first large-scale study (more than 12,000 couples) to quantify the effects of age on a man's fertility. In the study, pregnancy rates fell by 10 percent by the time the male partner hit 35 and by 20 percent after age 45, no matter the age of the woman. Furthermore, the study found that beginning when men were in their mid-30s, miscarriage rates started to rise, enough to double by age 45, at which point about one in three couples with men age 45 or older had a pregnancy ending in miscarriage, regardless of the women's age.

### What You Can Do About It

Men and women can combat the effects of aging on fertility by paying attention to the remaining lifestyle choices, upcoming recommendations about nutrition and supplements, and specific self-help, medical, and Chinese medical treatments later in the book. These will help to improve the development of follicles, blood flow to the ovaries, and sperm count and quality and help to manage hormonal fluctuations, no matter what a couple's ages.

## CONTROL YOUR WEIGHT

Roughly 12 percent of all infertility cases can be traced to weight problems in women — split pretty much evenly between weighing too little and weighing too much, according to the ASRM. Seriously overweight women suffer from infertility at a rate approaching double that of normal weight women. Roughly the same is true for underweight women. Men, too, face fertility problems related to being overweight. Seriously overweight men are 50 percent more likely than normal weight men to be infertile. And it turns out that couples in which both partners are overweight are three times more likely not to be pregnant after a year of trying than are couples of normal weight. Just 10 percent over or under your ideal body weight is all it takes to make a difference in your fertility.

The Harvard Nurses' Health Study, a large, long-term research project on a variety of health topics, found that overweight women took twice as long to get pregnant as normal weight women. Underweight women experienced an even greater gap compared to women of normal weight — it took them four times as long to get pregnant. Being underweight or overweight increases the risk of miscarriage and other risks of pregnancy as well.

None of this bodes well for a nation such as ours: famously fat yet obsessed with being thin, thin, thin. A tangle of factors connect weight and fertility, and no one has teased them all apart yet. One important component is the estrogen made in fat cells: the more fat cells, the more estrogen. Increasing estrogen prevents ovulation (this is what birth control pills do). Seriously overweight women often have irregular and/or infrequent periods, thanks in part to this estrogen interference, as well as periods without ovulation or with inadequate ovulation.

Being overweight also increases androgens ("male" hormones) in women, impairing ovulation. In addition, those estrogen-producing fat cells are throwing off inflammatory substances that can reduce fertility. And excess weight comes with an increase in insulin levels, yet another contributor to the fertility issues overweight women have.

Women who are underweight — who don't have enough body fat — can't produce enough estrogen. The physical stress of being inadequately nourished lowers FSH and LH levels, which creates low estrogen. This chain reaction results in irregular cycles, follicles that can't develop properly, and inadequate or nonexistent ovulation.

Weight matters for men who want to conceive, too. Many cases of low sperm count can be blamed on excess weight. Overweight men have lower testosterone levels than men of normal weight. As body weight goes up, so does the rate of conversion of testosterone into a form of estrogen. An excess of estrogen results, which impairs proper functioning of the testicles, including the development of sperm.

In addition, researchers theorize that excess body fat in the groin area and thighs increases the temperature of the testicles, damaging sperm and impairing fertility through excess heat, just the way a hot bath or tight leather pants can. As body weight increases, the quality of sperm decreases (that is, the rate of genetic abnormalities increases and motility decreases). Couples in which the man is overweight also have a greater risk of miscarriage, probably because of sperm abnormalities.

Being overweight lowers the success rate of fertility treatments. For example, overweight women have a higher rate of miscarriage with ART pregnancies than do women of normal weight, and the higher the number of excess pounds, the higher the risk. In addition, overweight women are less likely to respond well to fertility drugs and so are less successful with IVF and other high-tech fertility interventions. Being overweight also increases the risks associated with surgery for infertility.

## What You Can Do About It

The vast majority (more than 75 percent) of women struggling with infertility caused by being overweight will conceive naturally once their weight stabilizes at a healthy point. Results are even more dramatic for underweight women: 90 percent of them can expect to conceive once they reach their ideal weight. If you are overweight, the loss of 5 or 10 percent of your body weight, ideally with the addition of some exercise, will significantly boost your chances of pregnancy, even if it doesn't bring you all the way to your "ideal" weight. If you are underweight, putting on only a few pounds can make the difference. If you are planning on IVF, losing any excess weight (or gaining a bit if necessary) before you begin is one good way to increase your chances of success. In fact, if you improve your weight, you might not even need IVF. Most doctors don't discuss weight with patients before proceeding with fertility treatments; if you know you are not at your ideal weight, you should make it your business to have that discussion before you sign up for any more invasive approaches to getting pregnant.

You are never going to have a stronger motivation to manage your weight than you do right now. Wanting to wear a smaller-size wedding dress or impress an old boyfriend at a high school reunion can't hold a candle to your desire to conceive a child. Not even your own health and well-being can. So take advantage! You know what you need to do: eat well and move more. If you are underweight, add some healthy fats and protein to your diet. Just a handful of nuts each day and half an avocado on your lunch salad can do the trick (we're not asking you to eat chips and cream sauces). Whether you need to gain or lose, now is the time to take action.

The nutrition plan in this book can help you attain your desired weight. If you need help with specifics such as portion control, you may want to consult any of the myriad diet books out there or a doctor or nutritionist. Just steer clear of fads, drastic dieting, and anything likely to produce only short-term results, such as fasting or meal replacement. The only way to succeed with weight control is to approach it as a lifestyle change, not a "diet," and to proceed at a healthy pace — a pound or two a week. (Losing weight too fast, like other stressors, can affect the hormones and, as a result, fertility. Anorexia and bulimia are the extreme examples, but even before you get that far, your body could be off balance enough to stop ovulating, even if you are still getting a period.) To maximize your fertility, find that healthy weight and maintain it.

It's never easy to get a handle on your weight, but if you are like most of our patients, ready and willing to do *anything* to have a baby, why not start now? Managing your weight has to be easier than undergoing surgery or enduring months and months of treatment with powerful chemical hormones and toxic drugs, with all the attendant short- and long-term side effects and risks. You'll also enjoy a long list of benefits to your general health, and if weight is the root cause of your fertility problem, normalizing it is the thing that's going to work best anyway.

## Case Study: Morgan

Morgan had been a semipro tennis player before taking up a fast-paced job on Wall Street. She was now 28 and as driven and determined to get pregnant as she had been about her career. But she hadn't had a period in months, and it had always been erratic in any case.

I (Sami) suspected that Morgan's estrogen level was too low, and testing established that she was not ovulating. Prescribing clomiphene (Clomid) to make her ovulate was an obvious choice, but I felt that her body may have been showing some wisdom in not allowing her to conceive. I feared that if I forced ovulation with drugs, she might not be able to sustain a pregnancy.

So I talked with her about taking some time to get her body ready to conceive before proceeding with any treatment. I recommended that she scale back on the amount and intensity of her exercise (she hit the gym daily at 5:30 a.m. and was still in close to competitive shape), and I talked with her about getting a little more fat in her diet. She controlled her diet as she did everything else in her life,

and she paid particular attention to avoiding fat for health reasons. But in doing so, she was actually missing some of the nutrition her body needed.

Morgan applied the same determination that had made her so successful in other areas of her life to changing her diet. She made sure to get some healthy fats at every meal, adding flaxseed oil to her salads, snacking on almonds and avocados, and eating salmon at least once a week. Morgan gained about four pounds doing this, which she admitted she found a bit frightening. But it brought her up to an appropriate weight for her height, so I knew that her body would be much better able to regulate its hormones and was ready to support a pregnancy.

At the same time, Morgan consulted Jill and began using an herbal formula to help rebalance her system. After three months, she ovulated on her own. But ovulation continued to be erratic, so Morgan decided she wanted some pharmaceutical help. I gave her Clomid at a very low dose. She immediately began to ovulate monthly and was soon pregnant.

## EXERCISE

The image of the top athlete who trains hard enough to stop getting her period is so familiar that many women are hesitant to exercise when they are trying to get pregnant. Some doctors don't want to recommend exercise to patients who are planning to conceive; some even warn against it. Although intense exercise can cause women to stop ovulating, the newest research shows that moderate exercise actually benefits fertility.

One finding to emerge from the Nurses' Health Study was a reduction in the risk of ovulatory infertility with exercise. Hitting the gym three to five times a week could bring the risk down by as much as 25 percent or more. Other, smaller studies also have concluded that exercise improves fertility.

Regular activity helps the body control blood sugar levels by burning off sugar in the blood. That means insulin can work as it is meant to, without going to the kinds of extremes that can interfere with ovulatory function and conception. Exercise also helps keep androgens at appropriate levels so they will help, not hinder, fertility. Exercise fights inflammation, too, decreasing the chances that it can get in the way of conceiving. And exercise relieves stress, which can improve fertility as well (see chapter 4).

Men's fertility also is affected by exercise: too much, too intensely has a negative effect (though men generally have a higher tolerance for it than women do). Moderate exercise is, however, a boon to good health, including fertility. Serious long-distance runners (more than one hundred miles per week) may have low testosterone levels while in training, enough to curb their sex drives and potentially decrease their fertility.

---

### Case Study: Larry

Larry and his wife had been trying to conceive for many months with no luck. They appeared to be about as healthy a couple as you'd ever meet—both were marathon runners. I (Sami) sent Larry for a semen analysis, which revealed that his sperm count was low. I couldn't find anything else in either of them that could explain their difficulties conceiving. My advice was to be patient until after Larry's upcoming race. Sure enough, once the stress of high-intensity training let up and the compression shorts spent more time in the drawer and less time on Larry, his sperm count went up to the normal range. Within a couple of months, he was officially a father-to-be and back in training.

Distance cyclers (more than fifty miles per week) may have reduced sperm production. (With bicycling, it's not just the stress of intense exercise but also the bicycle seat and even the bike shorts; see page 81). When not done to these extremes, exercise is a positive choice, and fertility is soon restored when men in particularly intensive training tone it down a bit.

### What You Can Do About It

There's no reason not to exercise when you are trying to conceive. Normal exercise will not impede fertility, and we all know it's a key component of weight control, making it key for optimum fertility as well. The bottom line is, *exercise is good for you.* So just do it! You are more likely to have fertility problems traceable to obesity and a sedentary lifestyle than to overdoing it physically.

Our general recommendation for exercising to maximize fertility is pretty much the same as for exercising to maximize overall health. Most people should try to get at least thirty minutes of moderate exercise almost every day—more if they are trying to lose weight—and vary their activity so they get aerobics, strengthening, and stretching out of the deal. If you haven't been exercising regularly or at all, now is an

---

### Case Study: Martha

Martha had no trouble getting pregnant the first time around. She and her husband wanted a second child, but after a year of trying, she still wasn't pregnant. (This "secondary infertility" is particularly perplexing to doctors.) Sure, Martha was three years older than she was the first time, but I (Sami) discovered that it was another change in her life that was causing the problem: she'd begun taking an intense aerobics class four times a week. The endorphin rushes from her intense workouts were lowering her progesterone level so far that although she was conceiving, she was actually miscarrying before she even knew she was pregnant. She was still getting her period regularly, so she never suspected she was overdoing it. I explained that there's a gray zone where the cycle doesn't obviously change, but intense exercise makes it harder to get pregnant and more likely that a woman will miscarry. As she thought this over, Martha realized that when she got pregnant with her first child, she'd been in the middle of a really busy stretch at work and had temporarily given up going to the gym.

So Martha scaled back. She didn't give up the class, but she did slow down a bit, and she never pushed herself to the point where she got that endorphin rush. That was all she needed to do. She easily got pregnant (and stayed pregnant)—twice!—with no further help from me.

excellent time to start. But start slowly and gradually build up so as not to stress your body. For women who are certain fertility types, some kinds of exercise are more appropriate than others. See part V for the Making Babies Rx for each type.

You can keep tabs on how much exercise is too much for you not by the number of minutes spent exercising but by the intensity. Exercise should make you feel good, physically and emotionally, not completely drained or exhausted. While you are trying to conceive, stay away from your peak exercise level. If you exercise to the point where you get that endorphin rush, the so-called zone, scale back. That rush is a sure sign you're overdoing it from a fertility perspective.

Estrogen levels decrease in women when they really push themselves physically — enough to potentially stop ovulation — so it makes sense for those who frequently exercise intensely for extended periods of time to cut back a bit. Now is perhaps not the time to go into training for a competitive marathon. Hormone levels and menstrual cycles will return to normal when women stop doing such intense exercise, so this is a problem with a simple solution.

In women with very low body weight, even less extreme exercise can negatively affect ovulation. Lean women need to be sure to keep "moderation" as their watchword when it comes to exercise. But that's good advice for all women wanting to conceive. When it comes to exercise, don't overdo it.

### Exercising Through Your Cycle

*Phase 1 (Menstruation)*
- Avoid strenuous aerobic exercise during your period.
- Try workouts with a meditative bent, such as yoga, tai chi, or qi gong.

*Phase 2 (Pre-ovulation)*
- Spend twenty to thirty minutes a day on aerobic exercise.

*Phase 3 (Ovulation)*
- Exercise gently; try swimming, walking, yoga, or qi gong. Avoid exercise that involves high impact, such as running or step aerobics. Exercise gets the blood moving, which

encourages good blood flow to the uterus, so it's particularly beneficial around ovulation.

### Phase 4 (Potential Implantation)

- Get moderate exercise to keep the qi and blood moving after ovulation, when an embryo may be trying to implant, but avoid intensely aerobic exercise or high-impact exercise, such as jogging or trampolining (unless you are sure you are not pregnant). Walking, cycling, swimming, yoga, and qi gong are all good choices.

## SLEEP

You may already know that sleep is important to your health, and surely you've experienced how vital it is to your state of mind. As it turns out, it is also key for fertility. Sleep helps restore and rejuvenate your brain and all your organ systems, including the reproductive system. Yet according to the National Sleep Foundation, 70 percent of Americans don't get enough sleep.

Over the long run, insufficient (in quantity or quality) sleep affects your mood and your immunity. Sleep deprivation also alters your hormone balance and encourages other fertility-disrupting lifestyle factors such as weight gain, overuse of caffeine, and tension with your partner. Lack of sleep can lead to irregular menstrual cycles and affect ovulation, making it harder to conceive. When researchers surveyed women in notoriously sleep-deprived professions — flight attendants and nurses working the late shift — half reported irregular cycles (compared to about 20 percent in the general population). Some had stopped ovulating altogether.

### What You Can Do About It

When you don't get enough sleep, you're adding to the list of stresses you and your body have to deal with. Six hours a night just isn't enough. Seven is better, and eight is better still. One of the most enjoyable ways to improve fertility is to spend more time in the sack — asleep! If you have trouble sleeping, even once you've made room for it in your life, seek advice on strategies for getting a good night's sleep.

## AVOID TOXINS

Tens of thousands of chemicals are used in this country every day, with about a thousand more debuting each year, almost all of which were unknown as recently as fifty years ago. The vast majority have never been studied for their effects on our reproductive systems. According to the Environmental Protection Agency (EPA), at least fifty of the most commonly used chemicals do have an impact on our reproductive systems, but only four are regulated because of it.

These toxic substances contaminate our air, soil, and water—and from there potentially just about anything we come into contact with. Sometimes we breathe them in. Sometimes they are in our food. Sometimes they just soak in through our skin. And when they do, they can cause all kinds of health problems. Cancer is perhaps the most publicly recognized threat from toxins in our environment, but they also have a detrimental effect on fertility.

The average sperm count for an American man has plummeted over the past few decades—so much so that doctors have had to redefine "normal"—and environmental toxins are among the prime sus-

---

### Case Study: George and Eleanor

George and his wife, Eleanor, came to see me (Sami) because Eleanor had been unable to get pregnant. I couldn't find anything in Eleanor's medical history and physical that explained the holdup, so I suggested that George have his sperm count tested. He told me he'd had it done a year before (for unrelated reasons), and it had been normal. Still, with no other explanation available, he agreed to have it done again. The results showed that his sperm count had plummeted.

So now it was clear why Eleanor wasn't getting pregnant, but what had happened to George's sperm production? I asked him what was new in his life, and he said only good things: he and Eleanor had bought a vacation home, and he was

enjoying the country life there very much. None of my questions unearthed anything further, so we returned to the topic of the vacation home. When George mentioned that it had well water, I advised him to have the water tested. It turned out that his new retreat was also the source of his new trouble: the water was high in heavy metals and mercury. He'd been slowly poisoning his sperm.

George switched to bottled water while he figured out how to clean up the well. He also went to see a specialist to discuss treatment with chelating agents to remove the heavy metals from his system. Months later, his sperm count was back up to normal, and I had full confidence that a pregnancy would soon follow.

pects. The quality of sperm has dropped, too, while abnormalities have increased. Women's bodies are also affected, although those changes are more complex to track than sperm count and so have been less comprehensively researched.

In cases of unexplained infertility or repeated miscarriages, both men and women need to be evaluated for environmental toxin exposure. Even in the case of miscarriages, it's not just the woman's body that may be responsible. To take just one example, the wives of Vietnam veterans exposed to Agent Orange were found to have increased rates of miscarriage and infertility.

Common toxins — including pesticides; lead, mercury, and other heavy metals; bromodichloromethane (a ubiquitous by-product of the addition of chlorine to our drinking water); cadmium; cigarette smoke; and PCBs — have been linked to a wide range of fertility problems in both men and women, including low sperm count, poor sperm motility, increased sperm abnormalities, higher levels of DNA-damaged sperm, reduced semen quality, impotence, increased miscarriage, higher rates of endometriosis, failure in IVF, and some cases of otherwise unexplained infertility. These are just a few well-studied examples from a very long list.

Detailing the effects of all the chemicals that have been studied could fill a whole book, so here we focus on just two: dioxins and xenoestrogens. We chose these in part because they are among the most pervasive toxins and the most damaging to fertility. But they also are largely

---

## Case Study: Wanda

Wanda was in her mid-30s and had been trying to get pregnant for a year when she came to see me (Sami). After doing a medical history and physical, I determined that she wasn't ovulating and that fertility drugs could easily solve her problem. One thing from her history stood out, however: Wanda reported that she loved swordfish and ate it about three times a week. This gave me pause, given the reports of high mercury levels in swordfish, so I had Wanda's blood tested. Her results for mercury came back so high — seven times the normal level (which is 10) — that I had to report them to the health department. I told her I wouldn't give her any fertility drugs until her mercury level came back down. In fact, I advised her to ask her husband to use a condom until then, just to be sure she didn't get pregnant. I feared for the health of any embryo conceived in such a toxic environment.

Fortunately, the solution was simple: Wanda gave up swordfish. Her mercury level returned to normal over the next couple of months, and I started her on fertility drugs to help her ovulate. Ovulate she did, and within a couple of months, she was pregnant.

avoidable. You are in control of how much exposure you have—once you know where to look for them.

### Dioxins

Dioxins are toxic chemicals created as by-products in a huge range of industrial processes, from bleaching paper to manufacturing herbicides to incinerating medical waste. Dioxins interfere with the body's hormonal system. Exposure can alter the menstrual cycle and has been linked to an increased risk of endometriosis. It also has been implicated in the inability to maintain pregnancies. In men, high blood levels of dioxins are associated with lower testosterone levels, impaired sexual performance, lower-quality semen, and decreased sperm production and motility. Decreased testosterone, in turn, can mean less muscle mass (less strength), less bone density, more fatigue, and more depression to go along with the sexual dysfunction and infertility. Dioxins are also associated with a range of other harmful effects. (We're focusing on just the most relevant to the subject at hand.)

Now for the good news: you are in control of how much dioxin you are exposed to. The biggest source of dioxins in humans is beef, milk, and other dairy products, followed by poultry and other meat and eggs. You can inhale dioxins (and do whenever you get a whiff of cigarette smoke, for example), but mostly you get contaminated by what you eat. That's because dioxins are attracted to, and concentrated and stored in, fat—as in the fat in any animal product you eat and in the fat reserves in your body. This is another good reason to keep your own body fat down—a leaner you makes it harder for the dioxins to stick around.

### *What You Can Do About It*

Our advice is to limit your intake of animal products and to switch to organic meats and low-fat and lean varieties when you do eat them. You don't want to exclude fats in general from your diet, but animal fats—which provide saturated fats as well as dioxins—shouldn't be your main source.

### Xenoestrogens

Xenoestrogens are chemicals that mimic estrogen in the body, wreaking havoc with the proper performance of real estrogen. Male as well as female bodies produce estrogen, although women make much more of course.

Estrogen is crucial to the workings of our reproductive systems, but it also plays an important role in bone development, growth, circulation, metabolism, and more. Estrogen serves as a kind of messenger, and pretty much every cell in the body has an *estrogen receptor*—sort of a docking station for estrogen molecules to plug into to convey their information.

Xenoestrogens are close enough structurally to estrogen to attach to these same receptors and block the real estrogen from doing its work. In this way, xenoestrogens are a prime cause of hormone imbalance—including estrogen dominance—and the infertility that can result from it. They are also testicular toxins. Exposure to xenoestrogens has been linked to declining sperm count, decreased semen quality, increased DNA-damaged sperm, low sperm motility, and otherwise unexplained infertility in men. It has been linked to increased risk of recurrent miscarriages, endometriosis, ectopic pregnancy, and polycystic ovarian syndrome (PCOS) in women. And it can reduce libido.

### *What You Can Do About It*

Xenoestrogens are released into our environment and our bodies mainly from pesticides and plastics, although they can also be found in a wide range of everyday products, from paints to toiletries to spermicides. So the best ways to protect yourself are to buy organic and to be careful about how you use plastics, especially when it comes to food. Do not microwave food in plastic containers or covered with plastic wrap, and don't place hot food in plastic. The heat will allow some plastic molecules to make their way into your food.

The molecules that can leach out of plastic and into food are "plasticizers" known as *phthalates*. Phthalates are versatile chemicals used in a wide array of products. They are ubiquitous in plastics, and they are also used in many cosmetics and personal care products. Phthalates are used most commonly in fragrances, including scented lotions, shampoos, and soaps. One kind of phthalate can be found in nail polishes that promise to prevent chipping and breaking, as well as in other plastic products that need to be strong, such as tool handles. At the risk of an imperfect manicure, you can protect yourself and your reproductive tract from phthalates by reading labels carefully—some are now proclaiming the absence of phthalates—or simply by choosing unscented products.

While you are reading those labels on personal care products, look out for *parabens* as well. Parabens are commonly used as preservatives in cosmetics. They are absorbed into the body through the skin, so you don't want them in your facial cleanser, lipstick, or hair conditioner.

A final line of defense against powerful unnatural estrogens is to include *phytoestrogens*—plant estrogens—in your diet. Phytoestrogens also mimic estrogen in the body, but in a beneficial way: when they bind to estrogen receptors, more powerful xenoestrogens cannot. Flaxseeds and soy are the best sources of phytoestrogens. Nuts, sesame seeds, and legumes are good sources as well. Small amounts are found in many grains and some fruits, vegetables, and herbs, another argument for including a variety of whole foods in your diet.

We don't see infertility due to environmental toxins all that often. Or rather, we may see the effects, as in low sperm count, but never trace the origins all the way back to the root cause. But doctors should be considering these toxins as part of the whole picture when trying to decode fertility problems. Particularly if you are dealing with unexplained infertility or miscarriage, toxicology screenings for lead, mercury, cadmium, and the like should be part of your workup.

## STOP SMOKING

Nobody really needs more information to convince them that smoking isn't healthy, do they? No one should smoke, period, end of story. But in case you have the habit and you want to conceive, you should know that, in addition to all its other negative effects, smoking has been linked to infertility in couples where one or both partners smoke. Research shows that it slashes a woman's odds of conceiving by more than a third. One study found that women who smoke are almost three and a half times more likely than nonsmokers to take more than a year to conceive. Another study showed that smokers took twice as long to get pregnant as nonsmokers and were much less likely to be able to get pregnant at all. Smokers also have a greater risk of miscarriage.

Toxins in cigarette smoke is one of the main problems. Nicotine is just one of those toxins. It decreases blood flow to the uterus and placenta, which could cause implantation problems or miscarriage. Smokeless tobacco will do the same thing. There is evidence that smoking impedes the action of the tiny hairs (cilia) lining the inside of the fallopian tubes, interfering with their ability to sweep a fertilized egg along to the uterus. Smoking also meddles with women's hormonal balance and at the extreme can even bring on early menopause.

Smoking can decrease sperm count, make sperm more sluggish, increase the number of abnormal sperm, and impair the sperm's ability to penetrate an egg. In men, the more cigarettes smoked per day, the greater the impact on fertility is.

Smoking by men and women also significantly decreases the success rates of ARTs. Female smokers tend to have fewer eggs retrieved and fewer eggs fertilized in IVF, and intracytoplasmic sperm injection (ICSI) success rates drop in women whose partners smoke. Genetic changes in sperm related to smoking can also lead to ART failure.

## LIMIT CAFFEINE AND COFFEE

Caffeine can decrease the flow of blood to the uterus, which can interfere with implantation. Too much caffeine may increase the risk of clotting and miscarriage. Caffeine can also increase stress and anxiety levels. Studies on caffeine and fertility in general are inconclusive, but you'll do best to avoid it if blood flow or implantation problems or miscarriage is your main fertility issue. Some fertility types are more prone to negative effects of caffeine than others (see part V), but for almost everyone, up to 90 mg a day is generally safe. That's the equivalent of about one cup of regular brewed coffee, two cups of black tea, or three cups of green tea. The caffeine in colas and chocolate counts, too.

It's best to limit coffee, whether it's regular or decaf. Coffee is acidic and can make the body and the cervical mucus acidic, too. Several studies have concluded that coffee (with or without caffeine) diminishes fertility. A recent large Dutch study determined that four cups of coffee a day lowered a woman's chances of having a baby by more than 25 percent — comparable to the fertility damage done by smoking, being overweight, or having three or more alcoholic drinks a week. Some studies have linked coffee and miscarriage, and some have linked coffee and low sperm count. But not all studies have found a problem with coffee. So as with most things, we recommend moderation. If you drink a lot of coffee, cutting back may be a good idea, perhaps to just one cup in the morning. (We're talking about a normal six- to eight-ounce cup, not the huge super-grande "to go" cups that everyone seems to be carrying around these days.) Many of our patients have made the switch from coffee to tea, and that's another good option. If you find you are having fertility problems, you may want to eliminate coffee altogether.

### AVOID ALCOHOL

Many women avoid alcohol while trying to conceive, on the theory that since they won't drink at all while pregnant, they shouldn't drink at any time when they *might* be pregnant. But being cautious about alcohol while trying to conceive is not just about potential effects on the fetus. Alcohol affects fertility, too.

The research on this subject is something of a mixed bag. Some studies have found no link between moderate drinking and fertility issues. But some show that even low levels of alcohol can cut fertility by as much as one-half. For example, one large study concluded that women who had fewer than five drinks a week were twice as likely to get pregnant in a given six-month period compared to women who drank more. Another study demonstrated that men who drank alcohol regularly took twice as long to get their partners pregnant as men who didn't drink at all. In both sexes, the more alcohol consumed, the less likely conception is. Most studies agree: high alcohol intake significantly impairs fertility.

Alcohol is one of the most common factors affecting fertility in men. It is toxic to sperm, and overuse can reduce sperm quality, increase abnormal sperm, and lower motility. Men who drink have been shown to have lower sperm counts and lower testosterone than teetotalers, as well as decreased libido and increased risk of erectile dysfunction (ED). In women, alcohol can be a risk factor for ovulatory infertility.

Drinking alcoholic beverages has also been shown to decrease the success rates of ARTs, including IVF. According to one study of couples undergoing IVF, women who had one drink more per day than others tripled their risk of not getting pregnant in any given cycle and more than doubled their risk of miscarriage. When it was the man who had that extra daily drink, the risk of miscarriage was between two and *thirty-eight* times greater, depending on the timing of the drinking in relation to the IVF cycle. One month before IVF and during IVF were the most hazardous times.

Besides its direct effects, alcohol also interferes with the body's ability to absorb nutrients from food. That includes zinc, which is key for male fertility in particular. Alcohol interferes with the action of folic acid as well, which plays an important role in the maturation of an egg for ovulation. Finally, alcohol acidifies the body, including the cervical mucus. If the mucus gets too acidic, sperm can't survive in it, and so can't reach the egg.

### What You Can Do About It

Most people will need to moderate their alcohol intake, and some will need to cut back substantially or eliminate it altogether. Some women actually benefit from a glass of wine or beer now and then. In general, women should have no more than one small glass of wine or beer per day, and men no more than two small glasses or one mixed drink. For most people it's best not to have a daily drink while you're trying to conceive; reserve drinking for social occasions. See part V for specific advice about alcohol consumption tailored to your individual fertility type.

---

### Case Study: Annie and Kevin

By the time Annie and Kevin came to see me (Jill), they had been through one unsuccessful IVF and one IVF that had ended in miscarriage due to chromosomal abnormality. Annie seemed quite healthy to me, and I could see no good reason why she was unable to conceive. She told me that her husband, Kevin, had been diagnosed with poor sperm motility and morphology, but the doctors had reassured them that although this may have been the reason they couldn't conceive naturally, it shouldn't get in the way of IVF.

I thought a session with Kevin would be in order. In my office, he said that he guessed he drank rather a lot of alcohol, unwinding in the evening after stressful workdays with a gin and tonic and a couple of glasses of wine. He said that he would cut that out if I thought it would help, and he would overhaul his diet while he was at it. Five months later, he had a perfect semen analysis, and they immediately scheduled another round of IVF—with healthy sperm this time—for the next month. Annie and Kevin are now the proud parents of a healthy baby girl.

## BE MINDFUL OF MEDICATIONS

We all know that most drugs must be avoided during pregnancy, and many women avoid drugs while they are actively trying to get pregnant, too. That is a smart strategy. Your doctor should advise you about any medications (or herbs or supplements) you take that could be harmful to a developing embryo. But you should also know that certain prescription and over-the-counter medications can impair your fertility as well. This goes for both men and women. Giving up a medication may not always be the answer, depending on why and how you are using it. But if you take any of the following and want to get pregnant, you need to have a serious discussion with your doctor about your options.

- **Antibiotics.** Although antibiotics are often the key to solving fertility problems (by clearing up the infections that are causing infertility or miscarriages), some hamper sperm production. Be cautious with aminoglycosides, Minocin, nitrofurantoin, and sulfasalazine. In addition, certain broad-spectrum antibiotics, such as Augmentin, Keflex, ampicillin, and amoxicillin, can provoke an overgrowth of vaginal yeast, which can make fertile cervical mucus hostile to sperm. And even if a yeast infection doesn't do that, it can make timing intercourse more difficult, since it will be hard to detect when you are having fertile cervical mucus.

- **Antidepressants.** Selective serotonin reuptake inhibitors (SSRIs), such as Prozac and Zoloft, can depress libido in both men and women and cause erectile or ejaculatory dysfunction. People taking antidepressants may experience an effect on their hormone balance, but it is difficult to say whether the depression or the drug is at fault. There's evidence that antidepressants can affect semen quality, too, and lead to lower sperm count. SSRIs may also reduce the number of days of fertile cervical mucus.

  Older antidepressant drugs, the tricyclics, can impede fertility by increasing prolactin levels, which can suppress ovulation.

  The decision about whether to use an antidepressant

while trying to get pregnant is a difficult one, and you should never discontinue one without consulting your doctor. For some people, extreme stress (including depression) plays a major role in their fertility problems, and in those cases an antidepressant can actually be useful.

- **Antihistamines.** Some antihistamines, such as Chlor-Trimeton, Allegra, Benadryl, Claritin, and Zyrtec, can dry up fertile cervical mucus, so it is important to avoid them around ovulation.

- **Anti-inflammatories.** Heavy use of anti-inflammatories, including nonsteroidal anti-inflammatory drugs (NSAIDs), such as ibuprofen, Advil, Motrin, and Aleve, and COX-2 inhibitors, such as Vioxx and Celebrex, can stop ovulation. They can lead to luteinized unruptured follicle syndrome (LUFS), the failure of the follicle to release the egg. They can also reduce the amount of fertile cervical mucus produced.

- **Blood pressure medications.** Calcium channel blockers, such as Plendil, Cardene, Procardia, Cardil, Cardizem, and verapamil, can lower sperm count. (Look for generic names ending in "dipine.") Some blood pressure drugs can cause erectile or ejaculatory dysfunction. Verapamil and ACE inhibitors have been associated with increased prolactin, which can suppress ovulation.

- **Cough medicines and decongestants.** These can dry up fertile cervical mucus just as they do any other mucus. Be wary of pseudoephedrine and phenylephrine. (In some cases, thinning the cervical mucus *benefits* fertility; see page 271.)

- **Diuretics.** These can cause dehydration, leading to poor cervical mucus or low semen volume.

- **Painkillers.** These can inhibit prostaglandin release and delay ovulation, decrease libido, and cause ejaculatory dysfunction.

- **Sleeping pills.** These can decrease libido and cause ED in men, and they can decrease libido and arousal in women. It is important to note, however, that insomnia can cause low FSH, and therefore ovulation problems. So for some women, sleeping aids may be necessary; be sure to consult your doctor.

- **Steroids.** At high doses, steroids can affect the pituitary gland

and interfere with testosterone, FSH, and LH production. Anabolic steroids and testosterone can lower sperm count.

- **Drugs for peptic ulcer.** Cimetidine can lower sperm count in men and cause increased prolactin in men and women. Increased prolactin stops ovulation and impairs male fertility as well (see page 220).
- **Drugs for ulcerative colitis.** Sulfasalazine can lower sperm count.
- **Drugs for epilepsy.** Carbamazepine and valproate can lower sperm count. Dilantin decreases FSH. These drugs can decrease testosterone in men by suppressing LH, and they can suppress LH and estrogen in women.
- **Chemotherapy drugs.** These can lower sperm count. Talk to your doctor about any alkylating agents you may be taking, including cyclophosphamide, nitrogen mustard, and methotrexate.
- **Drugs for urinary function.** Nitrofurantoin (Macrodantin) can lower sperm count.
- **Antifungal medications.** These can lower sperm count. Ketoconazole can inhibit the production of hormones.
- **Propecia.** This can affect male reproductive hormones enough to weaken sperm production and function, especially in men with sperm counts that are low or borderline to begin with.
- **Migraine medications.** Ergots can restrict blood flow to the uterus, which can interfere with implantation, and are not safe when you want to get pregnant. While there has been no study of triptans in humans, research in other animals suggests that they carry a moderate increased risk of miscarriage.
- **Clomiphene (Clomid).** Ironically, this fertility drug acts as an antiestrogen and thus can reduce fertile cervical mucus.

## DON'T USE RECREATIONAL DRUGS

In case there's anyone out there who can't answer this for themselves, recreational drugs must not be used during pregnancy or while trying to get pregnant. They pose all the problems of pharmaceutical drugs and then some.

Authoritative studies have long established, for example, that marijuana disrupts the reproductive hormones. In women, marijuana use decreases FSH and LH and increases prolactin, thus interfering with the menstrual cycle and ovulation. In men, it decreases FSH, LH, and testosterone and increases prolactin, impairing sperm creation, function, and motility. Furthermore, marijuana affects the placenta and could prevent implantation or proper nourishment of an embryo or fetus.

Fortunately, all these effects disappear once there's no more exposure to marijuana. However, it is important to note that long-term exposure during adolescence — just as hormonal patterns are shifting to their permanent adult form — can be a factor in lasting fertility problems.

## MISCELLANEOUS

Excess heat can lower sperm count and quality and interfere with proper egg or embryo development, so you should avoid hot tubs, very hot baths, and saunas while trying to conceive. If you are a woman and you enjoy a bath, take your temperature under your tongue before and after a bath. If your temperature rises even 1°F, the bath was too hot and you stayed in it too long. Next time, cool it off a bit (warm should be fine), and don't sit quite so long. Men, you're definitely going to need to moderate the heat and bathe quickly; the testicles overheat in just a couple of minutes.

---

### Case Study: Meri and Dan

Meri and Dan had been trying to get pregnant for four years. They had seen a series of good doctors, under whose care Meri had taken some minor fertility drugs and had insemination, but still no dice. It turned out that one key question had been overlooked, and I (Sami) asked it in my basic evaluation on their first visit: do you take a bath or a shower? As it happens, their apartment did not have a shower, and Dan, age 52, enjoyed a nice hot bath every day. I asked him to stick a thermometer in the tub the next time he drew a bath and call me to give me the reading. He phoned the next day: 103°F. At that temperature, he was, in effect, cooking his testicles. From then on, he kept his bath at 98°F, and Meri was pregnant after three months with no further intervention.

---

You should also steer clear of electric blankets, which have been linked to increased risk of miscarriage and male infertility, and heated car seats.

Women should avoid flying. Long flights early in pregnancy have been shown to increase the risk of miscarriage. You should not put your entire life on hold while trying to conceive, but if you can, avoid airplanes for a few months.

Avoid scented tampons and vaginal douches. Both interfere with the production of fertile cervical mucus.

Men need to avoid bike shorts and any other tight pants or undergarments (such as jockstraps) that pull the testicles in close to the body. Your testicles are designed to hang away from the body, so that they can maintain a temperature just a little below your core body temperature to protect the process of sperm production and storage. Excess heat will kill or damage sperm.

Men also should avoid placing their laptops on their laps. The heat generated is enough to disrupt sperm production and fertility. A study of young men sitting with their legs together in order to balance a laptop showed that the temperature around the testicles rose 2.1°C before they even turned the computer on—at which point the temperature increased a total of 2.8°C. It was a small study, but given what we already know about the negative effects of heat on sperm count, it's enough to give us pause. Our advice is to keep your laptop away from your sperm-making equipment.

Men should moderate the amount of time they spend on their cell phones as well. Research presented at an ASRM conference in 2006 found that men who used their cell phones for four or more hours a day had lower sperm counts and lower sperm quality than men who weren't so devoted to their phones. More research is needed to confirm and explain the risk, but in the meantime, why take a chance? Hang up your cell phone once in a while or use a landline.

## Making Babies Action Plan

- ❑ Start a family when you are younger, if that's feasible.
- ❑ Make good lifestyle choices, especially as you grow older.
- ❑ Get to your ideal weight, or at least move in the right direction.
- ❑ Exercise regularly but moderately.
- ❑ Get enough sleep.

- ❏ Avoid environmental toxins.
- ❏ Don't smoke.
- ❏ Limit your caffeine intake.
- ❏ Limit coffee (regular and decaf).
- ❏ Drink alcohol in moderation, if at all. Because alcohol can impede conception, avoiding it is crucial around ovulation.
- ❏ If you take any medications, even occasionally, check for any potential fertility effects and avoid if possible.
- ❏ Avoid recreational drugs.
- ❏ Avoid overheating your testicles (or ovaries, although ovaries are harder to overheat than testicles). Skip electric blankets, hot tubs, very hot baths, saunas, laptops (if used literally on the lap), bike or compression pants or shorts, jockstraps, and tight briefs.
- ❏ Avoid heavy use of cell phones if you're a man.
- ❏ Avoid airplane flights, especially long ones.
- ❏ Avoid scented tampons and vaginal douches of any kind.

# CHAPTER FOUR

# De-stressing

**B**oth physical and psychological or emotional stress affect the body in all kinds of ways, not the least of which is fertility.

## THE FIGHT-OR-FLIGHT RESPONSE

You're probably already familiar with the fight-or-flight stress reaction—the increases in heart rate and blood pressure and the reduced blood flow to any part of the body not absolutely essential for staying alive. In the face of mortal danger, the body marshals all its resources in the interest of one thing: survival. This is an excellent plan for when we are indeed facing mortal danger.

The problem is, our bodies (and minds) are very bad at determining what's "mortal danger" and what isn't. We are likely to go into some variation of this emergency mode for the more everyday problems of today's world. The truth is, most of us live with at least some level of chronic stress, and not just as a result of the big things such as grief and unemployment but also from the ordinary pressures of deadlines and traffic jams and misbehaving children. Then, too, we stress ourselves in many ways without even thinking of it as stress, such as when we don't get enough sleep or we go on a crash diet. Wherever the stress comes from, if we don't know how to manage it, it takes its toll.

The familiar physical reactions to stress stem from the way it activates the adrenal glands, which overproduce adrenaline and cortisol and give us the butterflies, sweaty palms, galloping heartbeat, and other symptoms of stress. The excessive doses of adrenaline and cortisol also interfere with the production of other hormones, including FSH and LH, in both men and women. The decreases in FSH and LH in turn lower testosterone, estrogen, and progesterone, all of which are crucial in conception and implantation. In this way, chronic stress can stop ovulation (and menstruation) or decrease the production of sperm. Stress compromises the immune system as well — the cortisol again, which suppresses immunity. This can, among other things, leave you open to other fertility problems, from infections to inappropriate immune reactions.

While science is still sorting out all the whys and wherefores of the stress-conception connection, one thing is clear: people who are highly stressed have lower rates of conception. Stress decreases women's fertility in part because it can stop ovulation and menstruation altogether. Short of that, women under stress are less likely to get pregnant in any given cycle than are women not experiencing any particular psychological distress. Stressed women also face a higher risk of very early miscarriage.

Consider the study in which researchers "psychologically" stressed monkeys: 10 percent stopped menstruating. When the stress let up, the monkeys began menstruating again. Then the researchers created physical stress for the monkeys, either by having them exercise intensely for long periods of time or by limiting food intake. In each group, again about 10 percent stopped menstruating, and again the effect was reversed when the diet or exercise binge stopped. When researchers combined the psychological and physical stress, making already stressed monkeys eat less or exercise more, 75 percent stopped menstruating. It's hard to get pregnant if your whole reproductive cycle shuts down. It is reasonable to expect similar effects in humans. Most women will be able to handle a certain amount of stress without any impact on their fertility. But start layering stress upon stress, and the majority are going to run into problems.

Turkish studies have clearly demonstrated the fertility effects of stress in men as well. The research in this area has mainly been done on men with fertility problems, but this muddies the waters, since infertility all by itself is a major cause of stress. Scientists in Turkey took a different tack by recruiting healthy men with no fertility problems. As in so many cases, a pool of such men was readily at hand: medical students. Researchers collected semen samples from their volunteers at a time of stress (just prior to final exams) and again at a time of no extraordinary stress (three months later). The first (stressed) samples showed lower sperm counts, lower motility, lower semen quality, and a higher percentage of abnormal sperm compared to those taken later (not under stress).

Fortunately, full fertility was restored when the stress disappeared. We think that is the most important lesson to be drawn from this study: reducing stress can reverse fertility problems.

The stress effect shows up less formally as well. One of my (Sami's) colleagues noted that during the recent economic crisis, he's seen a significant decrease in sperm quality in his patients.

## AN EVOLUTIONARY IMPERATIVE

The way fertility shuts down under stress should not surprise us. Our bodies are obeying a larger evolutionary imperative. Consider the way animals in the wild have more or fewer babies depending on the cues they are picking up from their environment about personal and pack safety and access to resources. And we know that animals in zoos have trouble getting pregnant. They unconsciously evaluate the lack of space and limited resources, and their bodies respond by not allowing additions to the population. Zoo vets are experts at all kinds of ARTs, from insemination to IVF, as they try to get the animals under their care to reproduce in defiance of nature.

Humans react in ways similar to other animals. Birthrates decrease in times of war, for example. Evolutionarily, humans, like all animals, want to reduce reproduction whenever reproduction could interfere with (as opposed to bolstering) survival. Although most of us are not actually living in a war zone, our bodies may behave as if we are. Think about how news coverage is sensationalized to provoke as much fear as possible. Personal communication devices beep endlessly; our bosses and clients expect us to get back to them on the double. Advances in communications technology have not freed up our time, as predicted, but have enslaved us. In our deepest subconscious, this endless vigilance, this inability to switch off, feels like danger. Our bodies take evasive action, in part by reducing our ability to conceive.

We have several wonderful, accomplished, and resourceful patients who can't bring themselves to switch off their Blackberrys when, say, they receive an acupuncture treatment. Their approach to what should be a moment of calm appears to include e-mailing colleagues and talking on cell phones. And their bodies get the message loud and clear: no time or space here for a baby. For them, making their bodies understand that there *is* room can be the key to getting pregnant at last. These are extreme cases, but most of us are overscheduled and lacking in balance in essentially the same way. The bottom line is, you have to be in harmony with yourself; anything else is stressful.

## HORMONES, STRESS, AND ANIMAL BEHAVIOR

Say you're an African naked mole rat, but not just any naked mole rat: the queen of the colony. You are the only reproducing female in the whole group. If there's going to be any young, you're going to bear them. But there are all those other females living with you, and all those males ready and willing to mate—perhaps not as picky about their partners as you'd like. How are you going to make sure none of those rats, male or female, gets in on the reproduction action without your say-so?

You stress them all out—way out. You bully them into submission. You literally push them around, give them a good shove once in a while, just to show them who's boss. And in this way, you make sure their hormone levels drop low enough to decrease testosterone and sperm counts in the males and turn off the ovulatory cycle in the females, low enough even to prevent puberty.

In our fellow primates the marmoset monkeys, it's been shown to work pretty much the same way. Biologists call this *social suppression of reproduction*. The areas of the brain devoted to fertility and stress are pretty closely connected in mammals, so scientists think that what goes on in these animals, behaviorally and hormonally, can tell us a lot about how stress impairs human fertility as well. In fact, the naked mole rat study is not from the pages of some animal behavior textbook, but rather from the proceedings of the European Society of Human Reproduction and Embryology's annual meeting.

So even though you're not a naked mole rat, you might want to take a look at what's pushing you around. Get out from under it, and you'll be doing yourself and your fertility a favor.

## ANIMALS IN CAPTIVITY DON'T BREED WELL

Reproductive endocrinologists have a task not unlike vets at the zoo: to help people breed in captivity. And they are pretty good at it, too. But we all tend to be blind to the other option available to humans, if not to zoo animals: to leave captivity. Turn off the bad news and unpleasant images, learn to laugh more, and try to relax when you have the time. In fact, make the time!

So if you are having trouble getting pregnant, especially if no one can come up with a medical reason why, you should consider whether your body might be getting the impression that you are too unsafe, too underresourced, and too busy to provide for and look after a baby. Try to reverse those messages, letting your body know that you are fundamentally safe, that there is enough to eat, and that when you do have a child, you will be able to drop everything and play with building blocks on the floor for half an hour. We've seen many patients who have come to respect the way their bodies are connected to a larger evolutionary design slow way down and then become moms.

---

### Case Study: Joanne

Learning to manage her stress level was a key component of fighting fertility problems for Joanne, whom you read about in chapter 2. Her irregular periods and slow hormonal transitions made it hard for her to get pregnant until she pinpointed when she ovulated using a BBT chart. Even then, however, I (Jill) think she would have had trouble conceiving if she hadn't also finally dealt with how stressed-out she was.

I knew Joanne was stressed-out even before I met her. She had made several appointments to see me, only to cancel them all due to her busy work schedule. When she finally made it in, she told me how hectic and overscheduled her life was. Then she whipped out her cell phone to make several calls while I gave her acupuncture.

It took some doing to get her to set aside one minute every morning to take her BBT. And it was even harder to convince her to shoehorn regular acupuncture appointments into her calendar. And then it took all my powers of persuasion to get her to turn off her cell phone during the acupuncture.

Ultimately, though, Joanne began to appreciate the value of taking those brief breaks. She also began to notice some signs that she was a bit more relaxed even when she wasn't in my office. For example, she wasn't so irritable right before her period. The tightness in her body was softening as she felt better—and she was feeling better as that tightness softened. I can't say for sure what part this newfound sense of space played in her ability to conceive after six months of Chinese treatment and BBT charting, but I feel confident it was an important piece of the puzzle.

---

## WHAT YOU CAN DO ABOUT STRESS

We can't live a life without any stress at all, and we are designed to cope with, or at least endure, acute stress, at least up to a point. Chronic stress, however, will compromise your fertility (along with your health in general) if you don't find ways to manage or disperse it. You need to find out what works for you and do it. Adopt daily stress management habits; try yoga, meditation, guided relaxation, or simply taking a walk after work to unwind.

You should also take a look at yourself and your habits to see if you have any negative ways of handling stress that could be revamped. Many women, for example, undereat or overexercise in an attempt, conscious or not, to deal with stress; both can lead to fertility problems. Maybe you're trying to cope by drinking coffee all day or having a couple of glasses of wine every night, or by working like a fiend. Whatever the case, it is important to deal with the underlying stress directly, rather than layering on additional problems.

Dealing with infertility, no matter the cause, brings its own stress. Studies have shown the effectiveness of "mindfulness" practices and other specific approaches to handling the stress of being diagnosed with and treating infertility. For example, research shows that just sixteen weekly sessions of cognitive behavioral therapy geared directly toward issues around infertility can not only reduce stress but also restore ovulation and fertility in cases where stress is the cause of, as well as the response to, infertility.

## Case Study: Mariel and T.J.

Mariel was deeply frustrated, sad, and angry about her unsuccessful quest to get pregnant, although she didn't like to complain about it. It had been eight months, and as the pressure and resentment mounted, she and her husband, T.J., argued more than they used to—always right around the time Mariel was ovulating. Then they didn't feel like having sex—exactly when they should have been having sex to conceive—and another month would slip by with no pregnancy. It didn't take long to recognize the pattern, and when they did, Mariel and T.J. promised each other they wouldn't fight the next month. When the next month came around, they were at it again.

I (Jill) didn't find anything that should be keeping Mariel from getting pregnant, but I suggested that she and T.J. consult a psychotherapist. A short stint in couples counseling helped them understand how and why the stresses of trying and failing to conceive, and the fear of facing the same disappointment again and again, were leading them to such poorly timed clashes. They also learned some more constructive coping mechanisms. Not long after that, Mariel became pregnant. She went on to have a healthy baby and began planning for their second child.

## Stress Reduction Throughout Your Cycle

Chinese medicine holds that where you place your mind, the qi will follow. This section walks you through the phases of your cycle, looking at strategies that can support the connections between mind and body and emotions to maximize fertility at specific times. The sections that follow give specific visualization exercises and self-massage techniques for each phase of your cycle. Try to carve out some quiet "me time" every day to practice whichever of these approaches fits you best.

### Phase 1 (Menstruation)

- Your energy is naturally low at this point in your cycle, so focus on relaxing and resting so that your body can direct its energy to the regeneration that is beginning. Some cultures have a tradition of women withdrawing from society when they menstruate. Most of us don't have the time or inclination for that today, but it is still natural to feel more withdrawn during your period. If you feel a bit less sociable than usual, go ahead and stay at home and cocoon.
- The best way to handle the disappointment that your period has come is to accept, for now, that you are not pregnant and, with a positive attitude, begin making a plan for the next cycle.

### Phase 2 (Pre-ovulation)

- Estrogen tends to put you in a positive frame of mind and increase your feelings of well-being. We often hear from our patients that they feel a renewed sense of hope and optimism as their fertility efforts resume after their periods end. Many women find that their energy is high at this time. Some report that they feel sexier and more attractive. Take advantage of this time. The quest to conceive can get incredibly intense, so make the most of this little break. Some of the greatest benefits will come from enjoying low-intensity connected time with your partner, such as taking a walk together, going out on a date, talking about the future, and making love even though you are not yet at your most fertile.

### Phase 3 (Ovulation)

- Studies have shown that the increase in estrogen, FSH, and LH lead to a sense of overall well-being right around ovulation. This can be a welcome relief in a stressful situation, so try to note, appreciate, and build on it.
- You may feel more sexual desire as ovulation approaches. Heed its call!
- Many couples feel very anxious that they have only a small window of time in which to fertilize an egg. This pressure can take a toll on your relationship, leading to conflicts that get in the way of using that window wisely. It also can translate into performance trouble for men. The best advice is to feel confident that in having regular sex in the lead-up to ovulation, you are doing what needs to be done. Take care of any other issues that could stand in the way of conception — the ones within your control, anyway — then relax, knowing you've done your best. And remember, the window's not all *that* small, since sperm can survive in fertile cervical mucus for days, as they wait to catch the egg as it is released.

### Phase 4 (Potential Implantation)

- This can be the most anxiety-provoking part of your cycle, waiting to see if your period will come. Once ovulation has passed, the optimistic feelings and excess energy of the follicular phase diminish, and women tend to become pensive and reflective. Try to focus on staying steady, looking at this as a long-term process rather than a month-by-month one. Feel secure in knowing that you are doing the right things to reach your goal.

## Visualization Exercises

Spending a few minutes a day centering yourself and focusing positively on your body, your health, your cycle, and your fertility is a great way to tap into the Chinese medicine idea of qi following intention. Shifting your focus slightly with each phase of your cycle will keep your attention on where the action is at that time. But each time you perform this easy meditation and relaxation exercise, you'll begin and end the same way.

What to do:

- Sit on a chair in a comfortable position with your feet touching the floor.
- Inhale deeply, allowing your abdomen to expand. As you inhale, imagine breathing light into your body.
- Exhale, pulling your abdomen in. As you exhale, imagine breathing out light all around you.
- Continue breathing in and out this way until your body feels full of light and you can imagine yourself surrounded by light emanating several inches out from your body.
- Turn your attention inward, according to which phase you are in, as directed below. Continue for a few more minutes.
- Finish by imagining yourself under a waterfall. Envision the cleansing water passing over and through you, taking with it any problems, worries, or health issues.
- When you feel ready, slowly open your eyes.

### Phase 1 (Menstruation)
- Turn your attention inward, focusing on your uterus.
- Imagine the lining of the uterus sloughing off easily, leaving behind a smooth surface.
- Visualize the blood vessels leading to your uterus and blood flowing through them to replenish it with a new supply of blood.

### Phase 2 (Pre-ovulation)
- Turn your attention inward, focusing on your ovaries.
- Imagine ten to twenty small follicles growing on your ovaries.
- Visualize one follicle becoming dominant. See it receiving all the resources it needs from your body. See it growing. Feel the potential this follicle holds.

### Phase 3 (Ovulation)
- Turn your attention inward, focusing on the dominant follicle on your ovaries.
- Imagine the egg emerging from the follicle and being squeezed out until it is sitting on the surface of the ovary.

- Visualize the egg being gathered up by the little fingerlike structures at the end of the fallopian tube.
- See the egg in the lower part of the tube, being met by sperm.
- Imagine a sperm merging into the egg.
- Imagine the fertilized egg continuing its journey to the uterus.

### Phase 4 (Potential Implantation)

- Turn your attention inward, focusing on your uterus.
- Imagine the embryo arriving in the uterus and burrowing into the uterine lining.
- Visualize the embryo drawing nourishment from the uterus's rich blood supply.
- Turn your attention back to your ovaries and see the ruptured follicle that the egg left behind. Imagine this follicle secreting progesterone to maintain the pregnancy.

### Self-Massage

Arvigo Maya Abdominal Massage, based on an ancient Mayan technique of abdominal massage, was developed by Dr. Rosita Arvigo as a non-invasive way of gently repositioning internal organs and improving the flow of blood and lymph. It can be used for any disorder that involves congestion in the abdomen and pelvic cavity, but it is best known for the correction of a prolapsed, fallen, or tilted uterus, for the prevention and treatment of benign prostate enlargement in men, and for relief of many common digestive disorders. It can be especially useful for improving or restoring fertility. Following are some techniques you can use to support your body at each phase of your cycle. A qualified Maya Abdominal Massage practitioner can provide additional information, instruction, and guidance on self-care techniques, as well as professional massage. (The massage technique for phase 2 is from Dr. Arvigo, while the other three were developed by Nicole Kruck, LMT, certified Arvigo practitioner and self-care instructor.)

### Phase 1 (Menstruation)

This sacral self-massage can help you ease menstrual cramps. According to the Mayan massage tradition, this technique improves enervation of the reproductive organs. Chinese medicine considers it a way to move qi and blood.

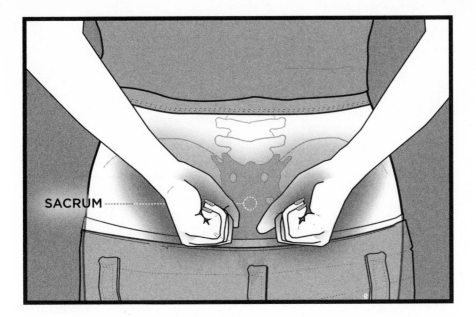

SACRUM

- Feel for your sacrum, the triangular bone at the base of your spine, between your hips. Make sure you find the sacrum and not the tailbone, which is smaller and beneath the sacrum.
- Make loose fists with your hands and bounce them directly on the sacrum. Use the same force you would for clapping. Use a rhythmic motion, one to two seconds apart, allowing the impact of each bounce to spread before the next one hits, like ripples in a pond.
- Continue for at least one to two minutes.
- This should always feel good. If you experience any discomfort or pain, make the impact lighter until you are comfortable. If you need to, pause, breathe, and begin again more gently. If it still doesn't feel good, try again in a day or so.

### *Phase 2 (Pre-ovulation)*

This massage supports follicle development and a healthy uterine lining and can help keep fallopian tubes open. You can begin using this technique every day as soon as your period ends, stopping two days before you expect to ovulate. After ovulation, stop any massage of the pelvis and sacrum until you know for sure that you are not pregnant. Wear loose clothing, trim your fingernails, and make sure your bladder is empty before you begin.

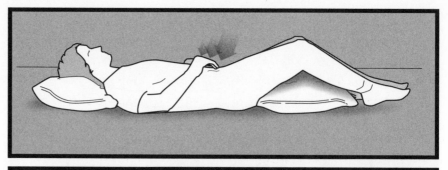

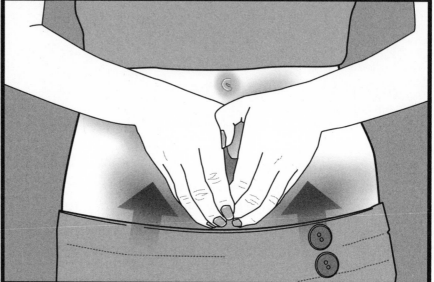

- Lie on your back with a pillow under your knees.
- Place your hands on your pelvis and breathe deeply for a few minutes until you feel relaxed.
- Find your uterus. The fundus (the top of your uterus) should be in the middle of your pelvis, below your navel and about one and a half inches above your pubic bone. It may feel like the tip of your nose or a balloon filled with water. You may also sense a slight internal tugging. (If you don't feel anything yet, don't worry — you will. The more you do the massage, the more easily you will discover what is under your hands.)
- Should anything feel uncomfortable, stop, breathe, and decrease your pressure.

- Place both hands on your pubic bone, with your thumbs hooked one over the other and your fingers close together, slightly bent and relaxed. You'll be creating a kind of scoop.
- Take a deep breath; visualize the breath coming into your pelvic area. As you exhale, sink the pads (not the tips) of your fingers as deeply as you comfortably can into the soft flesh. Without lifting your hands, continue with light but firm pressure, gently massaging, lifting up toward the navel two to three inches.
- Repeat the movement from the pubic bone toward the navel ten times.
- Now massage each side of the uterus. Bring your "scooped" hands slightly over to the right side of the pelvis. Maintain contact with the pubic bone with two or three fingers, placing the other fingers just inside the hip bone. Using the same technique as above, move your hands diagonally toward your navel. Repeat ten times.
- Do ten strokes on the left side as well.
- If your uterus is not centered in your abdomen (an inch and a half above the pubic bone, with equal space on the right and left sides), increase the massage strokes over the parts closest to the uterus. For example, if you find your uterus to be more on the right side of the pelvis, do ten extra strokes on that side.
- This should be a gentle and nurturing experience. If you begin to have discomfort, stop massaging, breathe, and try again with less pressure. If it is still uncomfortable, give it a day or two, then try again.

### Phase 3 (Ovulation)

This massage for the ovaries improves circulation to them, which supports smooth hormonal transitions and healthy ovulation. It is meant to be used for two or three days before ovulation. Start approximately four days before you ovulate and stop one or two days later. In other words, perform it after you're done with the uterine massage for phase 2. After ovulation, stop any massage of the pelvis and sacrum until you know for sure you are not pregnant.

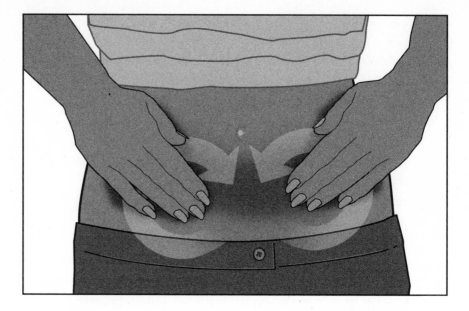

- Bring both hands to your pubic bone and spread out your pinkie fingers. The spread of your hands will cover roughly the space your ovaries occupy. You may even be able to feel them — sometimes they feel like grains of rice under your fingers. If you don't feel them, that's fine, too.
- Whether or not you feel your ovaries, hold the intention of placing your hands on top of them in your mind. Focus your thoughts on helping the ovaries receive optimal health.
- As shown in the illustration, massage the general area of the ovaries lightly, in small circles, using the pads of three or four fingers and gentle pressure as you would to stroke a baby.
- Massage for ten seconds, then rest for one second. Repeat for one to two minutes.
- This should be a gentle and nurturing experience. If you begin to experience any discomfort, pause, breathe, and try again with a bit less pressure. If it is still uncomfortable, try again in a day or so.

### *Phase 4 (Potential Implantation)*

This "warm hands" massage is for use after ovulation, when you don't want to be doing active massage of the pelvis or sacrum. This is a time

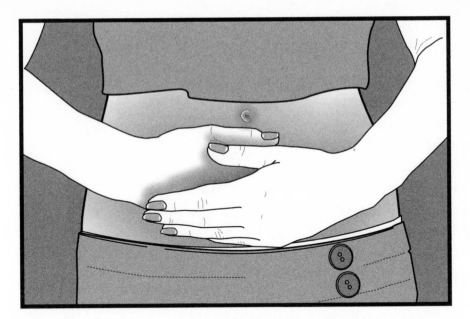

for more stillness, nurturing, and grounding, and this technique supports implantation by calming the nervous system, creating better circulation, and warming the uterus. You can also use it during any phase to promote relaxation and centering.

- Lie on your back with a pillow under your knees.
- Place your hands directly over your pelvis/lower abdomen.
- Take slow, deep breaths. Imagine the breath moving into and through your hands. Feel your hands move as your breath moves your body.
- Continue for five minutes.

# Making Babies Action Plan

- ❏ Recognize the stress in your life.
- ❏ Look for unproductive ways you may be trying to manage stress, such as the use of caffeine, alcohol, or stress eating, and seek new ways to manage your stress.
- ❏ Strive for balance in your life.
- ❏ Get the rest you need. Make sure you have some downtime.
- ❏ Try yoga, guided relaxation, meditation, or mindfulness practice.
- ❏ Exercise; it can be as simple as taking a walk around the block to unwind after work.
- ❏ Take care of your relationship.
- ❏ Make a plan to deal with your fertility problems, do what you need to do to follow it, and trust it to work for you.
- ❏ Consider psychotherapy to handle general stress or the stress of fertility problems. Cognitive behavioral therapy has been proven to be beneficial.
- ❏ Try visualization exercises to focus on your reproductive cycle.
- ❏ Try self-massage to support fertility.

# CHAPTER FIVE

# Eating to Conceive

Just as with the general lifestyle advice in chapter 3, many of the recommendations in this chapter are unlikely to be news to you. Eating well to maximize fertility is not much different from eating well to maximize good health in general. But what may come as a surprise to you is that some specific foods and types of foods, as well as some ways of eating, can have specific fertility effects. Diet can help correct hormone imbalances that may be at the root of fertility problems, and certain foods and drinks are known to decrease fertility. You'll find general eating advice in this chapter and recommendations tailored to your particular fertility type in part V.

The most potentially powerful fertility effect your diet may have is that it can make you healthy. As my (Jill's) Chinese medicine teachers taught me, a healthy body gets pregnant. It's something we've both seen play out in our own patients time and time again, and it is our simplest recommendation to you: Get healthy to get pregnant; get pregnant by getting healthy.

The Chinese have a saying: "Eighty percent is perfection." In that spirit, we urge you to aim to follow the Making Babies rules about 80 percent of the time. It just takes too much effort to follow them 100 percent of the time, 24-7, and if that is your goal, you'll be unlikely to stick with the program over the long haul. We hope you'll consider our recommendations for a healthier pattern of eating as guidelines, not strict orders. That's right, we're giving you permission to cheat. In fact, we want you to, at least once a week.

If following these guidelines is a drastic change for you, you should ease into them, building up to the full program gradually. This will help you stick with the program and avoid unnecessary stress on your body. As always, you should discuss changes like these with your doctor.

For those who want to "eat to conceive," we recommend fresh, seasonal, organic food in its natural state; whole grains; colorful fruits and vegetables; healthy fats; sufficient protein; alkaline foods; and plenty of water. Steer clear of trans fats, highly refined grains, processed foods, refined sugar, heavy metals, aspartame, and MSG. Finally, always keep a positive attitude toward food and eating.

## FRESH, SEASONAL, ORGANIC FOOD IN ITS NATURAL STATE

Eating good-quality food is one of the most important things you can do for your overall health. If you stick to this one rule, you will accomplish much of what follows by default. After all, there's no such thing as an organic Twinkie. "Fresh, seasonal, organic food in its natural state" by definition eliminates trans fats and simple carbs, and right away you're in compliance with two more of the most important recommendations of this program.

Eating organic allows you to avoid the pesticides, chemicals, synthetic additives, and other agents contaminating so much of our food supply and wreaking havoc on our health. These pose a long list of health risks. In terms of fertility, many agricultural chemicals, as well as the hormones given to animals raised for their meat, milk, or eggs, affect hormonal balance.

Furthermore, organically farmed crops are more nutritious, providing more of what a healthy body needs to thrive and be fertile. The soil they are grown in is nutrient-rich, and the crops are raised in such a way as to absorb those nutrients as nature intended. Research shows that the overall nutrition level of all our common foods has decreased over recent decades due to industrialized farming methods, which deplete the soil. Organic foods are actually able to nourish you better, and so you will be able to nourish new life.

Some studies even show that organic foods boost fertility. For example, the *Lancet* published a Danish study of organic farmers who lived mainly on the fruits of their labors (and so ate a diet free of pesticides). This study unexpectedly revealed that the men had sperm counts more than twice as high as those of the group of blue-collar workers to which they were compared.

Finally, in the traditional Chinese medical view, foods as well as people contain qi (energy). This qi is depleted as food is refined and processed. As I (Jill) explain to my patients, an ear of corn absorbs nutrients from the soil and energy from the sun as it grows. Cooked in its natural state, it passes on those nutrients and that energy to you. Once it has been processed into breakfast cereal, it has lost some of its nutrients and most of the energy it absorbed when it was a living thing. Breakfast cereal companies and other food manufacturers make up for this by adding nutrients back in, but just as that can't re-create the complex interplay of nutrients and micronutrients in fresh foods, it can't replace the energetic value either. Choosing whole, unprocessed foods ensures that you will get all the benefits of the foods' life force.

## WHOLE GRAINS

Most of the grains Americans eat have been refined. They cook faster and spoil more slowly that way. They are also digested faster, much faster, so they bombard the body with simple carbohydrates—the same way sugar does, metabolically speaking—making us feel lousy. We constantly cycle from brief "sugar highs" to long, low "sugar crashes"—the sharp peaks and valleys of energy with which most of us are all too familiar. Blood sugar and insulin levels go through the roof as the body tries to handle the rapidly digested carbs, ultimately creating insulin resistance and increasing our risk of type 2 diabetes and a host of general health issues. This cycle also increases the risks of hormonal and ovulatory problems that impair fertility.

In addition, refining robs grains of most of their natural nutrition. The whole point of refining is to remove the germ (the part of the grain that, if fertilized, will reproduce) and the protective layer of nutrient-rich bran. As the outer shell of the grain is stripped away, so too are the fiber, protein, antioxidants, B vitamins, and phytonutrients that make whole grains so nutritious. Many of these same lost nutrients play key roles in fertility.

Refined and processed grains are also acidic in the body, which can wreak havoc with fertility, among other things.

With the popularity of high-protein diets, we've seen more and more patients who simply don't eat enough carbohydrates. You need some carbohydrates every day to maintain balanced hormone levels. (Women with polycystic ovarian syndrome, or PCOS, may need to cut back on carbs, however. See page 204.) Just choose your carbs wisely, focusing on complex carbs such as vegetables (even starchy ones such as sweet potatoes) and whole grains.

Explore a wide range of whole grains; there's a universe of them out there. Discover high-protein quinoa. Enjoy magnesium-rich millet. Try spelt. Switch to brown rice. Experiment with bulgur. Just remember that all grains should be cooked thoroughly to ensure easy digestion.

## IT DON'T MEAN A THING IF IT AIN'T GOT THAT JING

*Jing* translates as "reproductive essence." It describes our genetic inheritance and how it affects our longevity and ability to conceive. Healthy people have healthy jing and a healthy reproductive capacity — which they inherit from their parents and pass on to their children. Our jing helps us produce eggs or sperm.

This isn't just a human thing. All living things have jing, including plants that become our foods. Jing is mostly associated with foods designed to nourish new generations, including eggs, seeds, nuts, and sprouts.

Grains are full of jing. Grains are seeds, and like all seeds (and nuts), grains contain the fertilized germ cells and the nutrition to sustain a new plant: jing! You need whole grains to get the jing, because it is destroyed by refining.

Seaweed and algae are also considered to be full of jing, because they are so rich in trace elements.

Male or female, our jing is best supported by foods naturally full of jing.

## COLORFUL FRUITS AND VEGETABLES

Fruits and vegetables, including beans, are the other major sources of healthy, slow-digesting carbohydrates. Beyond that, they are packed with fiber, vitamins, minerals, antioxidants, and phytonutrients. We all know that getting our fruits and veggies is good for our health. But we're here to tell you that they're also crucial for fertility. We recommend eating a broad range of colorful fruits and vegetables every day.

What does color have to do with it? A plant's color signals its phytonutrient content, and the more intense the color, the more phytonutrients. The antioxidant beta-carotene is probably the most famous phytonutrient, and also the most important for fertility. It works to maintain hormone balance and prevent early miscarriage. The corpus luteum, which helps produce the progesterone necessary to sustain a pregnancy, has very high levels of beta-carotene. Research shows that cows deprived of beta-carotene develop ovarian cysts and are slow to ovulate, and their fellow mammals—humans—work much the same way. You get beta-carotene in your diet from yellow and orange foods (including carrots, cantaloupe, and sweet potatoes), as well as from broccoli and leafy greens such as spinach.

Lycopene is also important. It's been shown not only to prevent cervical and prostate cancers but also to increase sperm count. It's found in red fruits and vegetables, such as tomatoes, red peppers, and watermelon.

Green is good, too, especially cruciferous vegetables and leafy greens, including kale, chard, collard greens, dandelion leaves, cabbage, broccoli, arugula, spinach, bok choy, and seaweed. Not only are these foods rich in folic acid (see page 117), but they also contain beta-carotene, B vitamins, vitamin E, iron, zinc, magnesium, and selenium. In addition, they are full of fiber and important phytonutrients. Broccoli, Brussels sprouts, cabbage, turnips, mustard greens, kale, and the like contain a phytonutrient called di-indolylmethane (DIM), which helps both men and women metabolize estrogen better. For women, that means cruciferous veggies help combat the estrogen dominance that can lead to fibroids and endometriosis. In men, they improve the balance of testosterone with estrogen and allow more testosterone to circulate freely in the body. DIM helps eliminate active estrogen, breaking it up into particles, a process that can release testosterone bound to certain proteins. One daily serving of these vegetables is all you need to get the job done.

Round out your food color spectrum with blues and purples, including blueberries, blackberries, eggplant, plums, red cabbage, grapes, and red onions. They are rich in phytonutrients, particularly anthocyanins, which are anti-inflammatory as well as powerful antioxidants, both of which are benefits to fertility.

Vegetables with more neutral tones bring a lot to the table as well. The allium family, including garlic, onions, shallots, and chives, have antibacterial and antifungal properties that boost your immune system. Undetected infections are a major cause of unexplained infertility, so eat your alliums to help protect against infections.

Cook vegetables lightly to maintain the maximum amount of vitamins and enzymes, both of which can be destroyed by heat. Cooking

104 Getting Pregnant Naturally

makes veggies more easily digestible, so that your body can extract the nutrients it needs. Raw veggies are fine, too — where would we be without salads? — but you wouldn't want to go exclusively raw.

## HEALTHY FATS

First of all, you need to eat some fat. If you've been strict about keeping fat from crossing your lips, adding healthy fats back into your diet will be important for your fertility as well as your overall health. Your body needs dietary fat to make hormones, fight inflammation, and facilitate ovulation, among other things.

You do need to make smart choices about which fats you eat. And, of course, you need to eat them in sensible quantities. Eating too much fat or the wrong fats interferes with ovulation, spurs insulin resistance, increases the risk of endometriosis, and disrupts hormone production and balance, not to mention all the other ways it messes with your health. Healthy fats are good for everyone, and in particular for people who tend to be very thin, women in phase 4 of their cycle, and men with low semen volume.

Saturated fats from animal products harm your heart and contribute to insulin resistance, endometriosis, and PCOS. They are also where the dioxins (see page 71) hang out, so limiting them will protect you from dioxins as well. You do need some cholesterol in your diet to support fertility, and cholesterol is found where you find most saturated fats — in animal products. The body uses cholesterol in making hormones, including progesterone and testosterone, and if you don't have enough cholesterol, you won't have the right building blocks to make hormones.

Eliminate trans fats altogether, because, among other things, they can cause or exacerbate insulin resistance and ovulatory dysfunction and interfere with hormone production and balance. There is no safe level of trans fats in your diet. Eliminating trans fats is crucial for women with PCOS.

In a large, long-term study, researchers at the Harvard School of Public Health and Harvard Medical School found a link between increasing amounts of trans fats in women's diets and increasing instances of infertility. Women who ingested trans fats were 70 percent less likely to get pregnant than women who did not. Even as little as 4 grams a day of trans fats was enough to cause problems.

If you are eating only fresh, whole, natural foods, you don't have to give trans fats a second thought: they exist only in commercial, industrially prepared, and factory-manipulated foods. Watch out for commercial baked goods, crackers, cakes, and so on, as well as frozen meals and, the biggest transgressor of all, stick margarine. Trans fats now must be listed on food labels, so read them. Avoid anything with "partially hydrogenated vegetable oil," which is the source of trans fats. Many manufacturers are reformulating their products to eliminate trans fats, but it's worth noting that revamped products often rely on saturated fats. Be sure to check the labels carefully so that you know what you are eating.

Pruning these bad guys from your daily diet will leave room for healthy, beneficial fats. Unsaturated fats are the way to go: olive oil, nuts and seeds (and their oils), and avocados are the most nutritious sources. These are important for everyone, especially for women with PCOS.

Essential fatty acids (EFAs) also are crucial. EFAs are, as stated right there in their name, essential, and your body can't make them. EFAs are a vital component of every human cell, so they have many health benefits. For our purposes, we want to call attention particularly to their vital role in balancing hormones and supporting the opening of the follicle to release the egg. Once you are pregnant, they are equally important for nourishing a developing embryo.

The key EFAs for fertility are the omega-3 and omega-6 fatty acids. Omega-9 fatty acids are good for you, too, but not technically "essential," because your body will manufacture them if you have enough 3s and 6s. You also get 9s in olives, avocados, and nuts.

Omega-3 fatty acids have a broad range of benefits, including increasing blood flow to the uterus, thereby increasing the chances of implantation and pregnancy. They also fight inflammation and so can soothe menstrual pain and help with other problems that can interfere with conception. Increased blood flow also benefits the placenta, supporting optimum growth of a fetus and ultimately reducing the risks of premature birth and low birth weight.

The standard American diet is jam-packed with omega-6s, largely because they are plentiful in processed oils such as corn, sunflower, and soybean. We're getting way too much of a good thing. At the same time, most of us don't get enough omega-3s. Even more important than the absolute level of omega-3s in your diet is the ratio between omega-3s and omega-6s. Getting even amounts of each is most supportive of hormone balance. To achieve that, you'll need to play up omega-3s while de-emphasizing omega-6s.

Fish, flaxseeds, and flaxseed oil are the best sources of omega-3 fatty acids. Cold-water, fatty fish are your best bets, including cod, salmon, herring, mackerel, anchovies, and sardines. Walnuts are another good choice, as are eggs from chickens fed a diet rich in omega-3 fatty acids (check the labels). Omega-6 fatty acids are found in flaxseeds and flaxseed oil, olives and olive oil, some seeds and nuts, and chickens fed diets rich in EFAs. (See the box on page 126.)

## FERTILITY SUPER-FOODS

**Flaxseeds.** Along with a rich supply of omega-3 fatty acids, flaxseeds provide lots of B vitamins, magnesium, and manganese. They also contain really gentle phytoestrogens (plant estrogens) known as lignans, which block harmful xenoestrogens (synthetic chemicals in the environment with estrogenic properties) in the body. All in all, flaxseeds are powerful packages for balancing hormones and boosting fertility.

Aim to get about two tablespoons of flaxseeds every day. Grind them up, since whole flaxseeds are hard to digest and tend to pass through your digestive system whole, and you don't get much benefit from them that way. Try sprinkling them on hot or cold cereal or a salad, or blending them into a smoothie. Or use flaxseed oil as a salad dressing. (Don't bother cooking with it, as heat destroys many of the beneficial properties.)

**Sprouts.** Chinese medicine particularly prizes sprouting grains, legumes, and seeds. Sprouts are full of jing. The dynamic balance struck in the process of changing from seed to sprout is thought to be particularly nourishing to couples trying to develop their very own "sprouts."

If you prefer a more grounded explanation of the fertility benefits of sprouts, we've got you covered: eating sprouts encourages an alkaline (rather than an acidic) environment in your body.

**Goji Berries (Wolfberries).** Tiny, red Goji berries, a traditional Chinese herb also sold whole and dried to eat as you would raisins, are packed full of antioxidants. Look for them in your health food store. Studies have shown that they can increase sperm count and promote follicle growth in women who have trouble ovulating.

## PROTEIN

Our patients are split into two groups, each needing different advice when it comes to protein. The first group needs to be told to eat more protein. The amino acids that make up protein are vital for egg production and sperm maturation and for making hormones such as LH and FSH.

Animal studies link inadequate protein intake with poor-quality eggs, and there's no reason to assume humans are any different. You need at least two and a half ounces of protein every day. You can get it from meat, fish, eggs, and dairy products, of course, but there are plenty of vegetarian sources of protein, too, including beans, lentils, brown rice, quinoa and other whole grains, and nuts and seeds (especially sunflower seeds). Soy foods are another good source of protein, and soy protein powder can be the easiest way for vegetarians and vegans to boost their protein intake. If you are relying on soy as a major source of protein, you should be aware that the phytoestrogens in soy foods can adversely affect sperm count. Some women don't handle the phytoestrogens well either. If you are a Stuck type (see page 303), you should have no more than two servings of soy per week to make sure you don't run into any problems.

With the rising popularity of high-protein diets, we find ourselves advising our second group of patients to cut back on their protein — or to switch from animal to plant sources of protein at least some of the time. Too much protein can be as much of a problem as too little, depleting the body of calcium and creating excessive levels of ammonia. High-quality protein should be the goal. Beans, nuts, and seeds are nutritional powerhouses, packed full of not just protein but also iron and fiber. One of the largest long-term studies of women's health ever undertaken demonstrated that women who got more of their protein from plants and less from animal sources had fewer ovulatory fertility problems. Whether you need to get more protein, more animal protein, or less animal protein depends on your fertility type. See part V for more details.

Protein is digested and released into the bloodstream slowly, thus allowing for maximum absorption of amino acids. You can support that process by eating small amounts of protein at a time, so you don't overload your system.

## ALKALINE FOODS

Cervical mucus must be alkaline (as opposed to acidic) so that sperm can survive long enough to journey to the egg. What you eat has a big impact on the pH of your mucus. (High pH is alkaline; low is acidic.) In fact, if you eat well, you can keep your whole body alkaline, which is beneficial for your health in general. To keep your cervical mucus alkaline, focus on fruits, vegetables (especially green vegetables), sprouts, and wheatgrass, and lean less on acidifying meat, dairy, and grains. Alcohol and coffee acidify the body, which is part of the reason you should cut back on these. Artificial sweeteners have the same effect.

You can find comprehensive lists of foods that are alkaline and acidic in many books and on Web sites, and some of this information is contradictory. Try not to get bogged down in the details here. Like so much else, it is all about balance. If you're good about getting whole grains and veggies, cutting down on coffee and alcohol (see chapter 3), and keeping your portions of meat sensible, your system will generally be more alkaline than acidic.

## WATER

Water is one of the most important nutrients we consume. Seventy percent of the human body is water. It is vital to the functioning of each and every system, and it plays a key role in transporting hormones, developing follicles, and maintaining optimum consistency and quantity in both semen and cervical mucus. (Women, be especially sure you're well hydrated during phases 2 and 3 of your cycle so that you'll produce fertile cervical mucus.) Water also helps us absorb nutrients and eliminate toxins, both of which are important for fertility and overall good health.

Women with cervical mucus that is too thick to promote conception may simply be dehydrated. The same goes for men with low semen volume. In these cases, simply drinking more water can restore fertility.

Aim for six 8-ounce glasses of water a day to maintain adequate hydration (eight glasses for Dry types). Consider limiting yourself to filtered water, to eliminate chlorine. Most tap water is chlorinated, and about half of bottled water is nothing more than bottled tap water, so it's chlorinated, too. Chlorinated water contains chemical compounds called trihalomethanes (THMs), which have been linked to increased risks of miscarriage and certain cancers.

You can substitute juiced raw vegetables, fruits, or cereal grasses (such as wheatgrass); herbal tea; or green tea for some of the water.

Caffeinated or alcoholic beverages are dehydrating, so if you partake, you can't count them toward your water quota. In fact, you should probably add a bit more water to make up for the dehydrating effects.

If you've been chronically dehydrated—as so many of us are—it will take some time for your body to get used to all the liquid coming in. Build up to the recommended amount gradually over a couple of weeks to ease the transition.

## THAT MUST BE WHY THEY CALL IT FERTILI-*TEA!*

In my (Jill's) family, putting on the kettle and brewing a cup of tea was the solution to just about anything. So it's no surprise to me that tea is good for fertility, too.

If you don't want to take my word for it, ask the researchers at the Kaiser Permanente Medical Care Program of Northern California in Oakland who studied 210 women as they were trying to get pregnant. Women who drank tea every day—even just half a cup—were twice as likely to conceive as women who never drank tea. Women who were getting similar levels of caffeine from other sources (mainly soda or coffee) did not experience a similar boost in fertility.

Scientists suggest that tea might promote fertility in two ways. First, the hypoxanthine in tea might be necessary for the follicular fluid that helps eggs mature and get ready for fertilization. Second, powerful antioxidant polyphenols in tea might help prevent the chromosomal abnormalities that can cause an embryo to miscarry or fail to implant. Like all antioxidants, polyphenols benefit the immune system as well.

The study at Kaiser Permanente did not get into what kind of tea the women drank, but we recommend green tea to our patients. Green tea has up to ten times more polyphenols than black tea and only about half the caffeine. Three cups of green tea a day (or two of black tea) will keep you within our caffeine guidelines (see page 74). You'll also reap the same benefits from two or three cups of decaf tea.

## STEER CLEAR

Along with all the good things you should include in your diet, there are a few things you'll do best to avoid when you are focusing on fertility. Trans fats, as already discussed, are the biggest no-no, followed by highly refined grains and processed foods. You also should take it easy with alcohol. Here are some other foods you should watch out for.

Refined sugar and sugary foods cause sharp peaks and valleys in blood sugar levels, which in turn lead to hormone imbalance and, potentially, fertility problems. It goes like this: You eat a candy bar, your body rapidly digests the sugar, and you get a sugar rush. That part feels pretty good. But every time this happens, your pancreas goes into overdrive, producing insulin like crazy to try to get all the sugar out of the blood and into your cells, where it can be converted into energy. Then your blood sugar plummets, and you feel drained and exhausted. In an attempt to replenish your blood sugar, your adrenal glands secrete extra cortisol. (And, to the same end, you probably crave even more sweets.) Over time, excess cortisol weakens your adrenal glands to the point where they produce lower levels of sex hormones. And the repeated high demand for insulin leads to insulin resistance, which has been associated with infertility.

Heavy metals contaminating common foods create fertility problems, along with a host of other serious health consequences. Mercury, all too often present in certain kinds of fish (the biggest ones, at the top of the food chain), is a toxin that was never meant to find its way into the human body. When it does, it interferes with the action of zinc. That's a big problem, because zinc is crucial for the formation of healthy sperm and eggs. You should not eat swordfish while trying to get pregnant (or while pregnant or nursing) and must also avoid shark, tilefish, and king mackerel. You should limit your intake of fresh or frozen tuna, red snapper, and orange roughy to no more than twelve ounces a week. (Canned tuna is generally okay.) Cadmium gets into the body via foods grown in polluted soil and through pesticide residue on produce. It, too, interferes with zinc, and it's been implicated in increased miscarriage rates as well. Eating organic will help you avoid this problem.

The artificial sweetener aspartame has been linked to infertility and birth defects, as well as cancer. Everyone would benefit from avoiding it. While you're at it, skip all artificial sweeteners—they make the body too acidic.

Studies in rats have linked monosodium glutamate (MSG) with decreased fertility in both males and females, and from our point of view, that's more than enough reason to recommend avoiding it.

## NOURISH YOURSELF

It is well established that in times of famine (as in times of war), birthrates drop. This is true of all kinds of animals, including humans. When resources are scarce, the best strategy for group survival is not to have to share those resources with a growing population. We don't have to consciously decide this for our bodies; it happens on a much deeper level, and it is largely beyond our control.

Why bring this up? Tough though times may be, American society is clearly not experiencing famine; all our patients have access to all the food they'll ever need. But many people are so controlled about what they eat or on such strict diet-and-exercise regimens that it amounts to the same thing. Bodies receiving all the same signals they would if they were starving may well respond by not working to bring new life into the world.

So while you are busy planning how to eat to enhance your fertility, we want to leave you with some final words of advice: make eating a positive experience, a true nourishment of your body. At the most basic level, this means eating enough and eating foods rich in nutrients to convincingly portray the world to your body as a welcoming, sustaining place. You can maximize the effect by supporting proper digestion, so that all the good nutrients in your food can be put to use. Chew your food, don't eat on the run, eat in an emotionally positive environment, and don't multitask while you are eating. Eat foods worth eating, and treat each meal as a little oasis in your day. That's nourishing yourself.

### Eating Through Your Cycle

#### Phase 1 (Menstruation)

- Eat foods rich in iron—including meat, eggs, fish, kelp, spinach, broccoli, dried fruits, and sunflower seeds—to help your body replenish the blood it is losing.
- Include foods rich in vitamin C—including citrus, mangoes, cherries, potatoes, tomatoes, cantaloupe, strawberries, peas, and watercress—to help with iron absorption.
- Make sure you get plenty of protein from both animal and vegetable sources.

#### Phase 2 (Pre-ovulation)

- Eat well so that you'll be well nourished and able to nourish a maturing follicle. Protein is especially important.
- Choose foods rich in vitamin E, which is found in the fluid around the developing egg and is important for its

nourishment. Good sources include cold-pressed oils, sweet potatoes, avocados, leafy greens, nuts, seeds, and whole grains.

- Avoid alcohol now most of all.

### Phase 3 (Ovulation)

- Get plenty of B vitamins, which are particularly important to the release of an egg and implantation. Choose leafy greens, whole grains, eggs, and (if you eat it) meat.
- Eat foods rich in zinc, which is needed for cell division and helps with progesterone production. You can find it in meat, fish, poultry, wheat germ, eggs, and whole grains.
- Be sure to get vitamin C, which is found in high quantities in the corpus luteum and is thought to play a role in progesterone production.

### Phase 4 (Potential Implantation)

- Now is the time to get your fill of pineapple. The bromelain it contains has been shown to help implantation.
- To support implantation, eat plenty of warming foods and avoid cold, raw foods, or at least balance them out. For instance, if you eat a salad, warm up your meal by adding soup, a baked potato, or some steamed brown rice.
- If you have PMS, it is especially helpful to limit processed foods, refined sugar, alcohol, and coffee and to increase your fiber intake, all in the interest of helping your body eliminate estrogen more efficiently and less uncomfortably.

## Making Babies Action Plan

- ❏ Remember: "Eighty percent is perfection."
- ❏ Implement drastic changes gradually.
- ❏ Choose fresh, seasonal, organic food in its natural state.
- ❏ Choose whole grains and cook them thoroughly.

- ❏ Choose colorful — yellow, orange, red, green, blue, and purple — fruits and vegetables, especially cruciferous vegetables (such as broccoli, Brussels sprouts, cabbage, turnips, mustard greens, and kale) and members of the allium family (garlic, onions, shallots, and chives). Cook vegetables lightly.

- ❏ Include some fat in your diet. Avoid all trans fats and limit saturated fats. Get some healthy fats every day (unsaturated fats and EFAs, such as omega-3 fatty acids from olive oil, nuts, seeds, avocados, fish, and flax).

- ❏ Get at least two and a half ounces of protein every day from meat, fish, eggs, dairy, soy, beans, whole grains, nuts, or seeds. It's fine if you get more than that, as long as you don't go overboard. Most people should aim for more plant and less animal protein. Eat protein in small servings.

- ❏ Lean more on alkaline foods (vegetables, fruits, sprouts, and wheatgrass) and less on acidifying foods (meat, dairy, grains, alcohol, and coffee).

- ❏ Aim for six 8-ounce glasses of water (or other healthy fluids) each day.

- ❏ If you like it, drink tea. Two cups of black tea or three of green tea will not put you overboard in terms of caffeine. Or drink decaf tea.

- ❏ Avoid highly refined grains and sugars and processed foods of any kind.

- ❏ Don't use aspartame or any artificial sweeteners, and avoid MSG.

- ❏ Support good digestion.

- ❏ Don't strictly limit what kinds of food or how much food you eat.

- ❏ Make eating a positive activity.

# CHAPTER SIX

# Fertility Nutrients

The first and most important thing we want to say about fertility, nutrition, and supplements is that the very best nutrients don't come in capsule form. The best way to nourish your body is to eat well, not to swallow a collection of pills. Specific nutrients are most powerful in foods, where they come prepackaged with a complex array of precisely balanced macro- and micronutrients. So we encourage you to follow our guidelines for eating well in chapter 5.

But even the most conscientious diners on the best diets cannot be sure of getting all the nutrients they need to have the absolute best chance of conceiving. This chapter recommends a basic program of supplements to ensure you don't have any gaps and to provide higher amounts of certain key nutrients you're not likely to get from diet alone.

There is a lot of talk out there, especially in Internet chat rooms, about supplements that boost fertility. Unfortunately, much of it is uninformed or misguided, and there is simply no evidence they do anything at all for fertility. There's plenty of research on the nutrients we recommend and wide support for their ability to prevent and sometimes treat common fertility problems. If we haven't covered it in this book, that means we haven't found any good reason to include it. You'll find a summary of what supplements you may want to take, along with dosing information, at the end of this chapter in the Making Babies Action Plan. We provide slightly different recommendations for men and women, to meet their different fertility needs. Taking these supplements during your three-month "pre-mester" will give your body plenty of time to soak up optimal levels of these key nutrients and have you in excellent shape for conception.

## TAKE YOUR VITAMINS: THE MULTI

Anyone trying to conceive should take a good-quality multivitamin every day. This includes would-be fathers. Women should look for a pre-natal vitamin, which is likely to have close to our recommended levels of the various nutrients. The Making Babies Action Plan at the end of this chapter includes a rundown of the specific nutrients you should look for when choosing a multivitamin.

Studies show that regular use of a multivitamin decreases the risk of ovulatory infertility. Multivitamins have been shown to benefit men's fertility as well, increasing sperm count, quality, and motility; decreasing immune system interference with fertility; and increasing pregnancy rates, even in couples where the man is diagnosed as "subfertile." The University of Surrey study mentioned in chapter 3 found that 80 percent of couples diagnosed with infertility who made positive changes in their lifestyles and diets and took nutritional supplements got pregnant.

The key ingredients to look for in a good fertility-enhancing multivitamin are described in this section. The rest of the chapter discusses other key supplements you might want to take in addition to your multi. Many of these beneficial nutrients are antioxidants, which protect sperm and eggs from genetic damage, support proper implantation and embryo development, and fight inflammation (which can impair fertility in various ways) and other specific disorders, including endometriosis, blocked fallopian tubes, and infections.

### Vitamin A

This antioxidant is vital for the production of both male and female sex hormones and for follicle building. It is important for progesterone production and so supports the buildup of the endometrium. Vitamin A also helps increase sperm count and motility, improve the sperm membrane and form, and protect the sperm from oxidative stress (the latter being exactly what you need an antioxidant for).

Your body requires two varieties of vitamin A—preformed and beta-carotene. Preformed vitamin A is an important fertility nutrient and is crucial to embryo development, but in extreme doses it can actually cause fetal abnormalities. So pregnant women and women planning to conceive need to be very careful about preformed vitamin A. There's plenty of preformed vitamin A in the average American diet to meet your requirements. It's widely available in meat, dairy, fish, eggs, and fortified cereals, so you don't need any in your supplements. If you avoid supplements, you'll never reach a dangerous level (more than 10,000 IU a day).

Beta-carotene is a plant compound that the human body converts into vitamin A on an as-needed basis. It does not carry any of the risks associated with preformed vitamin A. Look for beta-carotene in your supplements. In addition, you can safely get as much beta-carotene as you want from fruits and vegetables.

Keeping vitamin A to smart levels is one important reason we urge people *not* to double up on prenatal vitamins or to take any supplements that haven't been recommended by their health care practitioners. Most prenatal vitamins provide at least part of their vitamin A content as beta-carotene, but some over-the-counter brands and regular multivitamins contain excessive amounts of preformed vitamin A. Be sure to read the labels carefully.

A final caution relating to vitamin A: pregnant women and women trying to conceive need to stay away from the prescription acne drug isotretinoin (sold under the brand name Accutane and others) and the topical ointment tretinoin (Retin-A). Both are related to retinol, a compound of vitamin A.

## EAT IT! GOOD SOURCES OF VITAMIN A AND BETA-CAROTENE

**Vitamin A**
Meat
Dairy
Fish
Eggs
Fortified cereals

**Beta-Carotene**
Dark green vegetables (peas, broccoli, spinach)
Orange fruits and vegetables (sweet potatoes, carrots, apricots, winter squash)

### Vitamin B Complex

B vitamins are important for the release of the egg and for implantation and embryonic development, making them particularly important in phases 3 and 4 of a woman's cycle. Here's a look at the fertility effects of specific members of this nutrient family.

A deficiency of **thiamine (vitamin B$_1$)** has been linked to anovulation (lack of ovulation).

**Riboflavin (vitamin B$_2$)** is important in estrogen metabolism.

**Pantothenic acid (vitamin B$_5$)** is vital for fetal development.

**Vitamin B$_6$** helps the body produce progesterone and metabolize excess estrogen. It can lower elevated prolactin levels and is important for male sex hormones. Deficiency has been shown to cause infertility in animals. Studies of humans have shown that women who have trouble conceiving can enhance their fertility by taking vitamin B$_6$.

**Folic acid (vitamin B$_9$ or folate)** is in all prenatal vitamins. Proper levels dramatically lower the risk of neural tube defects (spina bifida) in embryos. Folic acid is very important in DNA replication. Regular use of folic acid supplements (in addition to a multivitamin) lowers the risk of ovulatory infertility. It also helps mature the egg before ovulation and helps the ovary respond to FSH. Men should take folic acid, too, because it improves sperm count, quality, and function. One study gave men suffering from fertility problems a combination of folic acid and zinc supplements, and their sperm counts increased by 74 percent.

The body uses **vitamin B$_{12}$** when synthesizing DNA and RNA (a key part of the reproductive process, since sperm and eggs are essentially little packets of DNA). B$_{12}$ helps improve low sperm counts, increase motility, mature sperm, and decrease abnormal sperm. B$_{12}$ is found exclusively in animal products, so vegetarians and especially vegans can be deficient and should be sure to take a supplement (and not just while trying to conceive).

## EAT IT! GOOD SOURCES OF VITAMIN B COMPLEX

| Thiamine (Vitamin B$_1$) | Riboflavin (Vitamin B$_2$) |
| --- | --- |
| Whole grains | Milk |
| Beans and legumes | Eggs |
| Nuts | Fish |
| Brown rice | Spinach |
| Egg yolks | Liver |
| Poultry | Asparagus |
| | Broccoli |

| **Pantothenic Acid (Vitamin B$_5$)** | **Folic Acid (Vitamin B$_9$ or Folate)** |
|---|---|
| Wheat germ | Leafy green vegetables |
| Salmon | Liver |
| Sweet potatoes | Asparagus |
| Strawberries | Oatmeal |
| Cashews | Avocados |
| Legumes | Legumes |
| Nuts | **Vitamin B$_{12}$** |
| **Vitamin B$_6$** | Meat |
| Leafy green vegetables | Shellfish |
| Whole-grain cereals | Dairy |
| Meat | Eggs |

### Vitamin C

The body uses vitamin C in making hormones and for ovulation. Vitamin C is an antioxidant, so it helps to prevent damage from free radicals. That includes protecting sperm from oxidative damage that can harm both the sperm and the DNA within them. Some sperm DNA damage can make it difficult to conceive. If conception does take place, abnormal sperm DNA can increase the risk of miscarriage.

Vitamin C benefits sperm count, quality, motility, and morphology. Vitamin C also reduces the tendency of sperm to clump together in a woman's body, a common cause of infertility.

Vitamin C has a key role in keeping ovaries healthy and in creating and maturing follicles. It is a key component of the fluid surrounding and nourishing the egg in the follicle, and it is highly concentrated in the corpus luteum and so is key to the release of progesterone, both of which make vitamin C particularly important during phases 2 and 4 of a woman's cycle. It has also been shown to fight endometriosis and inflammation, which can impair fertility, and to improve progesterone levels and reduce early miscarriages in women with luteal phase defect (LPD; see page 200). Studies have found that women using fertility drugs to stimulate ovulation respond better when they take vitamin C.

Women planning to conceive should *not* take high supplemental doses of vitamin C (more than 1,000 mg a day). Too high a dose can cause cervical mucus to become acidic enough to kill sperm. Excessive doses can also dry up cervical mucus.

---

### EAT IT! GOOD SOURCES OF VITAMIN C

| | |
|---|---|
| Green vegetables (especially spinach, asparagus, and peas) | Mangoes |
| | Kiwifruit |
| Citrus fruits | Grapes |
| Strawberries | Alfalfa sprouts |
| Cantaloupe | Tomatoes |
| Cherries | Potatoes |

---

### Vitamin D

Vitamin D is an antioxidant, so it helps protect sperm and eggs against genetic damage. Vitamin D also supports the production of estrogen. In some cases, bumping up vitamin D intake to adequate levels can restore ovulation in women with polycystic ovarian syndrome (PCOS; see page 202).

You can get vitamin D from your diet or from supplements, but the best way to get it is from the sun. Be sure to get out in the sun for a little while every day *before* you put on your sunscreen or your big floppy hat. The body turns ultraviolet light into vitamin D. Optimal timing depends on your skin type; for most people, about twenty minutes of sun a day is good, at minimum ten to fifteen minutes twice a week, with paler skin requiring less exposure than darker skin.

Very high levels of vitamin D can be toxic. You may see recommendations for up to 2,000 IU daily, but we think that is too high for regular use. We recommend between 800 and 1,000 IU daily. (It's fine to combine that with sun exposure.) Your doctor can test the level of vitamin D in your blood to make sure you are getting what you need. If you are taking vitamin D supplements, be sure you are also getting sufficient magnesium and calcium. Without them, vitamin D can leach minerals out of your bones instead of supporting bone health, which it does as long as it is well balanced.

**EAT IT! GOOD SOURCES OF VITAMIN D**

| | |
|---|---|
| Shellfish | Fortified milk |
| Oily fish | Sunshine |

### Vitamin E

Vitamin E is a powerful antioxidant, fighting inflammation and helping to protect DNA from free-radical damage (among other things). It also supports the buildup of the endometrium and is important in follicular fluid, so it's particularly important in phases 1 and 2 of a woman's cycle. Animal studies have linked vitamin E deficiency with infertility. Studies in humans have shown that vitamin E supplements are beneficial in treating infertility in both men and women.

Vitamin E improves ovulation, supports proper embryo implantation, and reduces the risk of early miscarriage. It improves sperm count, quality, and motility; helps keep the sperm membrane healthy; and protects sperm from free-radical damage. Studies show that vitamin E supplements improve the sperm's overall ability to penetrate an egg. In fact, IVF success rates are higher for couples in which the man takes vitamin E supplements.

Vitamin E is easier to absorb in its natural form (d-alpha-tocopherol) than in the synthetic version (dl-alpha-tocopherol), a subtle but important difference. Read the label carefully to make sure you get the type your body can use to the best advantage.

Vitamin E has anticoagulant properties, so you'll need to reduce your dose if you take aspirin (or low-dose aspirin) daily or heparin. Talk with your doctor to establish the best dose for you.

**EAT IT! GOOD SOURCES OF VITAMIN E**

| | |
|---|---|
| Alfalfa sprouts | Eggs |
| Lettuce | Sweet potatoes |
| Wheat germ | Avocados |
| Cold-pressed oils | Nuts and seeds |
| Leafy green vegetables | Whole grains |

## Calcium

Calcium plays a key role in ensuring good sperm motility. Without sufficient calcium, sperm lack the ability and energy to penetrate an egg. Calcium also is needed for blood clotting and hormonal balance, both of which are important to fertility.

---

### EAT IT! GOOD SOURCES OF CALCIUM

Milk

Dairy

Shellfish

Sardines

Leafy green vegetables

Sesame seeds

Tofu

Flaxseeds

Almonds

---

## Copper

Copper is an essential mineral. It helps with production of DNA and RNA, but perhaps its greatest contribution to fertility is in allowing you to use zinc (see page 124). Copper deficiency is rare, but if you take a supplement containing zinc, you should be sure it also contains a small amount of copper to ensure that your body gets enough. Excessive amounts of copper are toxic, however. Be aware that both smoking cigarettes and taking oral contraceptives can increase the amount of copper in your blood, sometimes to too high a level.

---

### EAT IT! GOOD SOURCES OF COPPER

Nuts

Legumes

Molasses

Raisins

Shellfish

Organ meats

Whole grains

---

## Iron

Iron plays a key role in DNA replication and in the maturing of the egg in advance of ovulation. Research shows that women who get enough iron cut their risk of ovulatory infertility by about one-half. It is also helpful to have enough iron during your period, to compensate for the blood lost. (Menstrual blood loss is the reason women require more iron than men.)

More than half of women don't get the 10 to 15 mg a day of iron they need. Your diet should include plenty of sources of iron, and a supplement may be smart as well. Too much iron can have negative effects, however, so we recommend taking a separate iron supplement only if you have a proven iron deficiency. Almost all prenatal multivitamins contain iron; those amounts are generally modest but enough for most people.

Vitamin C improves iron absorption, so be sure to get your share of that as well, especially in the first half of your cycle.

## EAT IT! GOOD SOURCES OF IRON

| | |
|---|---|
| Red meat | Beans |
| Poultry | Tofu |
| Eggs | Nuts |
| Fish | Seeds (especially pumpkin seeds) |
| Leafy green vegetables | Oatmeal |

### Magnesium

A deficiency of magnesium has been linked with female infertility. Magnesium supports progesterone production and increases the blood supply to the uterus. It is important for egg production. Some research shows that magnesium, when taken along with selenium, helps lower the risk of miscarriage, so make sure your multi contains both.

## EAT IT! GOOD SOURCES OF MAGNESIUM

| | |
|---|---|
| Leafy green vegetables | Millet |
| Kelp | Bananas |
| Tofu | Dried apricots |
| Rye | Avocados |
| Buckwheat | |

## Manganese

Manganese helps break down estrogen, and this can benefit fertility when there's too much estrogen in the body, such as after using birth control pills or when the body has an imbalance of estrogen in relation to progesterone. Manganese deficiency is rare in humans. Excessively high levels — which welders, for example, can have from environmental exposure — can cause male infertility. There's no reason for a separate supplement; check the label of your multivitamin to be sure you're getting the right amount.

---

### EAT IT! GOOD SOURCES OF MANGANESE

| | |
|---|---|
| Carrots | Legumes |
| Broccoli | Nuts |
| Leafy green vegetables | Ginger |
| Whole grains | |

---

## Selenium

Selenium is another useful antioxidant that helps protect against birth defects and miscarriage. It is important for egg production.

Selenium deficiency has been linked to male infertility, while selenium supplementation in men has been shown to improve pregnancy rates. Selenium improves sperm formation, quantity, structure, quality, motility, and function. The epididymis, the tube through which sperm pass from the testicle through the penis, needs selenium to function properly.

Very high doses of selenium can be toxic. Smaller (but still significant) doses taken regularly over long periods of time also can cause problems, the most common being hair loss and brittle hair and nails. Serious problems are almost always the result of industrial exposure, not supplements. To get the benefits without risking the side effects, take 50 to 100 mcg.

---

## EAT IT! GOOD SOURCES OF SELENIUM

Whole grains

Tuna

Wheat germ

Eggs

Garlic

Brazil nuts (Their selenium content is so
high, however, that you should eat no
more than two a day.)

---

### Zinc

Zinc is in short supply in the modern diet, and we find that although it is vital for proper growth and cell division of a fetus, many of our patients are not getting enough.

Zinc is a component of more than three hundred enzymes that are involved in all sorts of processes, including key roles in fertility. It is important for healthy follicular fluid, egg production, and proper processing of estrogen and progesterone. Zinc's importance is highlighted during phases 2 and 4 of a woman's cycle. Zinc deficiency has been linked to an increased risk of miscarriage, probably because of chromosomal changes in the egg or sperm.

Zinc may be the most important trace mineral for male fertility. It is found in high concentrations in male sex organs and sperm. Zinc is necessary for making the outer membrane and tail of the sperm and for sperm to mature properly. Zinc deficiency has been linked to low sperm counts, and zinc supplements have been shown to improve sperm count, motility, form, function, quality, and fertilizing capacity.

Exposure to stress, cigarette smoke, pollution, and alcohol can deplete zinc. Eating foods rich in zinc will support good fertility. If you are taking zinc supplements, you need to take copper as well to prevent copper deficiency (excessive zinc depletes copper).

---

## EAT IT! GOOD SOURCES OF ZINC

Eggs

Whole grains

Nuts and seeds

Cheese (especially cheddar and Parmesan)

Shellfish (especially oysters and shrimp)

Fish

Sardines

Duck, turkey, chicken, and lean meat

## OTHER KEY SUPPLEMENTS

Once you've found the right multivitamin, there are just a few more elements to a fertility supplement program you may want to work in. We think most people should take an EFA supplement along with their multivitamin. As for the rest, pretty much anyone can benefit from any or all of them. If you don't mind a big collection of pill jars in your cupboard, please feel free to use them. But to streamline the supplements you use while still maximizing your results, see part V to find out which ones are best for your specific fertility type. Here we describe the roles each element plays in fertility.

### Essential Fatty Acids (EFAs)

EFAs, most famously the omega-3 fatty acids, are crucial for healthy regulation of hormones throughout the body. They are also key to the health of your cell membranes. Choose a supplement with a balance of omega-3 and omega-6 fatty acids, and make sure you're buying a supplement that has been screened for toxins.

**Women:** This is the most important supplement after the prenatal multivitamin. Ideally, women should take EFAs for at least three months before they conceive to allow time for them to be fully incorporated into all the tissues.

EFAs help ensure that follicles have all the resources they need. They are key to cell membranes and growth in the ovaries. They help form body tissue, including tissue in eggs and in a developing fetus, and are essential for brain development in the fetus. Fish oils, a prime source of EFAs, are natural anticoagulants (clot-busters) and so may be particularly useful to anyone who has had recurrent miscarriages. (Use with caution, however, when combining with other blood thinners.) EFAs have been shown to improve endometriosis and therefore fertility.

Adding a plant source of EFAs to your intake, such as evening primrose oil, which is chockablock with omega-6 fatty acids, can help with PMS symptoms.

**Men:** EFAs are necessary to the production of healthy sperm. They improve sperm membranes and protect sperm from oxidative stress. Inadequate intake of EFAs has been linked to poor sperm quality, abnormal sperm, poor motility, and low sperm count, largely because of their role in membrane structure.

## Eat It! Good Sources of EFAs

**Omega-3 Fatty Acids**

Fatty fish (salmon, herring, sardines, mackerel)

Walnuts

Flaxseeds

Eggs (especially those from chickens that have been fed greens rather than corn)

Grass-fed beef (as opposed to standard grain-fed beef)

Dairy from grass-fed cows

**Omega-6 Fatty Acids**

Flaxseeds and flaxseed oil

Hempseeds and hempseed oil

Grapeseed oil

Pumpkin seeds

Sunflower seeds (raw)

Pine nuts

Pistachios

Olives

Olive oil

Black currant seed oil

Evening primrose oil

Chicken

### Coenzyme Q10 (CoQ10)

This antioxidant is in every cell in the human body. It promotes good blood circulation, so much of the research on CoQ10 looks at heart disease. But good blood flow is important to fertility as well. The body also uses CoQ10 as it produces energy at the cellular level. CoQ10 is difficult to get in significant amounts from food, so we recommend a supplement if you want to boost your levels of this nutrient.

**Women:** CoQ10 improves pelvic blood flow, especially to the uterus, so it is particularly helpful in phase 1 of a woman's cycle. Studies have shown that women taking CoQ10 had higher fertilization rates in IVF with intracytoplasmic sperm injection (ICSI) than women who weren't taking the supplement. Research links CoQ10 deficiency with miscarriage.

**Men:** CoQ10 has been proven to be beneficial in treating male infertility. It is found in seminal fluid, where it helps protect sperm from damage and improves motility. Studies have shown that use of a CoQ10 supplement can increase sperm count and motility.

### L-arginine

L-arginine is an amino acid that helps improve blood flow to the pelvis. It has been shown to help fertility in both men and women. L-arginine is found in protein-rich foods, so count this as one of the good reasons to get sufficient protein in your diet. It's also a good excuse to eat more chocolate. People who have the herpes virus, including cold sores, should not supplement with L-arginine because it could stimulate an attack.

**Women:** According to at least one study, women diagnosed with infertility who take L-arginine can significantly increase their odds of getting pregnant. Another study showed improved IVF outcomes when women classified as "poor responders" to fertility drugs took L-arginine.

**Men:** L-arginine is essential for sperm production, formation, and maturation. The head of the sperm contains high levels. L-arginine has been shown to improve sperm count, quality, and motility, although it is less beneficial when the initial sperm count is extremely low (less than 10 million per ml).

---

### EAT IT! GOOD SOURCES OF L-ARGININE

| | |
|---|---|
| Peanuts | Dairy |
| Walnuts | Pork and beef |
| Brazil nuts | Chicken and turkey |
| Legumes | Seafood |
| Chickpeas | Grains (especially oats and wheat) |
| Coconut | Chocolate |

---

### L-carnitine

This amino acid is an antioxidant that helps your cells produce energy. Research has shown that the use of L-carnitine supplements increases success rates in both natural conception and intrauterine insemination (IUI).

**Women:** L-carnitine is not an important fertility supplement for women.

**Men:** L-carnitine is essential for proper maturation and functioning of sperm. It is secreted in the epididymis, where its antioxidant properties help protect sperm from damage. Supplementing with L-carnitine can improve sperm count, quality, and motility in men with documented deficiencies in those areas. In fact, the best results are seen in those with the lowest motility to begin with. Supplements can bring motility up to normal. The higher the level of L-carnitine in the sperm, the higher the sperm count will be and the more motile the sperm. With a deficiency of L-carnitine, sperm development, function, and motility are all drastically reduced.

---

### EAT IT! GOOD SOURCES OF L-CARNITINE

| Meat | Dairy |
|------|-------|

---

### N-acetyl cysteine (NAC)

This antioxidant reduces inflammatory reactions. No food supplies NAC directly, but the body makes NAC from protein, and you can take NAC in supplement form.

**Women:** If there's inflammation of the endometrium, it can't support implantation and maintain a healthy embryo. NAC can help prevent this problem.

**Men:** NAC can improve the sperm membrane, protect sperm from oxidative damage, and help increase sperm count.

### Glutathione

Glutathione is another useful antioxidant. It isn't found directly in any foods, nor is it absorbed well from supplements. The body uses NAC to make glutathione. It can also be made from substances in undenatured, bioactive whey protein. Consider using either NAC or whey as your glutathione supplement. Eating the foods listed also will help your body boost glutathione levels.

**Women:** Studies have shown lower glutathione levels in women who experience recurrent, very early miscarriages.

---

### EAT IT! GOOD SOURCES OF GLUTATHIONE

| Asparagus | Broccoli |
|-----------|----------|
| Garlic | Avocados |
| Spinach | Whey protein (must be undenatured) |

**Men:** Glutathione helps ensure properly formed sperm. It's been proven beneficial in treating male infertility.

### Royal Jelly

Royal jelly is what bees in a colony feed to their queen to help her produce hundreds of eggs a day. Think of it as the bee equivalent of a fertility drug. Royal jelly supplements contain a complex blend of amino acids, vitamins, enzymes, EFAs, and sterols (which are a component of hormones). Royal jelly should not be used by anyone with an allergy to bee stings or any bee products.

**Women:** Studies have shown that royal jelly can positively affect menstrual irregularities, improving fertility compromised by unpredictable cycles.

**Men:** Research has shown that royal jelly can increase sperm production.

### Chlorophyll

Chlorophyll, the basis of all plant life, can arrest the growth and development of unfriendly bacteria, and it can build up red blood cells. In severely anemic animals, studies have shown that red blood cell counts return to normal after just four or five days of chlorophyll supplementation. The high magnesium content in chlorophyll also boosts enzymes that restore the sex hormones. In fact, American farmers have been known to give their cows wheatgrass to restore fertility.

You get chlorophyll whenever you eat green vegetables, but a liquid chlorophyll supplement (available at health food stores) provides much more than you could ever eat, because it is so concentrated. Better still, if you can manage it, drink a shot glass of juiced wheatgrass each day. That is one of the best sources of living chlorophyll. Other cereal grasses such as barley grass and rye grass will give you the same benefits.

---

### EAT IT! GOOD SOURCES OF CHLOROPHYLL

Green vegetables

Wheatgrass juice (or barley grass or rye grass juice)

**Women:** Chlorophyll helps build up the uterine lining.

**Men:** Chlorophyll is not an important fertility supplement for men.

### Para-aminobenzoic Acid (PABA)

PABA has been proven to correct certain aspects of autoimmune conditions that can affect fertility. People with autoimmune issues should consider supplements.

---

## EAT IT! GOOD SOURCES OF PABA

| | |
|---|---|
| Eggs | Molasses |
| Rice | Organ meats |
| Wheat germ | Leafy green vegetables |
| Wheat bran | |

---

## CHOOSE YOUR SUPPLEMENTS WISELY

Please don't go overboard, gobbling up handfuls of supplements with every meal. You *can* get too much of a good thing. High doses of nutrients can stress your body, throwing it out of balance, even if the doses are not high enough to be toxic. Remember that a healthy, organic diet will supply most people with what their bodies need. A balanced diet with five to eight servings of fruits and vegetables a day will provide plenty of antioxidants. If you are eating well, taking a multivitamin, and supplementing with omega-3 fatty acids, you can rest assured you are well nourished for optimal fertility. Your fertility type will suggest which, if any, additional supplements might make a good addition to your regimen (see part V).

For optimal pre-conception nourishment, look for a prenatal vitamin and mineral supplement with all the components included in the Making Babies Action Plan in this chapter. Depending on what you find, there may be a few other ingredients in there, too, which is usually fine. Don't expect to find anything that matches exactly all of our recommended doses. Consider our recommendations as guidelines. If your supplement has a little less than we recommend, remember that you are getting nutrients from your diet, too. If it has a little more, remember that as long as you don't take really large doses, a little more of a good thing won't hurt you.

Select a supplement meant to be taken three times a day, usually with a meal. A once-a-day formula may seem more convenient, but it will dump an excessively high amount of the active ingredients into your system all at once. As a result, some are not absorbed, and some won't be there when you need them. (Plus, it's sure to be a really big pill to swallow.) Take your vitamins with food to avoid getting an upset stomach and to facilitate the absorption of fat-soluble vitamins such as D and E.

Buy supplements from a reputable health food store or ask your doctor for recommendations. Health care providers have access to vitamins that are not available in stores and are generally of high quality.

The Food and Drug Administration (FDA) lays down guidelines for the manufacture of vitamins and herbal products called good manufacturing practice (GMP). Good vitamin manufacturers abide by these guidelines. Dietary supplements are not officially monitored, and there's a risk that what they actually contain varies from what's listed on the labels. Supplements should be tested for toxic substances, such as lead or mercury, and other kinds of contamination. Contact the labs that make the supplements and ask them about GMP, how they test their products, and what they test them for. A reliable company will be able to answer your questions. Another option is to consult ConsumerLab.com, an organization that tests vitamins. You need to purchase a membership to have access to its findings, but you may find its seal of approval on some labels.

And, of course, you should always read the labels. Ingredients for supplements should be from natural sources whenever possible. Look for notification of testing for contamination or toxins. Look for hypoallergenic products if you have sensitivity issues (avoid wheat, yeast, and corn). And make sure you're using a fresh product. Use it before the expiration date, and if there is no expiration date, buy something else.

If you see an herbalist, show him or her any supplements you take. The herbalist can tell you if there's any overlap between your supplements and your herbs and help you adjust as necessary.

# Making Babies Action Plan

## PRENATAL MULTIVITAMIN FOR WOMEN

For optimal pre-conception nourishment, look for a multivitamin and mineral supplement with the following components. Select a supplement meant to be taken three times a day, usually with a meal, not a one-a-day formulation.

| NUTRIENT | DAILY DOSE | NOTES |
| --- | --- | --- |
| Vitamin A (beta-carotene) | 5,000–8,000 IU | |
| Vitamin B$_1$ (thiamine) | 0.8 mg | |
| Vitamin B$_2$ (riboflavin) | 1.1 mg | |
| Vitamin B$_5$ (pantothenic acid) | 3–7 mg | |
| Vitamin B$_6$ | 25–50 mg | |
| Folic acid (vitamin B$_9$ or folate) | 800–1,000 mcg | |
| Vitamin B$_{12}$ | 100 mcg | |
| Vitamin C | 200–500 mg | High doses (1,000 mg a day or more) can dry up fertile cervical mucus. |
| Vitamin D | 1,000 IU | |
| Vitamin E | 100 IU | Get the natural form (d-alpha-tocopherol), not the synthetic (dl-alpha-tocopherol). Talk with your doctor before taking with blood thinners or daily aspirin. |
| Calcium | 300–600 mg | |
| Copper | 2 mg | Any time you use a copper supplement, you should balance it with zinc. |
| Iron | 10–15 mg | |
| Magnesium | 250–400 mg | |
| Manganese | 1–2 mg | |
| Selenium | 50–100 mcg | |
| Zinc | 15–25 mg | Doses higher than this can interfere with copper absorption. Anytime you use a zinc supplement, you should balance it with copper. |

## OTHER FERTILITY SUPPLEMENTS FOR WOMEN

| NUTRIENT | DAILY DOSE | NOTES |
|---|---|---|
| Essential fatty acids (EFAs) | 1,000–5,000 mg | Look for mixed EFAs with a balance of omega-3 and omega-6 fatty acids. The supplement should be screened for toxins. Talk with your doctor before taking with blood thinners. |
| Coenzyme Q10 (CoQ10) | 30–100 mg | |
| L-arginine | 500 mg | Don't take if you get cold sores or have herpes. |
| N-acetyl cysteine (NAC) | 600 mg | |
| Glutathione | — | Get from NAC or whey protein. |
| Royal jelly | Follow package instructions. | Don't take if you have an allergy to bee stings or bee products. |
| Chlorophyll | Follow package instructions. | |
| Para-aminobenzoic acid (PABA) | 300–400 mg | |

## PRE-CONCEPTION MULTIVITAMIN FOR MEN

For optimal pre-conception nourishment, look for a multivitamin and mineral supplement with the following components. Select a supplement meant to be taken three times a day, usually with a meal, not a one-a-day formulation.

| NUTRIENT | DAILY DOSE | NOTES |
|---|---|---|
| Vitamin A (beta-carotene) | 5,000 IU | |
| Vitamin $B_1$ (thiamine) | 1.2–1.5 mg | |
| Vitamin $B_2$ (riboflavin) | 1.3 mg | |
| Vitamin $B_5$ (pantothenic acid) | 5 mg | |
| Vitamin $B_6$ | 50 mg | |
| Folic acid (vitamin $B_9$ or folate) | 400 mcg | |
| Vitamin $B_{12}$ | 100 mcg | |
| Vitamin C | 500–1,000 mg | |

| NUTRIENT | DAILY DOSE | NOTES |
| --- | --- | --- |
| Vitamin D | 800–1,000 IU | |
| Vitamin E | 400 IU | Get the natural form (d-alpha-tocopherol), not the synthetic (dl-alpha-tocopherol). Talk with your doctor before taking with blood thinners or daily aspirin. |
| Calcium | 250–300 mg | |
| Copper | 2 mg | Anytime you use a copper supplement, you should balance it with zinc. |
| Iron | 2 mg | |
| Magnesium | 250–500 mg | |
| Manganese | 1–2 mg | |
| Selenium | 50–100 mcg | |
| Zinc | 50 mg | Anytime you use a zinc supplement, you should balance it with copper. Doses higher than this can interfere with copper absorption. |

## OTHER FERTILITY SUPPLEMENTS FOR MEN

| NUTRIENT | DAILY DOSE | NOTES |
| --- | --- | --- |
| Essential fatty acids (EFAs) | 1,000–5,000 mg | Look for mixed EFAs with a balance of omega-3 and omega-6 fatty acids. The supplement should be screened for toxins. Talk with your doctor before taking with blood thinners. |
| Coenzyme Q10 (CoQ10) | 100 mg | |
| L-arginine | 500 mg | Don't take if you get cold sores or have herpes. |
| L-carnitine | 1–2 mg | |
| N-acetyl cysteine (NAC) | 600 mg | |
| Glutathione | — | Get from NAC or whey protein. |
| Royal jelly | Follow package instructions. | Don't take if you have an allergy to bee stings or bee products. |
| Para-aminobenzoic acid (PABA) | 300–400 mg | |

# PART THREE

# The Five Fertility Types

# CHAPTER SEVEN

# What Is Your Fertility Type?

With the general precepts of this program out of the way, let's talk about what's really important in your quest for natural fertility: *you*. Not every approach to improving fertility will work for every person, no matter what most fertility clinics seem to think. Nor should it: we are all individuals and should be considered as such when we receive any kind of health care. The operative question isn't "What works?" It's "What works *for me?*"

This is exactly where Western medicine so often gets tripped up, tending to a one-size-fits-all style of treatment. It also happens to be the core strength of traditional Chinese medicine: considering the whole person as an individual, as well as how he or she fits into universal patterns. This can create its own problems, as Chinese medicine can get complex to the point where it may be impenetrable to all but the experts. So what we've tried to do is combine the strengths of the two systems, then distill the result down into something accessible and practical. Our aim is to make the information and its application as clear and simple as possible, so you can use your time and energy efficiently in arriving at a plan that will suit you best.

To that end, we've pooled our clinical experience to create five fertility types to help you identify the general pattern at work in your body: Tired, Dry, Stuck, Pale, and Waterlogged. These types were inspired by the patterns used in traditional Chinese medicine, although here they are pared down to focus on the most telling details relevant to fertility. When we sat down to review this system, we discovered (happily, but not really to our surprise) that almost all Western diagnoses divide neatly into these categories. So we're pleased to present a system that can unify East and West, to give you direct access to the best each has to offer for your particular situation.

The following short chapters, presented roughly from most to least common fertility type, describe the types in some detail and then provide simple checklists of common signs and symptoms of the types to help you figure out which type you are. But before we turn you loose on that project, we want to back up for a minute to explain a little more about traditional Chinese medicine.

We're operating under the assumption that you have a basic intuitive understanding of the mechanisms and underlying principles of Western medicine. Chinese medicine is something else altogether, offering a very different worldview.

Years ago, I (Jill) struggled with a chronic medical condition, swallowing antibiotics for six months with no improvement. My doctor said he was out of options and finally sent me to a Chinese medicine practitioner. Just a couple of weeks of acupuncture and Chinese herbs sorted out the problem. This experience turned my world upside down. It was a completely different paradigm than I'd ever been exposed to. That it worked at all was, frankly, a bit hard for me to believe, even though I'd experienced it myself in such a profound way. But I was drawn to understanding it better. I started reading everything I could get my hands on and asked a lot of questions. The more I learned, the more I wanted to know, and ultimately I went back to graduate school for a master's degree in Traditional Oriental Medicine.

While in school, I went to a lecture by a doctor who changed my life again. She was trained in China both in conventional gynecology and in acupuncture and herbology, and she talked about what Chinese medicine could do that Western medicine could not. She also explained what Western medicine could do that Chinese medicine could not. This vision of collaborative medicine excited and inspired me, and I've strived for that complementarity in the way I've worked ever since.

Fertility issues are especially well suited to this kind of combined approach. Infertility is often the result of a series of little imbalances in various body systems that, taken together, add up to one big problem. Chinese medicine is all about striking balances and gentle fine-tuning, so it's very effective in dealing with fertility problems. Herbs and acupuncture work in the body in subtle ways, just as the hormonal system itself functions. So, for example, traditional Chinese medicine has ways of stabilizing an irregular cycle that are hard to replicate in Western medicine. Then again, when you reach the limits of what Chinese medicine can do — when you have a surgical problem or something that needs a stronger push, or when Western testing offers a shortcut to confirming a diagnosis — it's good to have the strengths of Western medicine at hand as well. If you have fibroids impeding your fertility, for example, traditional Chinese medicine might be able to shrink them a bit, but it can't make them disappear. For that, you need a surgeon. Neither the Eastern nor the Western way is superior, but combining them is often better than relying on each alone.

I regularly consult with conventional doctors about our shared patients. I want to keep the doctors apprised of what I'm doing, and I want to understand their plans fully. I want to be sure our efforts will work well together. There are herbs I won't prescribe, for example, if I know a woman is taking drugs that function in a similar way. Most doctors are very receptive to working with me, and I believe that's because I speak their language. I was trained in hospitals and have taught in hospitals; I've worked alongside doctors most of my career. So I don't call up and say, "I'm treating so-and-so for kidney yang deficiency with blood deficiency." I translate for them just as I translate for my patients, talking about hormone imbalances and how herbs and acupuncture can level them out.

In this book, we hew to the same path, putting everything in the context of Western medicine so as to be most accessible to people entrenched in the Western perspective. We want readers to be able to grasp it easily and to be able to talk to their doctors about it. We also want them to be able to speak just as intelligently with an acupuncturist or herbalist, so the discussion of each type includes a brief section on how Chinese medicine views it.

Doctors' biggest complaint about alternative medicine is that it is too open-ended. I set time limits and assessible goals for my treatment so that everyone — the patient, the doctor, and myself — can judge how it is progressing. I'll say, for example, that I expect specific signs of hormones coming back into balance (less painful periods and improved sex drive perhaps) as treatment progresses through three menstrual cycles. I might suggest that the doctor do testing along the way to confirm that hormone levels are coming into balance.

My Chinese medicine teachers would say that healthy people have healthy babies. They taught me that if you don't know what exactly is causing infertility (or any condition), you should treat any area of imbalance you see. This is one definition of a holistic approach. I take everything into account, including a bunch of things that aren't obviously linked to reproduction—home life, state of mind, digestion, skin tone, back pain, and much more. Any imbalance in the body produces a symptom, and any symptom signifies an imbalance. Restoring balance is the path to health, and enjoying overall health is the best path to making a baby.

## THE FERTILITY TYPES

TIRED

DRY

STUCK

PALE

Which brings us back to the fertility types. Your goal is to find your balance within your type, whatever it may be. But the way you identify your type has mostly to do with the ways in which you fall out of balance. Symptoms occur when something in your body tips one way or the other, and those symptoms are the hallmarks of your type. They may be annoying or downright unpleasant, but consider them crucial notes to yourself, messages from your body about where you need to restore balance in order to restore optimal health.

Your type (Tired, Dry, Stuck, Pale, or Waterlogged) pinpoints the pattern of what's going on in your body as you prepare to conceive. It points you toward the conception strategies that will be most useful to you, as well as the fertility problems you are most likely to encounter. Each type has its own distinctive icon that marks the relevant sections for you throughout the upcoming chapters.

WATERLOGGED

Perhaps it goes without saying, but a complete individual medical diagnosis, whether Chinese or Western, is much more precise than any book-based system could be. A Chinese medical diagnosis in particular is very subtle and complicated. Chinese medicine emphasizes the interconnectedness of everything; practitioners are taught to look for patterns of dysfunction rather than specific symptoms. Any one symptom must be considered in relation to the whole person. So if you are interested in getting a full Chinese diagnosis, you should consult a licensed, board-certified acupuncturist (see chapter 19). Presumably, you already know the importance of working with your own conventional doctor as well.

Our focus in this book is on strategies you can implement on your own, at home. When it comes to information and advice that requires the involvement of a health care practitioner, we want to help you understand your situation, in layperson's terms, and prepare you to speak intelligently with your health care provider about it. We all have to be our own advocates if we want to be sure to get the best health care. We have to be responsible for ourselves as we go through the system. Our goal is to give you all the tools you need—information, vocabulary, self-knowledge—to negotiate the health care system successfully. If you want to be sure you have all the tests you should have, to rest easy that all your options have been considered, and to have access to the treatments that are best for you, you're going to need to know what they are and how to talk to your doctor about them.

This is an especially challenging task when you are taking advantage of two systems of care (not to mention the fact that both partners in a couple need their own individualized care). But though the systems may be separate, they are also complementary. You may just need to build the bridge between them if your doctor and/or acupuncturist isn't fully able to do so. This book uniquely prepares you to do exactly that.

## HOW TO FIND YOUR TYPE

The first step is to figure out your fertility type. That will be your key to unlocking all this book has to offer.

All the new information that's about to come at you may seem overwhelming at first, but don't worry; you don't have to memorize all the types or even keep them all straight in your mind. You do need to read about all of them to identify your type, but once you do that, you can put all your focus on just the information that applies to you. The whole typing process will, in the end, narrow the field of information you need to concern yourself with. But for now, don't try any shortcuts. Don't stop reading when you get to one familiar-sounding type. You may find another that fits you even better farther on.

Each of the next five chapters begins with a general description of the type, then describes what it looks like in women and in men, including the commonly associated fertility problems. (Full information on those fertility issues appears in chapters 14–18, with the fertility type icons marking each one so that you can easily find those most relevant to you.) Each chapter then lists the most common combinations with other types and the hallmark signs of each combination. Next up is a brief explanation of the type from a Chinese medicine perspective, then an example of a real patient who is that type. At the end of each chapter are checklists to fill out, summarizing all the key characteristics of the type, with special sections for women, women who keep a BBT chart, and men.

A BBT chart will give you a lot of information that can help determine your fertility type and identify specific fertility issues. Your doctor or other health care practitioner may find useful information there as well. But it isn't necessary to keep a chart to find your type or to benefit from this book. If you have trouble figuring out your type, doing a BBT chart may clarify things. Those of you who don't want to bother keeping a chart, just skip that section of the checklists.

In the checklists, you will find a lot of detailed statements about your menstrual cycle and your period. Chinese medicine puts a lot of emphasis on the quantity and quality of blood flow during the period, as well as the color, whether there are any clots, and more. Your answers will reveal much about your reproductive health in general and help you arrive at a diagnosis. My (Jill's) Chinese teachers taught me that the period should start like a river, become a sea, and end as a stream. It should start with a flow, not spotting, become stronger, and then ebb away smoothly, again without spotting. Where your cycle differs from this description helps point the way to a diagnosis.

As you read through the descriptions of all the types, you will probably recognize yourself in one (or possibly two) of them. Complete the checklists to determine which type fits you best. For most people, one will clearly be the winner; you might even figure it out from reading the general description. Or you may have a lot of checks on several lists; the one with the most points is your type. If you end up with a tie (or within a few points of a tie), you may be a combination type. If you take the full descriptions into account, whichever one seems more like you is your *dominant* type, but you'll be best served by following the advice for both types. If there's a conflict, follow the advice for your dominant type. An acupuncturist can help you sort out the nuances of mixed patterns, and we certainly encourage you to pursue that if you are so inclined. But it won't be necessary to do so to benefit from this book.

You can also go to www.makingbabiesprogram.com and complete

the online quiz to quickly and easily discover your fertility type. But you should still read through the descriptions—at least the ones that apply to you—to learn all you need to know about that type.

## Making Babies Action Plan

❏ Consider seeing a Chinese medicine practitioner for a full Chinese diagnosis.

❏ Use this book to learn how to be an effective advocate for yourself with any health care practitioner you consult and to help coordinate between practitioners.

❏ If you have trouble identifying your type, consider keeping a BBT chart to clarify things.

❏ Pay attention to the details of your menstrual cycle for what they can reveal about your health, reproductive health, and fertility type.

❏ Complete the checklists in each of the next five chapters to determine your fertility type (Tired, Dry, Stuck, Pale, or Waterlogged) so you'll be able to follow the Making Babies advice most suited to you.

❏ Go to www.makingbabiesprogram.com and complete the questionnaire there to determine your fertility type.

❏ Familiarize yourself with the icon for your type so you will be able to easily identify which of the remaining sections of the book are most important for you.

# CHAPTER EIGHT

# Tired

Tired people are a bit like flat tires. The deflation is not a permanent condition, but as long as they are out of air, they just can't be their usual selves.

Tired people are, above all, tired. They often feel weak or lethargic to boot, as if they lack the energy to tackle what life throws at them. They are quite comfortable in the role of couch potato. The most important symptoms indicating the Tired type are poor metabolism, hypothyroidism, and feeling cold.

Tired people are often cold. They are sensitive to the cold and may have a strong aversion to it. They feel chilly even when those around them are warm. They complain especially of cold hands and feet. They may have poor circulation.

Tired people need a lot of sleep but feel groggy in the morning and often have dark circles under their eyes. Because they're generally run-down, Tired people seem to catch every bug that comes around and take longer than most to bounce back from it. They are prone to various aches and pains, particularly low back and knee pain.

Tired people often have pale or sallow skin. They get out of breath and sweat easily and feel unfit. Many complain of "brain fog"—they have trouble concentrating, have little motivation, and feel generally dull.

Tired people can have a sluggish digestive system and experience a range of digestive complaints. They are particularly prone to loose stools first thing in the morning, bloating, and gas. Their appetite is often poor. Tired people are extremely sensitive to sugar, so they often use it to give themselves energy. But they get trapped in a negative cycle, craving carbs when they are tired and then, when they indulge, riding a roller coaster as their blood sugar surges and crashes. Many Tired people put on weight easily, particularly when they are fatigued or under stress, and many are chronically overweight. They tend to retain water, but many urinate frequently and have lots of clear urine.

These symptoms reflect a broad hormone imbalance affecting the reproductive hormones but also encompassing the thyroid, adrenal, and pituitary glands. Weaknesses in these systems affect metabolism and circulation, which in turn affect fertility.

Tired people often have a low libido — they simply have no energy for sex and often find it hard to get aroused. The lack of motivation can seriously hamper their attempts to conceive.

## WOMEN

Tired women tend to have metabolic problems, such as being hypothyroid.

Tired women may have a long menstrual cycle with slow or late ovulation (long follicular phase), or they may have a short cycle with a short luteal phase. They often have very heavy but short periods, or very heavy flow on the first two days. The blood is often watery and pale. Some Tired women have long periods (more than five days). Tired women may experience a range of symptoms with their periods, including fatigue, poor circulation, or digestive problems, particularly loose stools.

Tired women are most likely to run into problems during phase 3 (ovulation) of their cycle. Sometimes Tired women ovulate late. They tend to have symptoms at ovulation as well, including spotting, abdominal bloating, and the same symptoms they have with their periods. Some Tired women get spotting before their periods begin.

Tired women are prone to low progesterone levels, sometimes to the point where they have luteal phase defect (LPD; see page 200). In more extreme cases, Tired women can suffer from recurrent miscarriages or vaginal or uterine prolapse.

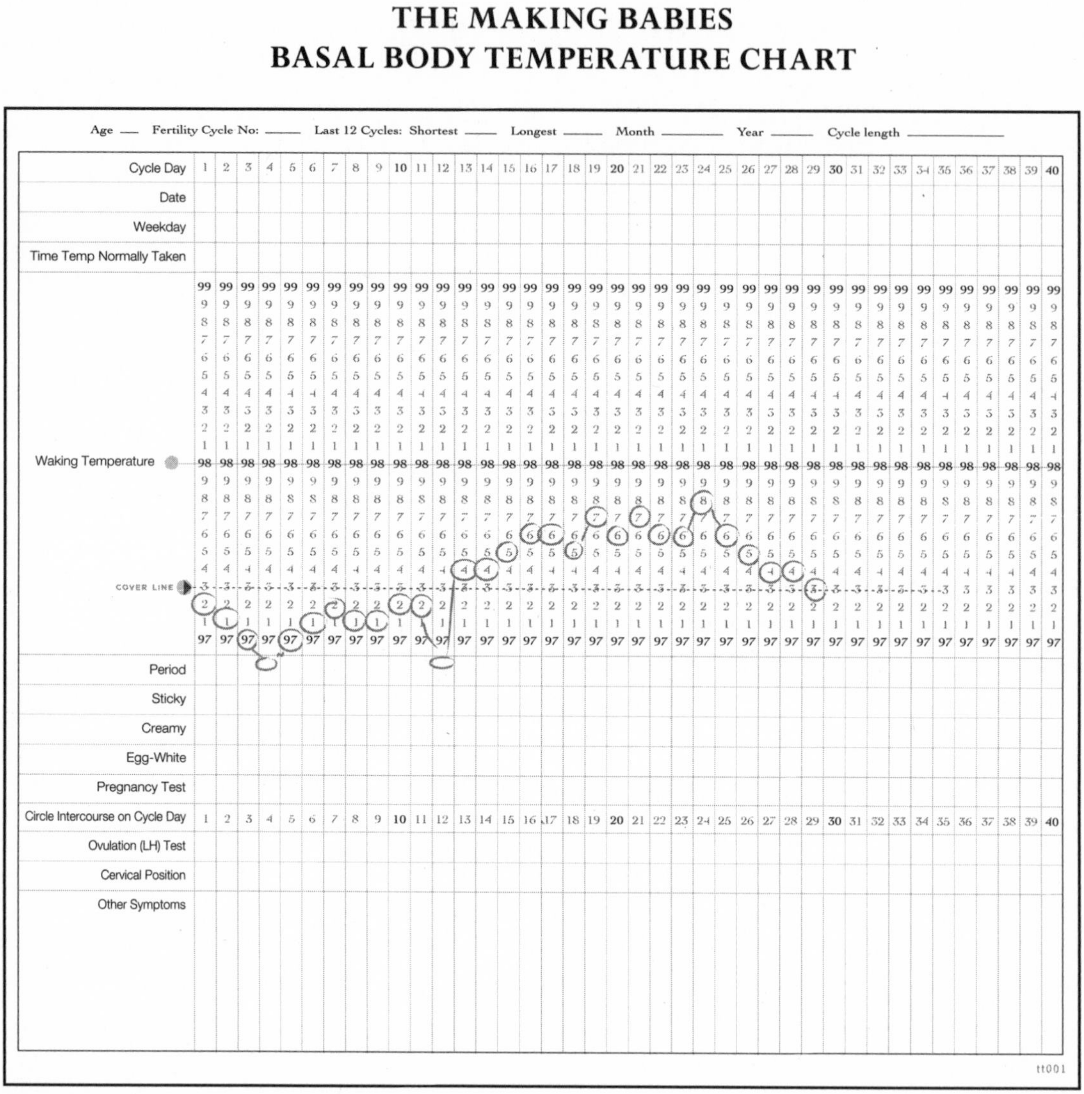

# THE MAKING BABIES
# BASAL BODY TEMPERATURE CHART

**Fig. 11:** Tired type with very low temperatures.

# THE MAKING BABIES
## BASAL BODY TEMPERATURE CHART

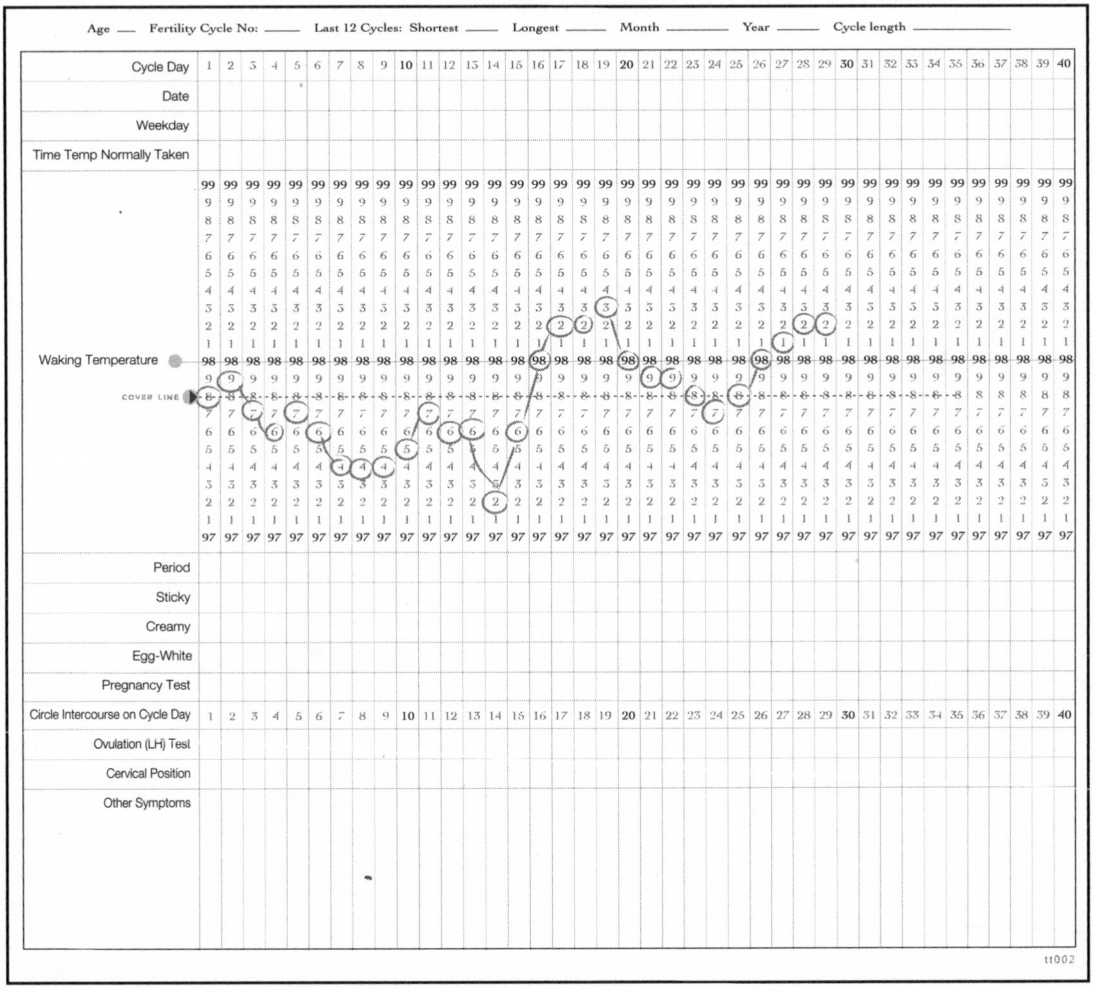

Age ____  Fertility Cycle No: ____  Last 12 Cycles: Shortest ____  Longest ____  Month ____  Year ____  Cycle length ____

| Cycle Day | 1 | 2 | 3 | 4 | 5 | 6 | 7 | 8 | 9 | 10 | 11 | 12 | 13 | 14 | 15 | 16 | 17 | 18 | 19 | 20 | 21 | 22 | 23 | 24 | 25 | 26 | 27 | 28 | 29 | 30 | 31 | 32 | 33 | 34 | 35 | 36 | 37 | 38 | 39 | 40 |
|---|---|---|---|---|---|---|---|---|---|---|---|---|---|---|---|---|---|---|---|---|---|---|---|---|---|---|---|---|---|---|---|---|---|---|---|---|---|---|---|---|

Date

Weekday

Time Temp Normally Taken

Waking Temperature

COVER LINE

Period

Sticky

Creamy

Egg-White

Pregnancy Test

| Circle Intercourse on Cycle Day | 1 | 2 | 3 | 4 | 5 | 6 | 7 | 8 | 9 | 10 | 11 | 12 | 13 | 14 | 15 | 16 | 17 | 18 | 19 | 20 | 21 | 22 | 23 | 24 | 25 | 26 | 27 | 28 | 29 | 30 | 31 | 32 | 33 | 34 | 35 | 36 | 37 | 38 | 39 | 40 |
|---|---|---|---|---|---|---|---|---|---|---|---|---|---|---|---|---|---|---|---|---|---|---|---|---|---|---|---|---|---|---|---|---|---|---|---|---|---|---|---|---|

Ovulation (LH) Test

Cervical Position

Other Symptoms

tt002

**Fig. 12:** Tired type with a temperature drop after ovulation.

# THE MAKING BABIES
# BASAL BODY TEMPERATURE CHART

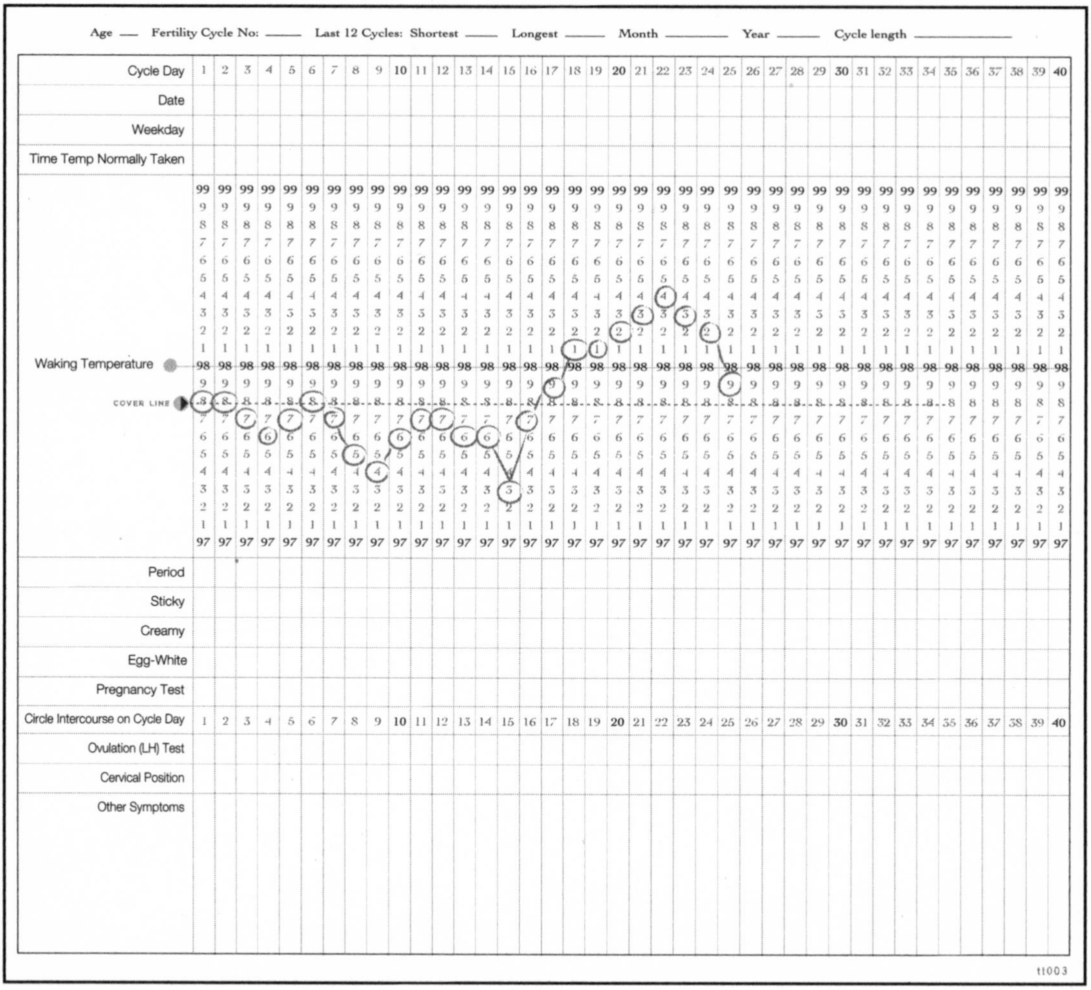

**Fig. 13:** Tired type with a short luteal phase.

## MEN

Tired men may have low testosterone levels. They can experience erectile dysfunction (ED). They also tend to have sperm with low motility and/or low sperm counts.

## COMMON COMBINATIONS

In this most common combination type, poor diet and lack of exercise contribute to problems with fluid metabolism, the buildup of fluids in the body, and the accumulation of mucus.

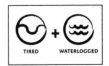

In these people, poor digestion leads to poor assimilation of nutrients from food, making them undernourished.

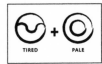

This combination type has digestive issues, especially premenstrually or with stress, often manifesting as loose stools when under pressure or, for women, diarrhea the day before their periods.

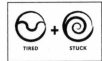

## CHINESE MEDICINE

Tired people are considered yang deficient, in part because they are qi deficient. Qi, sometimes described as life force or energy, isn't a specific physical thing. It describes several key bodily functions: movement, transformation, transportation, warming, protecting, and containing. When it comes to fertility, each of these functions comes into play. The ability to have an erection relies on qi, for example (movement). So does the ability to transform an egg and a sperm into an embryo (transformation). The body relies on qi to get an egg from the ovary to the uterus (transportation) and to create an environment of the right temperature in the uterus (warming). A healthy immune system is a function of qi (protecting) and a key to a successful and healthy pregnancy. The body also uses qi to keep things where they are (containing), including keeping a baby in the uterus.

## Case Study: A Real, Tired Woman

The first thing Audrey, age 42, told me (Jill)—after saying she'd been trying to conceive for six months—was that she was tired most of the time. She said she woke up feeling groggy in the morning and had another energy drop at midafternoon, to the point that she often felt she needed carbs in the form of chocolate simply to make it through to the end of the workday. Audrey's cycle was short—just twenty-four days—and her periods were very heavy but lasted only a couple days. She always had loose stools with her periods.

I gave Audrey an herbal formula to help balance her system, and after just two months she reported that she had more energy and was less groggy in the morning. Her cycle, though still short, had lengthened by a day, and her periods had lightened up a bit. After four months, her cycle stretched to twenty-six days, and she went most afternoons without ever thinking about chocolate. During the sixth month of treatment, she noticed that she no longer had loose stools and her cycle was up to twenty-seven days. She conceived two months later and delivered a healthy baby.

# Making Babies Action Plan

## ARE YOU TIRED?

### 5 POINTS EACH

- ❑ I have been diagnosed with a metabolic disorder.
- ❑ My metabolism is sluggish, and I gain weight easily.
- ❑ I have been diagnosed with hypothyroidism.
- ❑ I feel cold a lot of the time.

### 3 POINTS EACH

- ❑ I am often tired or lethargic, and I don't have much endurance or motivation.
- ❑ I need a lot of sleep.
- ❑ I am sometimes short of breath.
- ❑ I perspire easily with exertion.
- ❑ I am overweight.
- ❑ I often crave carbohydrates.
- ❑ I bruise easily.
- ❑ My libido is low.

**1 POINT EACH**

❏ I sometimes feel dull and have trouble concentrating.

❏ I catch colds easily.

❏ It takes me a long time to recover from an illness.

❏ My complexion is pale or sallow.

❏ My energy is low after I eat, and I get bloated.

❏ I sometimes have dark circles under my eyes.

❏ I often experience digestive complaints such as loose stools, abdominal pain, and flatulence.

❏ My first bowel movement of the day is often loose.

❏ My appetite is generally poor or erratic.

❏ I don't have much muscle tone; I feel weak.

❏ I am prone to low back or knee pain.

❏ I have poor circulation.

❏ I prefer hot weather/I hate the cold.

❏ I have cold limbs or cold hands and feet.

❏ Given the choice, I would prefer a hot drink.

❏ I urinate frequently, and the urine is very pale or clear.

❏ I retain water.

## FOR WOMEN ONLY

**5 POINTS**

❏ I have been diagnosed with low progesterone levels or LPD.

**3 POINTS EACH**

❏ I experience spotting before my period starts.

❏ My period is heavy but short; it seems to come all at once.

**1 POINT EACH**

❏ My menstrual cycle is long.

❏ I frequently have profuse vaginal discharge that has no odor, especially mid-cycle.

❏ I have a long period; it lasts longer than 7 days.

❑  I suffer from loose stools during my period or premenstrually.

❑  I get menstrual cramps that are relieved with heat (such as a heating pad).

## FOR WOMEN WHO KEEP A BBT CHART

### 3 POINTS EACH

❑  My BBT is generally low, sometimes so low that it is literally off the chart.

❑  I have a short luteal phase, less than 12 days; my period starts 11 days or less after my last day of egg-white mucus (possible LPD due to insufficient progesterone).

❑  My luteal phase temperatures are low.

### 1 POINT EACH

❑  My BBT is below 97.2°F in my follicular phase.

❑  My follicular phase lasts 16 days or more (late ovulation).

❑  I have no temperature change between my follicular and luteal phases (no ovulation).

❑  My BBT shifts slowly at ovulation, rising 0.2°F or 0.3°F a day.

❑  My BBT dips around ovulation, then slowly climbs 0.2°F to 0.3°F a day over 3 to 4 days to my post-ovulation BBT (body slow to react to increasing progesterone).

❑  My BBT drops too soon after ovulation (low progesterone). (After ovulation, BBT should rise within 1 to 2 days and remain high until just before your next period starts. If pregnancy occurs, it should stay high right through the early weeks.)

❑  My BBT rises slowly through the luteal phase (slow reaction to increasing progesterone).

❑  My BBT rises in the luteal phase but doesn't stay up for 12 days (premature drop in progesterone).

❑  My BBT forms a saddle-shaped pattern in the luteal phase — rising, falling, then rising again (due to a small surge in estrogen about a week after ovulation; this may be accompanied by an increase in cervical mucus, signaling failure to sustain progesterone).

❑  My BBT drops erratically during the luteal phase (possible LPD).

❑  My BBT drops 3 to 5 days before my period starts (possible LPD).

## FOR MEN ONLY

**3 POINTS**

❑  I have a low libido.

**1 POINT EACH**

❑  I have been diagnosed with poor sperm motility or a low sperm count.

❑  I sometimes have trouble maintaining an erection.

# CHAPTER NINE

# Dry

Dry people are a bit like a desert—so dry and hot that supporting new growth is difficult. But it is important to remember that in the right conditions, the desert will burst into full bloom.

The most notable physical sign of Dry people is that they have dry skin, dry eyes, and dry hair. Dry people tend to feel dehydrated; they are often thirsty. The most important symptoms pointing toward Dry type are night sweats, hot flashes, and vaginal dryness.

Dry people are also usually hot. They feel hot, though they are not feverish, often when other people don't. Dry people flush easily or have rosy cheeks. They have hot hands and feet. They are especially hot at night and may kick off the covers or want the window open even in cold weather.

Dry people find that their skin ages more quickly than average. They tend to be constipated. Dry people are generally thin, even wiry. They tend to have a low tolerance for stress. They can get restless, fidgety, jumpy, or anxious, and they often seem rather unsettled. Many Dry people have trouble sleeping, not sleeping soundly, waking up a lot during the night, or having intense dreams.

These symptoms generally increase with age—the older you get, the drier you get.

## WOMEN

Dry women's symptoms are due to an imbalance of reproductive hormones, especially low estrogen levels. They also tend to be short on progesterone, which creates trouble with the endometrium, and have elevated FSH.

Dry women may well run into trouble in phase 1 of their cycle. They often have a long menstrual cycle and short, light periods. They may have hot flashes and night sweats (especially premenstrually), as well as vaginal dryness. Some Dry women, however, especially those who are particularly hot, have a short cycle and heavy periods with bright red menstrual blood and mid-cycle bleeding. These women tend to have a high metabolic rate and sometimes even hyperthyroidism, which can cause unwanted weight loss.

Dry women may have a less predictable BBT than other types, especially in the follicular phase, and they often have trouble sustaining a high temperature in the luteal phase. Their BBT charts may vary from month to month, depending on what they've been up to—how well and how much they've been sleeping, if they've been under stress, or if they've had alcohol.

Because of their particular collection of symptoms, it's not unusual for Dry women to be told they are perimenopausal. Doctors may tell them they are too old (never mind their actual age), or their eggs are too old, to become pregnant. But Dry women are still ovulating and with proper treatment can come back into balance and be able to get pregnant.

Dry women may be diagnosed with an ovarian function problem. They tend to have a longer follicular phase in their menstrual cycle. This happens when follicles grow slowly because there is an imbalance of FSH and, consequently, not enough estrogen, and eggs take longer to mature. So these women may ovulate late or irregularly. An egg from a delayed ovulation may be of poor quality, or the corpus luteum created after the egg has been released may not work adequately, secreting insufficient progesterone. This leads to a thin endometrium, creating problems with implantation and the ability to nourish an embryo. Dry women are susceptible to recurrent miscarriages.

Some hotter Dry women tend to ovulate early. When one of these eggs is fertilized, it may have extra chromosomes and little chance of survival. This happens especially in perimenopausal women when FSH is too high.

Dry women are often prescribed fertility drugs because of ovulation problems, but they usually don't respond well to them, typically failing to produce many eggs and suffering from more side effects than other women. Dry women who take fertility drugs may be pushed even more severely out of balance. The Dry symptoms may appear, or existing Dry symptoms may intensify. In rare cases, fertility drugs can push a Dry woman over the line into premature menopause. With proper treatment not involving fertility drugs, Dry women can get pregnant, or such treatment can prepare a woman's body to handle fertility drugs and support it through the process.

In Dry women, dehydration can lead to insufficient cervical mucus, which can impair fertility. A Dry woman's cervical mucus may be too acidic or too thick for sperm to survive in.

## THE MAKING BABIES
## BASAL BODY TEMPERATURE CHART

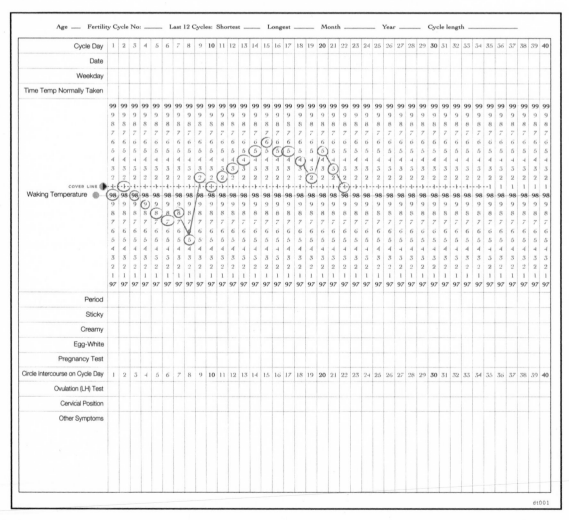

**Fig. 14:** Dry type with a short follicular phase.

# THE MAKING BABIES
# BASAL BODY TEMPERATURE CHART

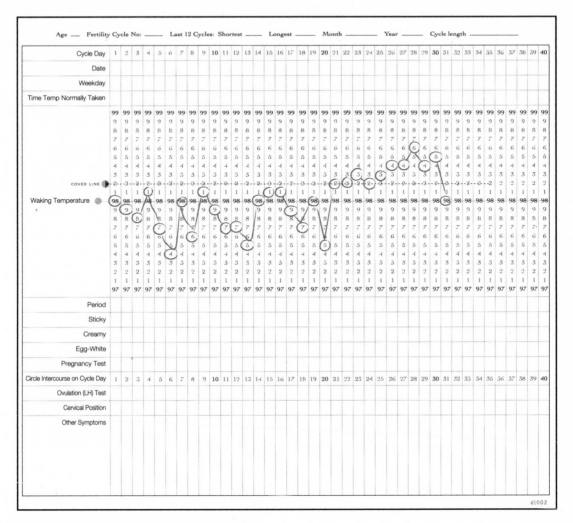

**Fig. 15:** Dry type with a long follicular phase.

# MEN

Dry men may experience frequent urination or dark urine in small amounts. They tend to have a strong libido but sometimes suffer from premature ejaculation or ED.

Dry men often have scanty ejaculate—basically, not enough liquid in the semen—which can create fertility problems. Dry men also may have low sperm counts.

## COMMON COMBINATIONS

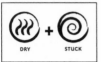

Over time, Pale people tend to become Dry people.

Dry/Stuck women often have perimenopausal symptoms such as hot flashes and night sweats, especially around the time of hormonal transitions, including just before their periods.

## CHINESE MEDICINE

The Chinese medicine diagnosis that is the hallmark of the Dry type is yin deficient or weak yin. Yin describes the functions of the body that are cooling, nourishing, moistening, and substantial. Without enough yin, the body both dries out and gets hotter.

Yin is what keeps us feeling young. It naturally depletes with age, but some people use up their yin faster than others. It all comes down to energy-consuming lifestyle choices. Burning the candle at both ends, whether for work or play, takes a toll because it consumes yin. Those who don't allow enough time for rest and to replenish resources are the most likely to suffer from lack of yin. It's an extremely common phenomenon given the world we live in; being overstretched is the norm. We don't get enough sleep, we eat poorly or on the run, we breathe polluted air, and we exercise in isolated, short, intense bursts. And we age prematurely, as our yin seemingly evaporates.

This phenomenon is well known in Chinese medicine but entirely absent from Western ways of thinking about infertility. It is so common and so treatable—and has such a huge impact on fertility and the success rates of the most common fertility treatments—that it's the one thing Chinese medical doctors most wish other doctors knew.

### Case Study: A Real, Dry Man

Mike and Imogen had opted for IVF pretty much as soon as they had trouble getting pregnant. Although Mike was diagnosed with a low sperm count and poor sperm quality, their IVF doctors assured them that the number of sperm was not that important, so they went ahead with IVF—three times—and still no pregnancy.

Imogen came to see me (Jill) first. Thorough

medical tests had turned up nothing problematic, so the fertility clinic was officially stumped. To me, she seemed to be in good shape for getting pregnant. So I advised her to keep doing whatever she had been doing.

Mike was a different story. Chinese medicine considers a low sperm count to be an indication of a deeper imbalance. Much of what he told me about his lifestyle fit that view. Between work and his busy social life, he kept a crazy schedule. He loved his job but felt overwhelmed by it. His diet was erratic, and he fueled himself throughout the day with coffee. To wind down in the evening, he always had a glass of whiskey, sometimes several glasses. He rarely got more than six hours of sleep at night and was too tired to exercise. Nonetheless, he was slim.

As Mike sat across from me, his cheeks were flushed, even though it was cool in my office. He said that his wife ribbed him about being a furnace, especially at night. He said that his skin always felt dry and that he was always thirsty.

Mike was a Dry type, partly based on the general tendency of his body and partly because of working and playing so hard. Given a little time, I thought, he could improve the amount and quality of his sperm. I recommended that he cut back on his alcohol consumption, try to eat right, and find some room in his life for exercise. I also prescribed herbs known to increase sperm count and to curb the tendency to be too hot, along with weekly acupuncture treatments.

Mike gave up whiskey, got down to one cup of coffee a day, and started going to the gym on his way home from work in the evening. He cut out processed food and junk food and kept up the acupuncture because, he said, he found it relaxing. He reported feeling much better all around. Imogen called to thank me for whatever I was doing, because she thought her husband was looking great. More important, after five months, a semen analysis showed Mike's sperm count to be back up to normal.

Mike and Imogen booked another appointment with the IVF doctor. Before they started the treatment cycle, however, they conceived naturally, and nine months later they welcomed a beautiful baby girl into their family.

## Making Babies Action Plan

### ARE YOU DRY?

**5 POINTS**

❏ I have experienced night sweats.

**3 POINTS EACH**

❏ My skin, hair, and/or nails are dry.
❏ I have dry eyes.
❏ I often feel hot.

❑  I sometimes feel feverish in the afternoon.

❑  I wake up during the night.

### 1 POINT EACH

❑  I am often thirsty.

❑  My mouth and throat often feel dry.

❑  I tend to be constipated.

❑  My bowel movements are hard and dry.

❑  I prefer colder weather.

❑  Given the choice, I would prefer a cold drink.

❑  My hands and feet tend to be hot or sweaty.

❑  My chest sweats, especially at night.

❑  I flush easily or have a red face.

❑  I often feel anxious or uneasy; I am a worrywart.

❑  I am thin.

❑  I am restless and fidgety.

❑  I am tired a lot.

❑  I am a restless sleeper.

❑  I have vivid dreams.

---

## FOR WOMEN ONLY

### 5 POINTS EACH

❑  My vagina often feels dry and unlubricated.

❑  I have been diagnosed with low estrogen levels.

❑  I have experienced hot flashes.

### 3 POINTS EACH

❑  My cycle is short, and my period is heavy and bright red.

❑  I have very little cervical mucus.

### 1 POINT

❑  My cycle is long, and my period is short and light.

## FOR WOMEN WHO KEEP A BBT CHART

**1 POINT EACH**

❑  My BBT is on the high side throughout my cycle.

❑  My chart changes a bit from month to month.

❑  I have an unsteady BBT or temperature spikes in the follicular phase.

❑  My follicular phase lasts longer than 13 to 14 days (low estrogen, low FSH, or reduced sensitivity to FSH).

❑  My follicular phase is shorter than 12 days (early ovulation).

❑  I ovulate late.

❑  I have spotting at ovulation.

❑  I see no clear temperature change between the follicular and luteal phases (no ovulation).

❑  My luteal phase is short (less than 12 days); my period starts 11 days or less after my last day of egg-white mucus (possible LPD).

❑  My luteal phase is long (more than 14 days).

❑  My luteal phase temperatures are high (above 98.4°F).

❑  My luteal phase temperatures are erratic.

## FOR MEN ONLY

**3 POINTS EACH**

❑  I have poor semen volume.

❑  Sometimes I ejaculate prematurely.

**1 POINT EACH**

❑  I have been diagnosed with a low sperm count.

❑  I have a strong sex drive.

❑  I sometimes suffer from ED.

# Stuck

Stuck people are stressed-out, but they internalize their stress. Like pressure cookers, Stuck people build up tension under a seal so tight nothing escapes. The stress builds and builds within them until they simply have to let off steam or explode. A pressure cooker has an escape valve to safely release the steam. Stuck people usually don't have a good escape valve, or they don't have a good working knowledge of how to use it, and instead they unconsciously try to release pressure in ways ranging from more subtle (sighing or grinding their teeth) to more extreme (losing their temper or lashing out).

Stuck people usually express stress physically, even when they are not always aware of the connection. They often complain of tension headaches or a nervous stomach. They are prone to high blood pressure, and some rely on stimulants and/or sedatives, sometimes to an unhealthy degree. Their muscles are really tight—tight enough to ache—especially over their ribs and on the sides of the body, or in the back, neck, and shoulders.

Stuck people show tightness in the digestive system. They can have bowel movements that can be either long and thin (like a ribbon) or compact and small. The Stuck cycle of bottling up and then exploding sometimes translates into alternating constipation and diarrhea.

The key symptoms pointing to the Stuck type in women are premenstrual mood swings, breast tenderness, fibroids, and endometriosis.

Stuck people tend to have poor circulation. They often have hormone imbalances. Stuck people are tightly wound, tense, and volatile. They tend to anger easily and be highly critical, especially of themselves. They may feel overwhelmed. The good news is that Stuck people can find their own personal release valve to restore a healthy balance. Some combination of movement and meditation usually works best, such as tai chi or yoga, or simply walking mindfully.

# WOMEN

Stuck women may well run into problems with their periods. They tend to experience three notable things in particular: dull or stabbing pain, periods that stop and start, and menstrual blood that is dark and clotted or brown and old-looking. They may have very heavy flows, although some Stuck women have very light periods.

Stuck women often have an irregular menstrual cycle that is as unpredictable as they are. They are likely to run into problems during phase 3 of their cycle (ovulation). They tend to have a long follicular phase and late ovulation, may experience pain at ovulation, and are likely to have PMS symptoms, including breast tenderness, mood swings, and digestive disturbances (all signs of difficulty with transition). Poor circulation leads to painful periods and mittelschmerz pains at ovulation.

Many Stuck women experience the effects of estrogen dominance, or too much estrogen in the body in relation to progesterone. These effects include irregular periods, PMS, fibroids, endometriosis, and fibrocystic breasts.

Stuck women tend to have obstructions in the reproductive system, including endometriosis, fibroids, uterine polyps, and cysts. They may also experience painful intercourse—not exactly conducive to conceiving.

Most Stuck women's symptoms are expressions of hormonal patterns disrupted by stress, with alcohol, poor diet, and environmental toxins potentially exacerbating the problem. The body has a hard time transitioning as hormones change throughout their cycle. Either hormone levels spike or the body is overly sensitive to normal levels. Stuck women are most likely to experience symptoms at times in their cycle when hormones are shifting—for example, when progesterone drops before the period starts.

Stress affects the pituitary hormones in particular. It raises prolactin levels, for example, causing an irregular menstrual cycle and interfering with LH. Some Stuck women experience luteinized unruptured follicle syndrome (LUFS), in which the body behaves as if ovulation has occurred when it really hasn't (see page 212). This happens when there's just enough LH to form a corpus luteum but not enough to release an egg.

# THE MAKING BABIES
## BASAL BODY TEMPERATURE CHART

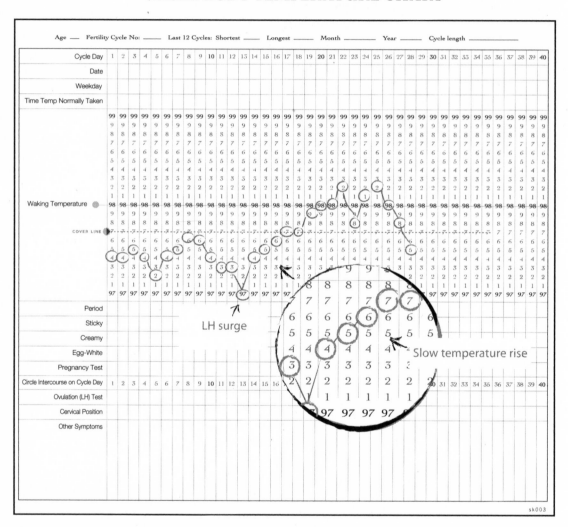

**Fig. 16:** Stuck type with a slow thermal shift after ovulation.

# THE MAKING BABIES
## BASAL BODY TEMPERATURE CHART

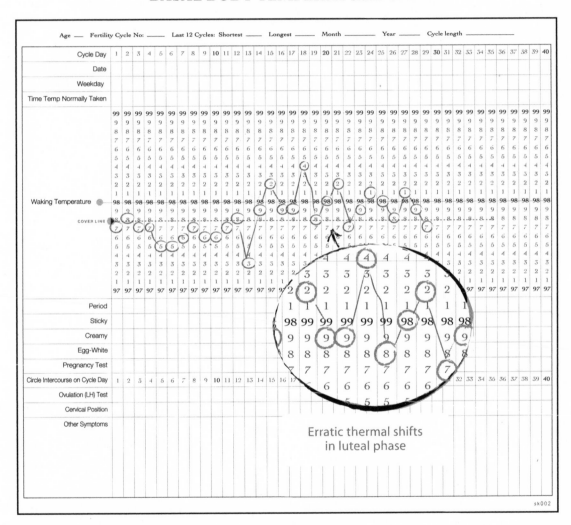

**Fig. 17:** Stuck type with a sawtooth luteal phase.

# THE MAKING BABIES
# BASAL BODY TEMPERATURE CHART

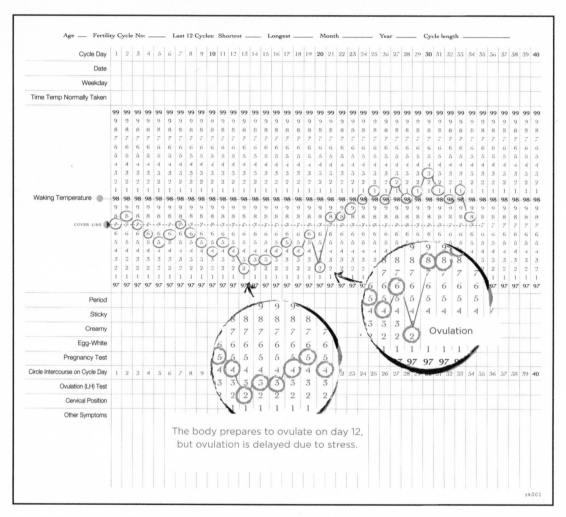

**Fig. 18:** Stuck type with delayed ovulation due to stress.

## MEN

In Stuck men, the most common fertility problems are conditions that obstruct the passage of sperm, such as testicular varicoceles (see page 144). Stuck men also may have stress-related impotence or experience pain in the testicles or penis. They may have a hyper or erratic sex drive. Some experience premature ejaculation or ED. Stuck men are also prone to misshapen sperm.

Stuck men are stressed and may choose to self-medicate with alcohol or recreational drugs, all of which have negative effects on fertility.

## COMMON COMBINATIONS

This combination usually reveals itself in a variety of digestive symptoms, such as gas and loose stools, either at times of stress or when the body is negotiating hormonal shifts (such as at ovulation). Stuck/Tired women are prone to developing fibroids and endometriosis due to metabolic slowness and blood stagnation.

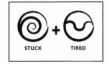

People with this combination are more likely to get weepy than to have angry outbursts. If you think this might be you, ask yourself what happens just before your period starts. Some women are likely to bite the head off of anyone who crosses them, but Stuck/Pale women are more likely to start crying over sappy commercials on TV.

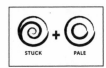

Stuck/Dry people are systemically hot, with red eyes and signs of inflammation. Stuck/Dry women may suffer from premenstrual night sweats or pimples. Stuck/Dry women often have too little cervical mucus, or mucus that is too acidic. Their BBT tends to be too high, which may reflect a high metabolic rate and possibly hyperthyroidism, especially if it is accompanied by agitation, insomnia, or weight loss.

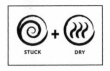

This combination leads to stagnation of mucus and fluids, causing inflammatory conditions and infections, such as repeated vaginal yeast infections in women or epididymitis in men. Women with endometriosis and fibroids may be both Stuck and Waterlogged.

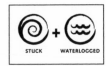

## CHINESE MEDICINE

In the view of Chinese medicine, all the tightness of a Stuck type stems from the poor flow of energy and blood through the body, or what is called qi and blood stagnation. Over time, this weak circulation leads to stagnation in the reproductive system as well. This leads to poor hormone transitions, resulting in PMS symptoms.

In men, this obstruction of flow can cause impotence. In women, qi stagnation can lead to problems with the ovary releasing the egg and to a lack of flexibility in the fallopian tubes. Blood stagnation can cause painful periods or a stop-and-start flow. Poor blood flow leads to denser and denser tissues, potentially creating the reproductive system obstructions that tend to show up in Stuck women—endometriosis, fibroids, polyps, cysts, and fibrocystic breasts.

In Chinese medicine, we see a correlation between the severity of pain and the degree of blood stagnation, ranging from minor breast tenderness to really bad menstrual cramps. Blood stagnation can also delay the period, creating a long cycle.

## Case Study: A Real, Stuck Man

I (Jill) diagnosed Dave as soon as he sat down in my office and sighed. That kind of sigh is such a common sign of the Stuck type, I thought I already knew something about the source of Dave's problems. But, of course, I needed to hear more from him to be sure.

Dave and his wife wanted to have a second child, but he had difficulty getting an erection and then would sometimes suffer from premature ejaculation. Dave was a man who was used to success. He was very driven, and he'd done very well for himself in his career. But he talked about how stressed-out it all made him. He slept poorly and had a nervous stomach. He'd get diarrhea the night before a big deal at work. His dentist had told him that he was wearing down his teeth by grinding them in his sleep. He said that he was ashamed of his hair-trigger temper and that he often shouted at his wife and young daughter. The remorse he felt afterward wasn't enough to prevent his outbursts, however.

Dave explained that he seldom spoke to his wife about any of his problems. It seemed to me that he was frustrated and very shut down. We talked about ways he could let off steam. He agreed to incorporate regular exercise into his daily routine. He didn't want to take Chinese herbs but did schedule weekly acupuncture treatments, which he came to love for how they relieved the tension in his body. I felt that Dave also needed an emotional outlet, because everything he was bottling up was exacerbating his physical problems, so I referred him to a psychotherapist.

As Dave returned each week for acupuncture, he reported that he was feeling better and that he thought his therapy sessions were helping him to express himself. After a while, his wife joined him for therapy, and together they worked on the forces creating turbulence in their marriage. Dave began to feel in control of his temper, and he adopted a much more balanced view of life. He was able to put fewer demands on himself and found that he was not so worried about work. His sexual problems got better, and he and his wife resumed their baby-making plans from a much healthier place.

Once Dave got himself on this better path, he no longer needed to come to see me. Several months later, I bumped into him on the street and met his wife for the first time. I was delighted to see that she was pregnant.

# Making Babies Action Plan

## ARE YOU STUCK?

**3 POINTS EACH**

- ❏  I am often irritable.
- ❏  I feel tense, overwhelmed, or just generally stuck.
- ❏  My bowel movements are thin and long like a ribbon.
- ❏  My bowel movements are like small pebbles.
- ❏  My ribs or flanks are painful or distended.
- ❏  I feel better or have more energy with exercise.

**1 POINT EACH**

- ❏  I am stressed-out.
- ❏  I sigh a lot.
- ❏  I grind my teeth at night.
- ❏  I have tense muscles.
- ❏  I have poor circulation.
- ❏  I feel as if I can't quite clear my throat.
- ❏  I have a nervous stomach and feel nauseous or get diarrhea when I'm stressed.
- ❏  I have cold hands and feet.

## FOR WOMEN ONLY

**5 POINTS EACH**

- ❏  I have discomfort, cramps, or pain with my period.
- ❏  My breast are sore premenstrually and also sometimes at ovulation.
- ❏  I have mood swings and/or irritability, especially right before my period.
- ❏  I have PMS.
- ❏  I have been diagnosed with fibroids or uterine polyps.
- ❏  I have been diagnosed with endometriosis.
- ❏  I have been diagnosed with elevated prolactin levels.

**3 POINTS EACH**

❏  I have an irregular menstrual cycle.

❏  My period stops and starts.

**1 POINT EACH**

❏  My period is very light.

❏  I have a very heavy menstrual flow.

❏  My menstrual blood is clotted and/or dark red or brown rather than bright red.

## FOR WOMEN WHO KEEP A BBT CHART

**1 POINT EACH**

❏  My BBT takes a few days to rise after the LH surge at ovulation (the body is slow to react to increasing progesterone). (After ovulation, BBT should rise within 1 to 2 days and remain high until just before your next period starts. If pregnancy occurs, it should stay high right through the early weeks.)

❏  My BBT has a sawtooth pattern during the luteal phase, fluctuating daily by 0.3°F or more (probably caused by stress).

❏  My BBT does not drop right away when I begin a new cycle.

❏  My BBT is unstable and unpredictable; it varies from month to month.

## FOR MEN ONLY

**3 POINTS**

❏  I have been diagnosed with a testicular varicocele.

# CHAPTER ELEVEN

# Pale

As you might expect, Pale people are pale. Their faces, and especially their lips, are where it's most obvious, although their nail beds show it, too. They also tend to be dry — dry hair, eyes, and skin, as well as brittle nails — though not as dry as Dry types. Their nails chip easily; they may have vision problems, such as blurry vision and tired eyes; and they may experience hair loss. The key symptoms pointing to the Pale type are a pale face and a light menstrual flow.

Pale people have trouble falling asleep, and so, not surprisingly, many complain of fatigue. It's not unusual for them to feel "shaky" from time to time and to experience a rapid heartbeat and perhaps dizziness when they stand up.

Pale people tend to be inflexible and prone to muscle injuries.

Some Pale people are undernourished: perhaps they don't eat enough, or enough healthy food; they eat too much junk food; the way they eat is not a good match for their body; or they don't properly absorb the nutrients from their food, even when their diet is good. Vegetarians, vegans, and people who limit the amount of meat they eat in whatever fashion are often Pale. Pale people may be diagnosed with anemia.

Pale people tend to be easily hurt or anxious and prone to weepiness.

## WOMEN

Pale women may well run into trouble in phase 1 of their cycle. They usually have light or short periods, with blood that is pale and watery rather than bright red. Sometimes their periods are late, or they may skip periods or have no periods at all (amenorrhea). Some Pale women get even paler during their periods. Symptoms such as pallor, fatigue, dry skin, and poor circulation may get worse during their periods as they lose blood. Some experience dizziness, especially if they stand up quickly.

Some Pale women complain of feeling really wiped out after their periods. They may also get cramps after their periods. Premenstrually, they may feel very needy or become weepy.

Pale women tend to have low estrogen, which means (among other things) that it takes longer for an egg to mature, or the follicle may be so

## THE MAKING BABIES
## BASAL BODY TEMPERATURE CHART

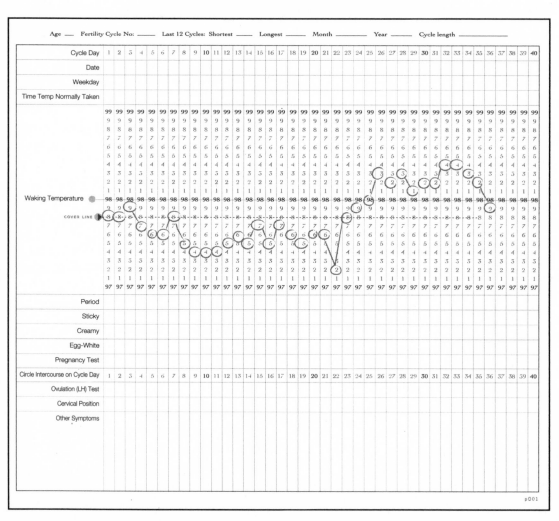

**Fig. 19:** Pale type with a long follicular phase.

undernourished that no egg is released at all. This same effect can occur if FSH levels are too low or the body has a reduced sensitivity to FSH.

Pale women may have a thin endometrium, making it difficult for an embryo to implant.

## MEN

Some Pale men have low semen volume, a low sperm count, and/or poor morphology. Some have a low or erratic libido.

## COMMON COMBINATIONS

The most common overlapping type for a Pale person is Tired. Pale/Tired people are undernourished because the digestive system is not working optimally and they have trouble extracting the nutrients from foods. They tend to have cold hands and feet because of poor circulation. (A lot of people with Raynaud's disease, a vascular disorder, are Pale/Tired types, for instance.) They get injured easily if they exercise without stretching.

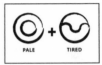

Pale/Stuck women get very tired and weepy whenever their body has to negotiate a hormonal transition such as ovulation. (You there, on the couch, bawling your eyes out over a sappy movie—this means you!) They may have light periods, PMS, and night sweats that intensify premenstrually.

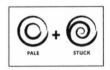

This combination becomes more likely as people get older, as many Pale people start to look a lot like Dry types over time.

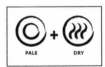

## CHINESE MEDICINE

Pale people are considered to have blood deficiency. This doesn't mean they don't have enough blood in the body, but rather that the quality of the blood leaves something to be desired. Furthermore, the concept of blood in Chinese medicine encompasses not just the stuff coursing through our veins and arteries but also the body's ability to nourish its tissues and organs. Looking at it this way, blood nourishes the endometrium, making it a hospitable home for an embryo to settle into. Blood deficiency results in a thin endometrium.

Blood deficiency can be caused by a tendency to anemia, which some people are born with. Blood deficiency also can be caused by a poor diet or by too much blood loss from heavy periods.

### Case Study: A Real, Pale Woman

Amy, age 31, was a pale, frail-looking woman who came to see me (Jill) because she was having trouble conceiving. She thought it was because of her irregular menstrual cycle. She often skipped a period, and when she had her period, it was light and lasted just two days. She also complained of being tired but found it hard to get to sleep at night.

I thought Amy was probably Pale, so I asked about her diet, since that is often a concern in Pale people. She'd had anorexia as a teenager, although she was over that now. She said that her diet was really healthy, mostly vegetables and whole grains, as she was a vegetarian. When I asked about her usual meals, however, I realized that apart from some soy milk and occasional tofu, Amy did not get much protein. Her diet was very low in iron.

We discussed various ways she could increase her intake of protein and iron. She decided to have a whey-based protein shake every morning and use a liquid iron supplement. I also prescribed an herbal formula to help rebalance her system.

Over the course of two months, Amy started to feel much more energetic and looked less pale. As her body gained strength, I used acupuncture to help improve her cycle, so she'd have slightly longer and heavier periods. The very next month, she ovulated on day 13 and had a twenty-seven-day cycle. The following month, she ovulated again on day 13 but had no period — because she had conceived. She continued with the additional protein and iron throughout her pregnancy and gave birth to a healthy baby boy.

## Making Babies Action Plan

### ARE YOU PALE?

**5 POINTS**

❏ My face is pale, especially my lips.

**3 POINTS EACH**

❏ My nail beds are pale, and my nails are dry and break easily.
❏ I get dizzy easily, especially if I stand up quickly.

**1 POINT EACH**

- ❑ I have blurry vision or floaters.
- ❑ I have trouble falling asleep.
- ❑ I am tired.
- ❑ My hair is thin and/or dry; I have been experiencing hair loss.
- ❑ I am a vegan or vegetarian.
- ❑ Sometimes I get palpitations.
- ❑ I often feel shaky.
- ❑ My muscles are tight, and it doesn't take much for me to injure them.

## FOR WOMEN ONLY

**5 POINTS**

- ❑ I have a light menstrual flow.

**3 POINTS**

- ❑ I have a short period (shorter than 3 days).

**1 POINT EACH**

- ❑ I sometimes miss a period or my period is late.
- ❑ My menstrual blood is pink rather than bright red.
- ❑ I get weepy and needy premenstrually.
- ❑ I have a dull pain after my period is over.

## FOR WOMEN WHO KEEP A BBT CHART

**1 POINT EACH**

- ❑ My BBT chart shows a long follicular phase (late ovulation).
- ❑ My BBT chart shows a long luteal phase.

## FOR MEN ONLY

**1 POINT EACH**

- ❑ I have been diagnosed with a low sperm count (low semen volume).
- ❑ Sometimes my libido is low.

# Waterlogged

Waterlogged people are something like sponges. Although sponges can certainly get waterlogged, they don't have to be that way. As in all things, the key is to find the right balance, somewhere between soggy and bone-dry, so that the sponge can best fulfill its purpose. Waterlogged types need to find their balance, too.

Waterlogged bodies do not metabolize fluids well, and this leads to congealed fluids that disrupt various bodily functions. Waterlogged people may develop edema, or swelling, as fluids accumulate faster than the body can process them out. Their body tends to react to irritation by producing excess mucus. Many Waterlogged people complain that they retain water or put on weight easily. The most significant symptoms pointing toward the Waterlogged type are polycystic ovarian syndrome (PCOS; see page 202) and being prone to yeast infections.

The buildup of mucus and fluids can make Waterlogged people feel really worn-out. It can slow them down and make their mind feel cloudy. Waterlogged people are prone to various kinds of inflammation, and many complain of painful joints; heavy, aching legs; or headaches that feel like a tight band wrapped around the head.

Waterlogged people also are prone to metabolic disorders and being overweight. They may have poor insulin metabolism, for example, which can lead to further hormone imbalances. To make matters worse, they often crave sugar, which can only aggravate their symptoms.

A lot of Waterlogged people find that their symptoms are worse on damp days. They react badly to mold both in food and in the environment. Excess mucus in the digestive tract means bowel movements that tend to be sluggish and unformed. If the bladder is affected, urine will be cloudy.

Waterlogged people tend to have a weak immune system. They are prone to chronic and acute infections, especially low-grade infections in the reproductive tract and yeast infections. They may have an infection and not even know it because they have no obvious symptoms. These hidden infections can impair fertility. Sinus infections, congestion, and drainage problems are common, as are allergies, asthma, and postnasal drip. Lung congestion may be a problem. Waterlogged people are prone to cystic acne, fibrocystic breasts, fatty nodules or tumors, and chronic swollen lymph nodes. Heart disease and diabetes are common in Waterlogged people. Chronic fatigue and fibromyalgia are relatively common in Waterlogged people.

Some Waterlogged people are worriers or pessimists, but the Waterlogged type also tends to be calm and dependable. These people are stubborn and resist change, and they are prone to overthinking things.

## WOMEN

Waterlogged women tend to have a long or irregular cycle with painful periods. Their periods may be scanty but thick, mucous, and clotted.

Waterlogged women are prone to chronic vaginal yeast infections and excessive vaginal discharge, although they may not have much fertile cervical mucus at ovulation. Waterlogged women often experience breast tenderness and bloating at ovulation. Premenstrually, they're likely to bloat again and experience water retention, weight gain, and breast tenderness.

Waterlogged women may produce cervical mucus at times other than around ovulation, which can make pinpointing ovulation difficult without a BBT chart or a testing kit.

Waterlogged women are prone to developing ovarian cysts at ovulation. These cysts create a hormonal pattern in the body that mimics pregnancy, complete with breast tenderness, nausea, and periods that don't start when expected.

Waterlogged women may have cervical inflammation blocking the cervix or fallopian tubes. They are also prone to endometriosis, uterine polyps, and fibroids, all of which can impede fertility. The walls of the fallopian tubes are normally coated with mucus, which makes them slippery and allows the egg to slide right along. But Waterlogged women produce excess mucus, to the point where it can block the tubes.

Many Waterlogged women are diagnosed with hormone imbalances, including PCOS and the insulin resistance typical of PCOS. Many are diagnosed with pelvic inflammatory disease (PID; see page 229), which can impair fertility.

## THE MAKING BABIES
## BASAL BODY TEMPERATURE CHART

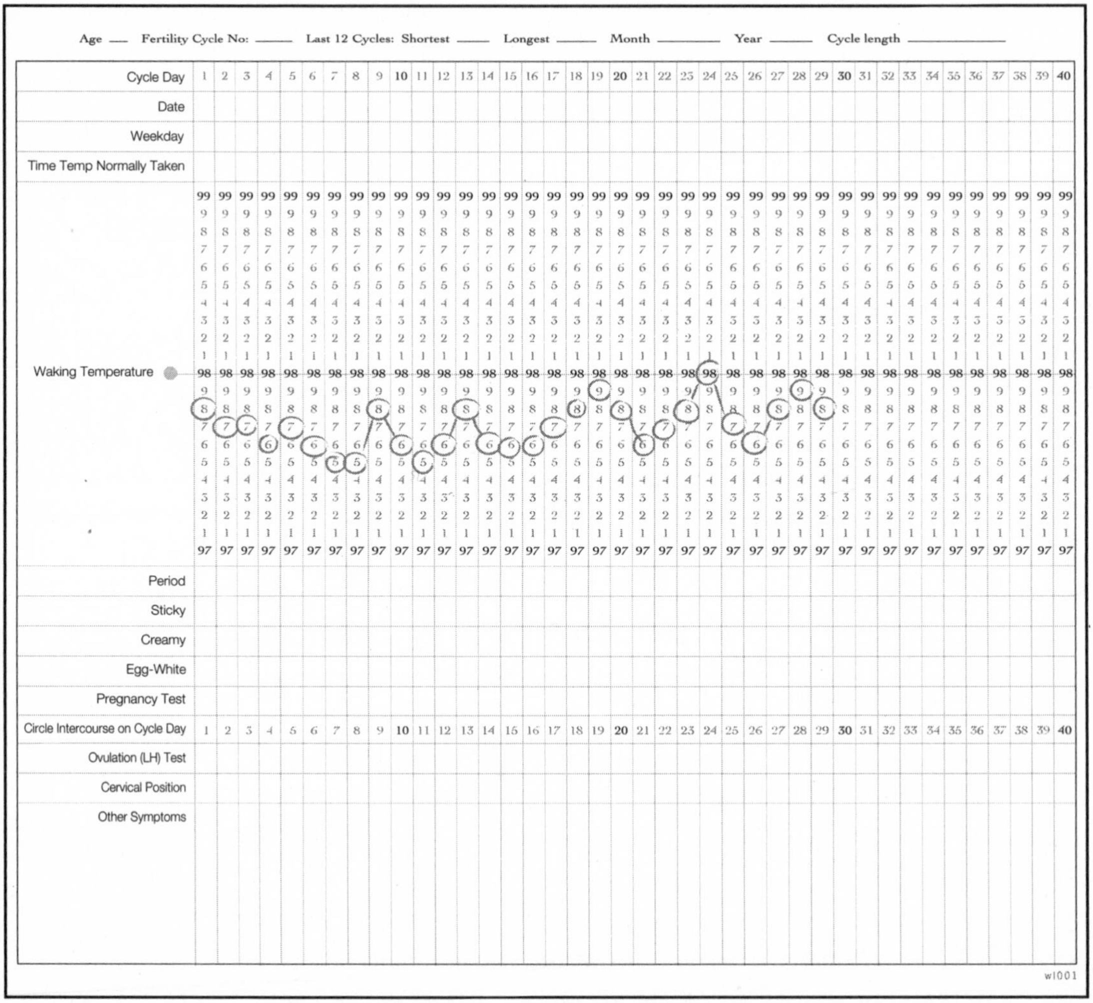

Age ____ Fertility Cycle No: ____ Last 12 Cycles: Shortest ____ Longest ____ Month ____ Year ____ Cycle length ____

| | | | | | | | | | | | | | | | | | | | | | | | | | | | | | | | | | | | | | | | | |
|---|---|---|---|---|---|---|---|---|---|---|---|---|---|---|---|---|---|---|---|---|---|---|---|---|---|---|---|---|---|---|---|---|---|---|---|---|---|---|---|---|
| Cycle Day | 1 | 2 | 3 | 4 | 5 | 6 | 7 | 8 | 9 | 10 | 11 | 12 | 13 | 14 | 15 | 16 | 17 | 18 | 19 | 20 | 21 | 22 | 23 | 24 | 25 | 26 | 27 | 28 | 29 | 30 | 31 | 32 | 33 | 34 | 35 | 36 | 37 | 38 | 39 | 40 |
| Date | | | | | | | | | | | | | | | | | | | | | | | | | | | | | | | | | | | | | | | | |
| Weekday | | | | | | | | | | | | | | | | | | | | | | | | | | | | | | | | | | | | | | | | |
| Time Temp Normally Taken | | | | | | | | | | | | | | | | | | | | | | | | | | | | | | | | | | | | | | | | |

Waking Temperature

| | | | | | | | | | | | | | | | | | | | | | | | | | | | | | | | | | | | | | | | | |
|---|---|---|---|---|---|---|---|---|---|---|---|---|---|---|---|---|---|---|---|---|---|---|---|---|---|---|---|---|---|---|---|---|---|---|---|---|---|---|---|---|
| Period | | | | | | | | | | | | | | | | | | | | | | | | | | | | | | | | | | | | | | | | |
| Sticky | | | | | | | | | | | | | | | | | | | | | | | | | | | | | | | | | | | | | | | | |
| Creamy | | | | | | | | | | | | | | | | | | | | | | | | | | | | | | | | | | | | | | | | |
| Egg-White | | | | | | | | | | | | | | | | | | | | | | | | | | | | | | | | | | | | | | | | |
| Pregnancy Test | | | | | | | | | | | | | | | | | | | | | | | | | | | | | | | | | | | | | | | | |
| Circle Intercourse on Cycle Day | 1 | 2 | 3 | 4 | 5 | 6 | 7 | 8 | 9 | 10 | 11 | 12 | 13 | 14 | 15 | 16 | 17 | 18 | 19 | 20 | 21 | 22 | 23 | 24 | 25 | 26 | 27 | 28 | 29 | 30 | 31 | 32 | 33 | 34 | 35 | 36 | 37 | 38 | 39 | 40 |
| Ovulation (LH) Test | | | | | | | | | | | | | | | | | | | | | | | | | | | | | | | | | | | | | | | | |
| Cervical Position | | | | | | | | | | | | | | | | | | | | | | | | | | | | | | | | | | | | | | | | |
| Other Symptoms | | | | | | | | | | | | | | | | | | | | | | | | | | | | | | | | | | | | | | | | |

wI001

**Fig. 20:** Waterlogged type with a monophasic chart reflecting no ovulation.

## THE MAKING BABIES
## BASAL BODY TEMPERATURE CHART

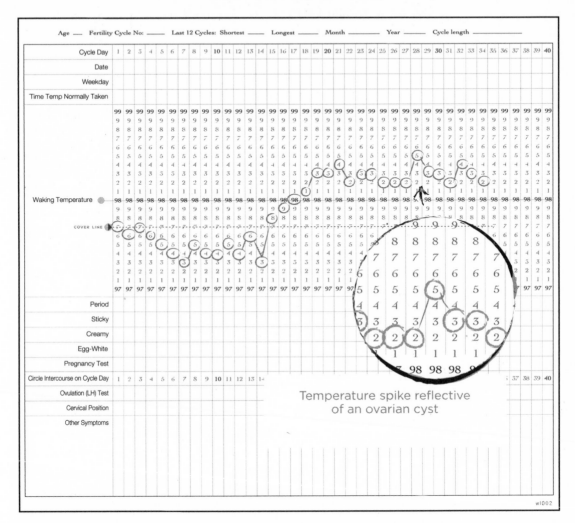

**Fig. 21:** Waterlogged type with a temperature spike when the period was due, reflecting an ovarian cyst.

## MEN

Waterlogged men are prone to low-grade infections of the reproductive tract. They may suffer from prostatitis, painful urination, testicular tenderness, or impotence. Or they may have chronic discharge from the penis or thick, congealed semen, both signs of infections that can impair fertility.

## COMMON COMBINATIONS

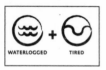

In this most common combination for Waterlogged people, a poor diet and poor assimilation of nutrients lead to problems with fluid metabolism and a buildup of mucus. Waterlogged/Tired people tend to have chronic conditions involving phlegm, such as sinus congestion and bronchitis. They often complain of abdominal bloating and gas, as well as a greasy taste in the mouth. Waterlogged/Tired women may have a chronic white vaginal discharge and general metabolic problems. Women with PCOS are often this type.

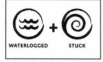

This combination is more common after a long history of mucus buildup. That accumulation of mucus is the Stuck part layered on top of the Waterlogged part and may result in blocked fallopian tubes and endometriosis. Waterlogged/Stuck women have all the Waterlogged symptoms plus the poor hormonal transitions of the Stuck type. Stuck symptoms such as PMS come in a Waterlogged variety, including premenstrual water retention and clotted, mucous menstrual blood. Mucus and mucus-related problems increase premenstrually as well.

## CHINESE MEDICINE

In Chinese medicine, Waterlogged people are considered to be experiencing an accumulation of dampness from the stagnation of fluids in the body. "Phlegm damp" or "damp stagnation" is a concept unique to Chinese medicine. It describes fluids congealing at certain sites or in certain systems in the body, to the point where normal function is disrupted.

Damp stagnation often develops in the wake of other issues—yang deficiency or blood stagnation, in Chinese terms. But it can also simply be the result of eating rich, sweet foods to excess. Such a diet damages the digestive system so that it can't properly break down foods and fluids. This creates fatty deposits that can eventually disrupt organ function. This is the link between damp stagnation and obesity.

In this type, the primary cause of hormone imbalance is this stagnation. Stagnant fluids lead to poor transitions of every kind, including the many tricky hormonal shifts involved in the menstrual cycle, conception, and implantation.

Waterlogged people usually take longer to respond to acupuncture and herbs than other types do. It can take months to clear the dampness.

## Case Study: A Real, Waterlogged Woman

Lorraine, age 38, had been trying to conceive for more than two years. Her periods were irregular, and her cycle tended to be long. When she tracked her cycle using a BBT chart, she discovered that her temperature was lower than normal and that she rarely ovulated.

Lorraine complained of seasonal allergies and chronic bronchitis each winter. She sounded wheezy and cleared her throat often.

Lorraine was overweight and complained that her metabolism was so sluggish, it seemed that she gained weight if she even looked at a slice of cake. She had recently seen a reproductive endocrinologist, who had diagnosed her with PCOS and prescribed metformin to control her insulin levels, in the hope that it would help regulate her other hormones so that she could conceive. The doctor also advised that Lorraine drastically limit her carbohydrate intake.

I (Jill) designed an herbal formula that could work alongside the prescription drug. Clinical research in China has shown that certain herbs are more effective than pharmaceuticals in inducing and improving ovulation in women with PCOS. The herbs also aimed at reducing her phlegmyness and preventing ovarian cysts. In addition, I gave her weekly acupuncture to help direct her cycle and promote ovulation.

Lorraine was very committed to her new diet and program. She soon started to lose weight and reported having much more energy. After two months of combined Eastern and Western treatment, she still had not ovulated, but her BBT was higher — a good sign. After four months, she ovulated. Her cycle remained long (never less than thirty-five days), but it became predictable, and after eight months of treatment she conceived.

## Making Babies Action Plan

### ARE YOU WATERLOGGED?

**3 POINTS EACH**

❏ I have trouble controlling my weight.
❏ My thinking often feels clouded.
❏ I have sinus problems, seasonal allergies, or a chronic cough.
❏ I have a tendency toward edema, or swelling.
❏ My hands or feet swell.

**1 POINT EACH**

- ❑ I often feel tired and sluggish.
- ❑ I get achy joints.
- ❑ My arms and legs feel heavy.
- ❑ My urine is cloudy.
- ❑ My mouth feels greasy.
- ❑ I feel bloated.

## FOR WOMEN ONLY

**5 POINTS EACH**

- ❑ I often suffer from yeast infections or have been diagnosed with PID.
- ❑ I have PCOS.

**3 POINTS EACH**

- ❑ I have been diagnosed with fibroids or uterine polyps.
- ❑ I have been diagnosed with endometriosis.
- ❑ I have painful periods, with mucus and clots.

**1 POINT**

- ❑ I experience clear, copious cervical mucus throughout my cycle or at erratic points in my cycle.

## FOR WOMEN WHO KEEP A BBT CHART

**1 POINT EACH**

- ❑ My BBT varies from month to month.
- ❑ My BBT forms a jagged sawtooth pattern, changing almost daily by 0.3°F or more.
- ❑ My BBT chart shows a long follicular phase.
- ❑ I'm not ovulating (anovulation).
- ❑ I'm ovulating unpredictably, on a different day during each cycle.
- ❑ My BBT doesn't change much or at all after ovulation. (I have a monophasic, as opposed to a biphasic, BBT chart.)
- ❑ My BBT rises slowly after ovulation; it takes a few days to come all the way up.

❏ My BBT chart shows a luteal phase longer than 16 days (I'm not pregnant) and a spike in temperature when my period should be starting (potential ovarian cyst).

## FOR MEN ONLY

**5 POINTS**

❏ I have a discharge from my penis.

**3 POINTS**

❏ My urination feels interrupted or incomplete.

# PART FOUR

# Common Fertility Problems and Solutions

# CHAPTER THIRTEEN

# What's Your Problem?

The next five chapters look at the most common fertility problems: hormonal and endocrine issues, structural or anatomical issues, infections, immune system issues, and general health issues. The chapters, and the sections within the chapters, are arranged roughly from most common to least common. That is, hormonal and endocrine issues are the type of fertility problems we see most frequently; luteal phase defect (LPD, the first entry in that chapter) is the hormonal issue we see most often. Different fertility types are prone to different fertility problems, so each section is marked with the symbol(s) for the most likely type(s) to be affected. You can skim through the chapters to find the sections of primary concern to you, depending on your type. Some issues can arise in all the types, and those are marked with the "nonspecific" symbol.

For each fertility issue, we cover the basics of what it is and how it affects fertility. Then we walk you through how it is diagnosed, how it is generally treated, and how it *should* be treated. If you've already been diagnosed, you can use these sections to understand your condition better and to learn strategies to improve your fertility in the face of the problem, both on your own and with your health care practitioner.

For those of you who do not have a specific diagnosis, the following chapters will help you focus on your potential problems, prepare you to speak with your doctor about confirming them (or ruling them out), and take action accordingly.

PALE

STUCK

DRY

WATERLOGGED

TIRED

NONSPECIFIC

## CHINESE MEDICINE

In most (though not all) of the fertility problems, Chinese medicine can be helpful, and we recommend acupuncture and herbs as appropriate.

Following is an overview of the general ways in which acupuncture and herbs work to improve fertility.

### Acupuncture and Fertility

Chinese women have experienced the fertility benefits of acupuncture for many generations, but it's only relatively recently that researchers have begun to study the phenomenon and document its positive results. Consider weekly acupuncture to prepare your body for pregnancy, help you conceive naturally, eliminate fertility problems, and/or support assisted reproductive technologies (ARTs; see chapter 25).

From the Chinese point of view, acupuncture needles stimulate qi and blood, as well as yin and yang. Building yin and blood aids follicle development; tonifying yin and blood increases blood circulation to the ovaries and uterus; moving qi promotes strong ovulation; and tonifying yang promotes implantation.

In Western medical terms, acupuncture can do the following:

- Influence hormonal pathways to stimulate hormone production, correcting subtle imbalances and helping to regulate menstruation and ovulation.
- Increase blood flow to the uterus, improving the quality of the endometrium (uterine lining) by thickening it and optimizing it for implantation.
- Increase blood flow to the ovaries, improving their function and nourishing the developing follicles, thus helping them grow. This is especially valuable as we age, because blood flow to the ovaries naturally declines as we get older. By menopause, ovarian blood flow is just one-fifth of what it was during our peak reproductive years.
- Build more follicles in ovaries not responding well to stimulation from pituitary hormones.
- Facilitate the smooth release of an egg and promote strong ovulation.
- Help with implantation by reducing uterine spasms.
- Relieve stress, decreasing the body's stress response, including tamping down the stress hormones that can interfere with fertility.

- Eliminate underlying inflammation that may impair fertility.
- Regulate the immune system, which can interfere with fertility when overactive.
- Increase sperm count and density in men with low sperm counts.
- Improve sperm quality and motility.

### Herbs and Fertility

Chinese medicine uses herbs to tonify blood, yin, and yang; support yin; move qi; and boost yang, qi, and blood. In Western terms, herbs can do the following:

- Encourage the building of a healthy endometrium.
- Encourage and enhance follicle growth and development.
- Increase cervical mucus.
- Gently stimulate the body to produce the necessary hormones. (Yin tonics, for example, help the body produce estrogen, whereas pharmaceuticals provide a direct estrogen supplement. The differing mechanisms of action allow these approaches to work well together or be effective on their own.)
- Increase blood circulation to the ovaries and uterus.
- Promote strong ovulation.
- Help reach and maintain an appropriately high BBT in the luteal phase, stimulating the production of more progesterone and increasing the likelihood that a fertilized embryo will implant.
- Lengthen a short luteal phase, thus improving implantation.
- Improve the quality and quantity of sperm.

## YOUR MEDICAL HISTORY AND PHYSICAL

When we think about going to the doctor, most of us focus on the physical exam. This makes a certain amount of sense — it is, after all, not something we can do for ourselves. A complete fertility workup most certainly needs to include a thorough physical — not the same physical you get at your annual exam (though you should be asked when you last had one of those), and not solely a gynecological, or even endocrinological, exam either. The form and focus it takes will vary a bit according to which type of specialist you are seeing, but fertility clues can come from anywhere in or on your body, and whoever is examining you should be checking you out from head to toe.

An equally crucial component of any diagnosis is a comprehensive medical history—for both partners. This is perhaps even more important than the physical itself, yet it is often skipped by fertility doctors. If a specific diagnosis is not considered important—usually because a particular treatment (fertility drugs or IVF) is a foregone conclusion—your doctor may take only a brief medical history or omit it altogether, especially for the man. But if you don't know the exact diagnosis, you may be missing a chance to solve the problem at its root and restore fertility, or at least to treat the symptoms accurately to improve fertility. The more subtle the diagnosis, the more likely it is to be missed with a hasty, careless, or foreshortened history.

A good detailed history should cover seven categories of possible causes of infertility: anatomical, hormonal/metabolic, infectious, autoimmune, genetic, environmental, and psychological. Your doctor should be asking you a host of questions about your menstrual cycle, gynecological health, hormones, sexual history, prior pregnancies, general health, mental health, stress level, family history, and diet and lifestyle choices. The interview should touch on age, weight, sexually transmitted diseases (STDs) and other infections, exercise habits, bathing habits, frequency of intercourse, sexual techniques and positions, timing of intercourse, quality and quantity of cervical mucus, and toxin exposure (lead, pesticides, solvents, petrochemicals, and heavy metals).

With all that you've learned in the previous chapters, you can understand why many of the questions I (Sami) use in my history (see the next section) are important. And, in fact, you'll be able to evaluate and address many of those issues yourself with the Making Babies program.

Many of my questions are intended to make sure all systems are go, to look for any chronic or serious problems, and to see that you are getting the health care you need, all in the interest of ensuring that you are generally healthy enough to have a baby. Many of the questions are designed not to elicit any particular answer, but rather to help establish a pattern or identify a recent change. I'm listening as my patients tell me that they "always" do this or "used to" do that. A departure from what is normal for any given patient points to an important area to focus on. For example, whether or not your periods are clotted may not tell me as much on its own as knowing that the clotting is relatively new for you — in which case I know that you may need testing to look for fibroids or uterine polyps. Or short periods may be normal for you now, but they used to be longer, which is a signal that your hormones may be decreasing with age. *Has there been a change?* is often the underlying question.

Some questions are not so much about diagnosis as about properly timing testing or treatment — for example, asking what day your last period began. Other questions can reveal subtler clues to fertility problems. If you took birth control pills but stopped taking them six months ago and still haven't gotten your period, perhaps being on the Pill had been hiding something, such as early menopause. Or perhaps your hormones are still suppressed, and stimulating ovulation might help. An unusually light menstrual flow could result from scar tissue in the uterus — for example, from a recent miscarriage, abortion, or D & C — creating Asherman's syndrome (see page 240). This might indicate that there's less normal endometrium to be shed and perhaps not enough for implantation.

We don't have room in this book to explore every detail of every condition that could be revealed by a really good history, but the next five chapters cover the ones you're most likely to experience. The point here is to show you how important it is that your doctor pay attention to all aspects of your health history and lifestyle. Clues to fertility problems can emerge from many different angles. It's important to work with a doctor who you trust will cover all the bases, and it's fair to ask how he or she evaluates each of these areas.

## A Thorough Medical History

Many of our patients have already been through the fertility medicine machine, and yet a shocking number don't know what they've been diagnosed with or why. They also have no idea what a thorough medical history for a fertility workup looks like. And why would they, if they've never had one?

The questions I (Sami) routinely ask new patients follow. If no one has ever run through a long list of questions like these with you, you haven't had a thorough medical history taken. And if you haven't had a thorough history taken and you don't have a good explanation for why you are not getting pregnant, you should not accept a diagnosis of "unexplained infertility." Infertility is not "unexplained" just because a doctor has not considered every possible avenue. If your doctor won't do this, you need to look for a doctor who will.

The significance of the answers to many of these questions will become clear as you read the next five chapters. For now, you don't need to worry about answering them or understanding what those answers may reveal. We just want you to know what a thorough history should entail.

### Fertility

How old are you?

How long have been trying to get pregnant?

What have you tried to get pregnant?

Have you figured out your most fertile day(s)? Do you know when you ovulate? How did you work that out?

Have you had any fertility treatments? If so, what, when, and where — and what happened? What was your diagnosis?

Have you ever taken any medications to help you ovulate? If so, what and when — and what happened?

Have you had your fallopian tubes evaluated by a doctor? If so, how and when — and what were the results? (Bring actual X-rays for review; don't rely on the report only.)

Have you had your hormones tested? If so, how, when, and where — and what were the results?

Do you have a single partner with whom you are trying to conceive? How long have you been together?

Has your partner had a fertility workup?

Have you or your partner conceived or had children with previous partners?

### Sexual History

How often do you have vaginal intercourse?

How is your libido? Do you find it difficult to get aroused?

Do you use anything other than the missionary position when you are trying to conceive?

How do you time intercourse?

Do you use a lubricant?

Do you douche?

Do you experience pain with intercourse? If so, is it on entry or on deep penetration?

Is premature ejaculation an issue?

What contraceptives have you used? Have you ever taken the Pill? If so, when and for how long? Have you ever used an IUD?

### Menstrual Cycle

How old were you when you first got your period?

What was your period like when you first got it? Do you remember having any problems, or did it go smoothly?

Is your period regular?

How long is your cycle? How long is your period? Is that the same as they have always been?

What is your flow like? Light or heavy? Clotted? Is the blood bright red or dark?

Do you have pain with your period? Where do you feel it? (In your back? In your abdomen?) Is it mild, moderate, or severe? When does it start? How long does it last?

Do you have staining before your period?

What day did your last period start?

Do you have breast soreness with your period? If so, do you experience it every cycle or just sometimes? Are there some months when your nipples are sensitive?

Do you get other signs of PMS, such as mood swings, headaches, food cravings, skin breakouts, loose stools, or nausea?

### Pregnancy History

Do your PMS symptoms sometimes last longer than usual?

Do you ever get a metallic taste in your mouth? Or do things taste or smell different to you some months?

Have you had previous pregnancies? If so, did you have any complications?

Have you ever had a miscarriage?

Have you ever had an abortion? Have you ever had a D & C for any other reason? If so, how many?

### Gynecological Health

Have you ever had an abnormal Pap smear?

Have you ever had a cervical biopsy, cauterization, or conization?

Have you ever had a sexually transmitted disease?

Do you get vaginal yeast infections easily or frequently?

Have you ever been diagnosed with chlamydia?

Do you have chronic or abnormal (brown or green color, foul odor, or otherwise unusual for you) vaginal discharge?

Do you have any sores on your genitals?

Have you ever been diagnosed with pelvic inflammatory disease (PID)?

Have you sought medical attention for pelvic pain of any kind?

Have you had ovarian cysts?

Have you had fibroids?

Have you had thyroid problems? (Enlarged thyroid? Thyroid cysts? Thyroid cancer? Over- or underactive thyroid?)

Are your breasts asymmetrical or scarred, or do they have any other abnormalities?

Have you been diagnosed with any anatomical abnormalities in your vagina, uterus, cervix, or ovaries or anywhere else in the pelvic area?

### Hormones

Is your skin excessively oily?

Do you have acne?

Do you have excessive hair on your face or elsewhere on your body, or hair in abnormal places? Have you had any changes to your hair (on your head or anywhere else on your body)?

Have you experienced any hair loss?

Are your breasts sometimes sore, tender, or hypersensitive?

Have you noticed any discharge from your nipples?

### General Health

How is your general health: good, fair, or poor?

Do you have any chronic health concerns?

    Do you have diabetes?

    Have you had tuberculosis?

Do you have high blood pressure?

Do you have ulcers?

How much do you weigh? How tall are you? Are you more than 20 percent over or under your ideal body weight? Have you had any recent weight change, gain or loss? If so, what was the cause?

Is your body type thin, normal, or obese?

Do you exercise? If so, how much? Doing what?

How many hours a day do you sleep?

Do you smoke or otherwise use tobacco?

Do you use any recreational drugs?

Do you take any medications regularly? Do you take any medications occasionally?

Do you use any herbs?

Do you take any vitamins or other supplements?

Have you been exposed to environmental toxins?

Do you know your blood type?

Are you taking steroids?

Do you urinate frequently or a lot? Do you get up at night to urinate? Do you have any other issues with urination (pain, bleeding, incontinence, etc.)?

Do you get frequent or regular headaches?

Do you have any allergies?

Have you ever been hospitalized? Have you had any major illnesses? Have you had surgery, especially surgery in the pelvic area or for pelvic pain? Have you had any complications as a result of any of these?

### Stress and Mental Health

How would you rate your overall mental health: average, above average, or below average?

Do you see a psychiatrist or psychotherapist?

Have you ever taken psychiatric drugs?

Are you anxious? Have you been diagnosed with anxiety?

Do you feel depressed or have you been diagnosed with depression?

Do your emotions or moods change dramatically, easily, or frequently?

Are you and your partner on the same page when it comes to
trying to conceive? Is your partner supportive?

How is your relationship? Are you getting along well in general?

Does your job situation stress you out?

### Family History

Have your parents or siblings had early (before age 60) stroke
or heart attack; lupus, rheumatoid arthritis, or other
immunological issues; diabetes; ovarian or breast cancer;
infertility or miscarriage?

Are your parents and siblings living? Are they healthy? If they are
deceased, what was the cause?

Did any close relatives have fertility problems or frequent
miscarriages? Did your mother take DES when pregnant
with you?

Have your siblings had any fertility issues, trouble getting
pregnant, or miscarriages?

### Diet

Is your diet balanced? How would you describe your overall diet:
good, fair, or poor? Is your appetite good, fair, or poor?

Do you follow any dietary restrictions (vegetarian, vegan,
macrobiotic, low fat, etc.)?

Do you eat fish? What kind(s)? How much and how often?

Do you eat shellfish?

Do you eat sushi or any raw fish or seafood? Do you eat raw meat
or unpasteurized dairy?

Do you eat meat? Do you eat red meat?

Do you eat lunch meat?

Do you have any food intolerances?

How much caffeine do you get in an average day?

Do you drink coffee and/or tea? If so, how much?

Do you drink alcohol? If so, what type, how much, and how often?

### Dads, Too!

It is critical for the would-be father to have a full workup as well. About
40 percent of all infertility cases can be traced back to issues with the

man. About the same percentage can be traced back to the woman, and about 20 percent are due to a combination of male and female factors or are classified as "unexplained." Yet we are still surprised at how often women seek our help when their partners have never been properly evaluated—or even evaluated at all. Men should see doctors who specialize in male infertility for their own thorough medical history and physical if there is even the slightest suspicion of a sperm or semen abnormality. For starters, men need to have a semen analysis to check on the fitness of their sperm—the quality as well as quantity. They also need to find out if they have malfunctioning hormones, anatomical defects preventing sperm from getting where they're supposed to go, or any problems making normally shaped sperm. Men, too, need to work with a doctor who will look at the problem from every angle. They should be asked many of the same questions that I (Sami) ask (not so much about their periods, though!), plus others focusing on male issues and anatomy.

## TESTING 1, 2, 3 . . .

Once you've had a complete history and physical, you'll need additional testing to pinpoint what exactly is going on. In fact, the history and physical are done in large part to determine which tests you may need. You don't want to have unnecessary tests, but you don't want to miss anything that might be useful either.

Some tests need to be done at certain times in your cycle, so you won't be able to get everything done right off the bat or all in one day. But you should schedule everything you need right away. If you orchestrate it carefully with your doctor, you should be able to complete all the tests within one or two months (during which time you can also be following the Making Babies program).

As you read through the following chapters, you'll learn which tests are required for each condition. A general battery of tests might include the following:

- **Postcoital test.** This test checks that the sperm are getting where they need to go and surviving the journey during natural intercourse. A postcoital test can alert you that you are using lubricants or positions that are interfering with conception, that you have "hostile" cervical mucus (perhaps due to infection, acidity, or thickness), or that you are making antibodies that are attacking sperm. Most things that commonly turn up in a postcoital test are easily rectified.

- **Hormone testing.** All the relevant hormones should be tested. For women, most tests need to be done at specific times in the menstrual cycle. On the second or third day of an idealized twenty-eight-day cycle, have blood hormone tests for follicle-stimulating hormone (FSH), estradiol, luteinizing hormone (LH), prolactin, and thyroid-stimulating hormone (TSH). Somewhere between day 21 and day 25, have a blood test for progesterone—or better yet, a series of tests on days 21, 23, and 25. Men need to have their hormones tested as well, including FSH, LH, and testosterone.

- **Testing for structural issues.** A pelvic sonogram may reveal anatomical issues. Women may need an X-ray of the uterus and fallopian tubes known as a hysterosalpingogram (HSG), or hysterogram for short. This must be done on day 7, 8, or 9 of your cycle, after the menstrual flow has stopped but before ovulation occurs. Hysteroscopy (see page 232) can help visualize any issues inside the uterus. It may also be necessary to have laparoscopic (outpatient) exploratory surgery to assess details of the pelvic organs that a hysterogram may not reveal. Men may need a testicular sonogram or genetic testing.

- **Immunological or chromosomal tests.** These tests might be required as indicated.

- **Cultures.** These tests are needed to check for infections in both partners.

## NOW WHAT?

Once you've been thoroughly evaluated, you should receive a diagnosis, which you should be able to find in the following chapters. Each section on each fertility problem includes the best things you can do to help yourself resolve the issue, along with information on how it's usually treated medically. Whatever your specific issue turns out to be, it should be improved by the advice in part V for your fertility type. If you have already begun your three-month Making Babies "pre-mester," you may experience improvement even before you have completed all the testing, have nailed down a diagnosis, and are ready to begin any necessary treatment. You will at least be moving in the right direction and will be in the best position to support and benefit from that treatment.

## Making Babies Action Plan

❏ Make sure you've had a comprehensive medical history taken.

❏ Make sure you've had a thorough physical exam.

❏ Schedule all necessary medical tests over a condensed period of time and at the appropriate times in your cycle.

❏ Make sure Dad has a workup, too.

❏ Correct or bypass any roadblocks to fertility you uncover.

# CHAPTER FOURTEEN

# Hormonal and Endocrine Issues

Hormones must be working in fine-tuned harmony for good fertility in both men and women. Many of the hormones associated with being either male or female actually play important roles in both sexes. This chapter covers the main hormonal issues people having fertility problems run into. They appear roughly from more to less common. The action plans at the end of the chapter pull together and summarize the information about medical testing that appears in each section.

## WOMEN

DRY

PALE

TIRED

STUCK

### Luteal Phase Defect (LPD)

A luteal phase lasting less than twelve days is too short for the endometrium to develop enough to properly support a fertilized egg. This is known as luteal phase defect. It's a common endocrine disorder, present in a significant portion of women having trouble conceiving and more than a third of women with repeated early pregnancy loss.

Low progesterone levels in the luteal phase are also an indicator of LPD. You might have a normal twelve- to fourteen-day luteal phase but still have progesterone levels that are too low. The result is the same: if there's not enough progesterone, the endometrium can't develop and function properly. Some studies have implicated LPD in poor follicle development and insufficient levels of FSH and LH.

If you ovulate very early (before day 10) or very late (after day 20), you may have LPD. Other signs of LPD include spotting before menstruation and symptoms typically associated with menopause. These signs could indicate other problems, too, so take note but don't rely only on them.

If your doctor suspects LPD, he or she should try to confirm the diagnosis in one or more of the following ways:

- Testing serial progesterone levels during a single cycle (seven, nine, and eleven days after you ovulate — in a typical twenty-eight-day cycle, testing on days 21, 23, and 25)
- Testing prolactin levels (elevated prolactin can lead to inadequate progesterone)
- Testing thyroid function with a TSH blood test
- Checking for polycystic ovarian syndrome (PCOS) with tests for fasting glucose, insulin, LH, and FSH levels (LPD commonly occurs as part of PCOS)

Sometimes a vaginal ultrasound may be recommended. Although it can determine endometrial thickness, it's not a good way to test for LPD. In the past, endometrial biopsy was commonly used to diagnose LPD, but this is no longer used much because it can be painful and is relatively expensive.

It is important to test progesterone on successive days because whether your levels are "high" or "low" is a relative matter. Testing on just one day will confirm only that you do produce progesterone. You need testing on three days to show whether it is trending in the right direction. If your progesterone levels are low, supplemental progesterone may be prescribed. In cases where that is not enough, the addition of a follicle-stimulating fertility drug such as clomiphene (Clomid) may do the trick. It may also be helpful to determine the reason for low progesterone. The usual suspects include stress, thyroid imbalance, and high prolactin.

### Chinese Medicine

Chinese medicine considers LPD an imbalance of the whole cycle, not just the luteal phase. (Western medicine recognizes this, too, when it combines intervention in the luteal phase — progesterone — with intervention in the follicular phase and at ovulation — clomiphene.) The luteal phase is governed by yang energy, which develops from the yin energy dominant in the follicular phase. The transformation from yin to yang happens through the movement of qi and blood at ovulation. An interruption in the flow at any point in the cycle can show up as LPD. Too little yin in the first half of the cycle leads to too little yang in the second half (typical of Pale and Dry women). Stagnated qi and blood at ovulation can slow the transformation from yin to yang (typical of Stuck women). Or there could simply be too little yang (typical of Tired women).

Once the proper dynamic is discerned, herbal formulas and acupuncture can be designed accordingly.

### *Help Yourself*

- Try chaste tree berry to help lengthen the luteal phase; take 16 drops of tincture (or follow package instructions) twice a day from ovulation until your period begins. It is especially useful if you have a slow transition from the LH surge to ovulation.
- Try red raspberry leaf (usually taken as a tea or tincture) to improve blood flow to the uterus. (Stop taking it when you become pregnant.)
- See a Chinese medicine practitioner for herbs and acupuncture.

TIRED

WATERLOGGED

STUCK

### Polycystic Ovarian Syndrome (PCOS)

Anovulatory disorders are among the most common sources of infertility in women. About 15 percent of infertility cases are due to a problem somewhere in the endocrine system resulting in anovulation. Obviously, if you are anovulatory—if a follicle doesn't release an egg at mid-cycle—you're not going to be able to get pregnant.

Polycystic ovarian syndrome is the most common anovulatory disorder and the single most common hormonal cause of female infertility. About 10 percent of women have PCOS. LPD often accompanies PCOS (see page 201).

In PCOS, hormonal dysfunction results in the ovaries not being able to fully mature an egg. Follicles begin to develop and build up fluid, but none gets far enough along to release an egg. As a result, there's no ovulation, and no pregnancy is possible. Instead, some of the semideveloped follicles turn into little fluid-filled sacs known as cysts. Without the progesterone matured follicles would make, menstruation is irregular or perhaps stops altogether. On top of that, the cysts make androgens, so-called male hormones (although they are normally made in women's bodies, too), which can prevent ovulation. It's a vicious cycle.

Some women with PCOS believe that they *are* ovulating, based on the fact that they have the expected rise in LH, but the LH rise causes high androgen levels. The androgens from the cysts send faulty messages through the hormonal system, and this ultimately results in a rise in estrogen. Increased estrogen in turn causes a rise in LH, but no egg is released.

Some women with PCOS do ovulate, but only late in their cycle, so the egg may be of poor quality. When these women do get pregnant, they face an elevated risk of miscarriage, possibly due to low progesterone or egg quality. Some don't respond well to fertility drugs. In some women, ovulation can be forced, but the quality of the egg released won't be improved. Women with PCOS who use fertility drugs also have to contend with a higher risk of ovarian hyperstimulation syndrome (OHSS; see page 323) because of the sheer number of follicles sitting in the ovaries awaiting stimulation.

Some women with PCOS have no symptoms. They may have a slightly irregular cycle, but they still ovulate. Although it may take them a little longer to get pregnant, they usually conceive without much ado. Most women with PCOS have irregular or missed periods, contributing to difficulty getting pregnant. Many have hair in unwanted places (face, lower abdomen, chest) or acne. Many have high blood lipid levels (including cholesterol), indicators of possible cardiovascular disease in the future. And most struggle with their weight; about half are obese. They are "apples"—the weight tends to collect around the middle—reflecting their elevated androgen levels.

These women's weight problems often stem from insulin resistance—a defect in the way the body processes sugar. This can ultimately disrupt hormone balance, interfering with the functioning of the ovaries and the menstrual cycle. Insulin is itself a hormone that the body uses to turn sugars in food into energy. Insulin resistance means that the body has stopped responding to insulin. The pancreas keeps making more in a futile attempt to get its message across, and blood sugar levels keep getting higher because the insulin can't process the sugars.

Eating well and exercising to manage weight are your best at-home strategies for maximizing fertility when you have PCOS. Our dietary advice for women with PCOS is markedly different from that for anyone else. We still recommend eating vegetables, fruits, whole grains, and lean protein. Along with their many healthful attributes, they help improve the body's use of insulin and processing of sugars, and they normalize blood sugar and hormone levels. And we still advise cutting out junk food, processed food, and added sugars. But women with PCOS will fare best on a low-carb diet, so they should put more emphasis on protein and healthy fats and limit carbs, even healthy carbs such as whole grains. This is not usually the best way to eat to get pregnant, but it works for people with this problem.

---

### Case Study: Sandra

Sandra has PCOS, but you'd never know it to look at her: clear skin; tall and slim, not an extra pound on her; not a shadow of hair anywhere but on her beautifully coiffed head. She's an editor at a fashion magazine, and she looks the part. She devotes extraordinary effort to her appearance, working out pretty much every day and being very disciplined about what and how much she puts into her mouth.

When Sandra wanted to get pregnant, however, she faced the same challenges as any woman with PCOS. But because she already kept her insulin levels so tightly controlled with an Atkins-style diet that was extremely low in carbohydrates, all it took was a small dose of Clomid to induce ovulation, and she conceived right away.

---

For many women with PCOS, eating this way and following the Making Babies program for their type will be enough to allow for a healthy pregnancy. (The majority of women with PCOS can get pregnant naturally.) If you need more help or want a faster intervention, there are several options you can discuss with your doctor. Since PCOS has essentially two faces, insulin resistance and hyperandrogenism, treatment should differ depending on which predominates.

If you have or suspect you have PCOS, get tested for testosterone and DHEAs (androgens) and for fasting blood sugar (glucose) and insulin levels. Most women with PCOS will test in the normal range in one and high in the other. A sonogram of the ovaries may reveal the "string of pearls" distribution of small follicles around the periphery of the ovary that is a hallmark of PCOS.

If your androgen levels are above normal, your best bet is probably clomiphene, to stimulate ovulation, along with the mild steroid dexamethasone, to suppress male hormone levels. Gonadotropins can also be used to stimulate ovulation, but they are more expensive, come with a higher chance of multiple births, and must be injected.

## Case Study: Lana

Lana was diagnosed with PCOS years ago, so she'd always known that when it came time to have children, she might need a little extra help. She'd been taking Clomid for a year and ovulating each month, but she still was not pregnant. Her regular doctor was out of ideas, so she came to see me (Sami).

My treatment plan hinged on one simple question: do you have hair growing in any unusual places? I didn't see any on her face, but when I asked, Lana complained about hair around her nipples and on her lower abdomen. This is a common sign of excess "male" hormones. I prescribed a very low dose of the steroid dexamethasone to be taken on the same day she took Clomid, to suppress the androgens that were interfering with conception, and that did the trick. In fact, it did it over and over again: Lana had six children (one at a time!).

If your insulin level is very high (insulin resistance), you'd be better off trying metformin (Glucophage), an oral medication usually used to treat type 2 diabetes. It controls insulin by increasing sensitivity to it, thus lowering blood sugar levels. In this way, it can eliminate the negative effects of too much insulin, including disordered ovulation. It should also help with weight loss. (It works best along with calorie reduction.) Your estrogen levels should be monitored over the course of your cycle to see if your body is responding to the metformin in such a way that allows it to develop an egg. If you do ovulate, you can maximize your chances of pregnancy by following the recommendations covered in chapter 2. If your estrogen levels don't rise and you have no proof that you are ovulating, you can add in clomiphene in your next cycle.

## Case Study: Melanie

Melanie had been under the care of a good infertility doctor for well over a year. She'd tried Clomid several times and injectable fertility drugs as well, but nothing seemed to work.

When she moved to New York and had to find a new doctor, she wound up in my (Sami's) office. The first thing I did was send her to have her insulin levels checked, which had not been done before. Her problem was ovulatory, so her previous doctor had been focusing on forcing her to ovulate. But I saw from her very high insulin levels that she was insulin resistant, so I took her off the Clomid and prescribed metformin instead, to stabilize her blood sugar levels. Within two months, she was pregnant, without fertility drugs.

IVF is often recommended for women with PCOS. But if the core problem is lack of ovulation, why not solve that problem directly and let nature take it from there?

Before we move on to the Chinese medical view of PCOS and self-help strategies, we want to make a pitch for seeking treatment for PCOS even after your fertility issues have been resolved. PCOS has long-term effects on your health, including increased risk of diabetes, high blood pressure, and heart disease at a young age compared to women of the same weight without PCOS, along with all the risks that come with being overweight, as so often happens with PCOS. Too often doctor and patient both consider fertility the primary concern and tend to let things slide once that's been addressed. Don't make that mistake.

### Chinese Medicine

PCOS is most commonly seen in Waterlogged women, and in particular in Waterlogged women who are also Tired, although it can affect other types as well, especially Stuck. The cysts on the ovaries are considered a result of stagnation caused by poor fluid metabolism. As with other stagnations, this can impede ovulation and cause a long follicular phase, or prevent ovulation entirely.

Acupuncture calms the entire sympathetic nervous system and relaxes the neuroendocrine system. This helps stabilize the hormonal system, eventually leading to normal ovulation.

Acupuncture can be used with, or instead of, drugs for ovulation induction. Clinical research in China has shown that certain Chinese herbs are even more effective at inducing ovulation in people with PCOS than the pharmaceutical blood sugar stabilizer metformin. Some herbs have been shown to reduce cysts, especially combined with blood-moving herbs to induce ovulation in a formula to treat the underlying condition.

---

### Case Study: Carolyn

Carolyn had PCOS and one blocked fallopian tube, so she wasn't surprised that it was difficult for her to get pregnant. But after five years of trying, including a few IVF attempts, she was really getting worried.

I (Jill) started her on herbs and acupuncture to regulate her periods and to get her to ovulate. I also suggested that she go on a very low-carb diet, because of the insulin resistance that is a part of PCOS, and give up coffee and alcohol. Over six months, Carolyn's overall health got better and better. She kept careful track of her newly regular cycle so that she and her husband could time sex carefully—which they must have done well, as she got pregnant on her own shortly thereafter.

*Help Yourself*

- Lose some weight if you need to. Studies show that losing just 10 percent of body weight can result in normal ovulation in women with PCOS.
- Cut down on animal fats and increase essential fatty acids (EFAs).
- Eat a wide range of fruits, vegetables, and low-fat protein such as chicken, fish, and beans.
- Balance your blood sugar by limiting your carbohydrate intake. Don't cut out carbs altogether, though, as that can lower serotonin levels and leave you feeling depressed. Instead, eat healthy carbs such as whole grains.
- Take N-acetyl cysteine (NAC) supplements to help reduce circulating testosterone, cholesterol, plasma triglycerides, low-density lipoproteins, and insulin. NAC included in a multivitamin is fine. Nutrient 950 with NAC by Pure Encapsulations is also good.
- Get plenty of antioxidant nutrients from foods and supplements. They fight inflammation, which can exacerbate PCOS.
- Get regular exercise to increase your metabolism. Aim for half an hour of brisk walking every day (or the equivalent).
- Practice stress management. Stress stimulates the production of more hormones, including testosterone, which makes PCOS worse. Try yoga, meditation, or a warm bath.
- Try false unicorn root (see page 295).
- See an acupuncturist for help restoring ovulation. European studies have shown that up to one-third of women with PCOS treated with acupuncture begin to ovulate again. Acupuncture balances hormones, including LH, FSH, and testosterone, setting the stage for normal ovulation.
- See an herbalist about creating a formula specific to your situation, to reduce cysts and balance hormones as needed.
- Allow at least three months of treatment before trying to conceive. Follicles exposed to excess androgens will be of poor quality and lead to a higher risk of miscarriage.

DRY

### Premature Ovarian Failure (POF)

It is estimated that about 1 percent of women have premature ovarian failure, but we both see cases of it regularly, and they seem to be getting more frequent. In POF, the ovaries stop functioning normally in women under age 40. Either the supply of eggs runs out way ahead of schedule or the eggs don't respond to FSH and so don't mature. Either way, estrogen levels drop, because the follicles stop releasing the hormone. POF is, in effect, much the same as menopause, and when estrogen levels fall, symptoms usually associated with menopause result: no menstrual period, hot flashes, night sweats, sleep problems, mood swings, vaginal dryness, and low sex drive. And almost all women with POF find it extremely difficult to get pregnant.

POF is usually diagnosed conclusively with a blood test to check estrogen and FSH levels. Estrogen will be very low, while FSH will be elevated. Normal levels of FSH are 5 to 12 mIU/mL. In women with POF, FSH often goes above 40 mIU/mL (just what you'd expect in natural menopause). The ovaries are no longer responding to FSH by producing estrogen (and developing fertile eggs), so estrogen levels drop, while the body keeps trying to get a response by making more FSH.

The causes of POF are often unclear. In some cases, it's inherited — 10 to 20 percent of women with POF have a family history of it. In others, a genetic cause such as Turner's syndrome or fragile X syndrome might be responsible. POF also can result from infections such as PID. Sometimes POF is linked to an autoimmune disease such as diabetes or thyroid problems, or to an endocrine (hormonal) disorder. Chemotherapy and radiation treatments for cancer can cause POF, as can several kinds of pelvic surgery. Removal of the ovaries is the clearest cause of POF.

---

### Case Study: Alexa

Alexa was only 32, but she hadn't had a period in two years. Her doctor regularly monitored her hormone levels with blood tests, and they consistently showed very low estrogen and FSH over 90 mIU/mL, indicating POF. The doctor recommended donor egg IVF as her only chance to carry a child.

Alexa came to see me (Sami) in search of a less drastic alternative. There was no way to know whether she still had follicles, so I explained to her that we could try low-dose estrogen, although it would be effective only if there were in fact follicles. Alexa agreed to try the treatment. She ovulated during her very next cycle, conceived via insemination, and nine months later delivered a healthy baby boy.

Hormone replacement therapy (HRT) is the usual treatment for POF. It can control the symptoms and address associated health risks, such as heart disease and osteoporosis, but it won't restore fertility. No conventional treatment will. Donor eggs are most often recommended to women with POF who want to get pregnant.

It is important to note that up to about 10 percent of women with POF who want to conceive might do so spontaneously. I (Sami) have had success with low-dose estrogen, which suppresses FSH. If there are follicles left, blood estrogen levels will rise with this treatment, followed by successful ovulation.

### Chinese Medicine

POF is more likely to occur in Dry women. The official diagnosis is usually yin deficiency with heat. Yin deficiency produces many of the same symptoms as POF: night sweats, hot flashes, vaginal dryness, scanty or absent periods, and so on.

---

## Case Study: Karen

Karen was in her early 30s and had been trying to conceive for a year when she came to see me (Jill) complaining of an irregular menstrual cycle, short light periods, insomnia, anxiousness, night sweats, flushing, vaginal dryness, and constant thirst. All of these symptoms are unusual in a woman of her age, and I advised her to see her ob-gyn to have her hormone levels tested.

Blood work revealed that Karen had low estrogen and high FSH. The doctor explained that she was going through premature menopause (that is, she had POF) and offered HRT to relieve her symptoms. Her only chance of getting pregnant, she was told, was with donor eggs.

But I thought I could help. Karen still had follicles, and her FSH was not *too* high. I was up-front with her, telling her I felt sure I could reduce her unpleasant symptoms but I couldn't say for sure whether Chinese medicine could help her get pregnant. We agreed to give it six months before she decided about HRT or donor eggs.

I prescribed herbs to boost yin and clear the heat from her body, a formula designed to help the body produce estrogen. Karen began to incorporate more soy into her diet, to capitalize on its estrogenic properties, and she took an EFA supplement. Within about three months, Karen was feeling less heat, was sleeping better, and felt that her mood had improved—signs that her estrogen level was rising. At that point, I started to give her weekly acupuncture. By the end of six months, her cycle had become more regular, and she had begun to ovulate.

Encouraged by this progress, Karen and I decided to keep going. It took another six months, but she did conceive. Unfortunately, she had a miscarriage at six weeks. She opted to continue treatment with me, and five months later she became pregnant again. This time she went on to have a beautiful little girl.

Herbs can coax hormone production. Acupuncture can promote ovulation from dormant or understimulated follicles once hormone levels have normalized. If there are no follicles left, however, neither acupuncture nor herbs will make a difference.

### Help Yourself

- Besides following the recommendations for the Dry type (see chapter 21), of which POF is an extreme version, see your doctor for medical help.
- See a Chinese medicine practitioner for help in boosting estrogen.
- See an acupuncturist to promote ovulation.

DRY

TIRED

### Early Pregnancy Loss

Some women think they are having fertility problems when really the issue is very early miscarriage—pregnancy loss that occurs before a woman even knows she is pregnant. You may be conceiving, and implantation begins, but the pregnancy doesn't develop properly. The body produces the chemical signal of pregnancy, human chorionic gonadotropin (HCG), but the pregnancy is never fully established and can't sustain itself. The woman gets her period right around the time she would expect to, perhaps a few days late. Medically speaking, this kind of extremely early miscarriage is sometimes referred to as *chemical pregnancy*.

Chemical pregnancy is quite common. Even when all systems are go and sperm meets egg, there are still a lot of ways for the process to go off the rails, including abnormality in the sperm, egg, or embryo; hormonal glitches; endometrial problems; infections; and structural problems in the uterus. The failure to grow, the failure to implant, or the abrupt stopping of growth happens normally. It's part of the plan and helps, ultimately, to conserve resources for a healthy pregnancy. It's why doctors don't worry if young, healthy women take up to a year to get pregnant.

There was a time when you probably wouldn't even have known if you'd had a chemical pregnancy. Now we have very sensitive blood pregnancy tests that can tell you you're pregnant even before you miss your period, and so you know when a pregnancy fails.

If this is happening to you repeatedly, your doctor can help figure out the source of the problem so that it can be treated. The first step is to determine whether you are in fact experiencing early pregnancy loss. The key is to have a *blood* pregnancy test when your period is just a day or two late. Blood tests can detect pregnancy by about ten days after ovulation. If your period comes right on time but you feel "different" (or if your cycle is unpredictable and you feel different), you should also get a blood test three to four days *before* your period is due to check for pregnancy.

Most women can feel physical signs of pregnancy from the earliest moments, even if they don't tune in to them as such, so note any departure from normal—*your* normal. In particular, be on the alert for breast fullness or nipple tenderness; increased frequency of urination or increased nighttime urination; unusual fatigue in the late afternoon or evening; or changes in smell or taste (some women get a metallic taste in their mouth when first pregnant). Any of these might be the same as your usual PMS symptoms, but if they are more intense or go on for longer than usual, they may signify pregnancy. Also keep an eye out for anything else that could explain the changes you feel. For example, if you've had an especially caffeinated month, increased breast tenderness could result from that alone.

Once you've established that you are conceiving but are not sustaining a pregnancy, your doctor should try to discover the underlying cause. The usual suspects are low progesterone (under 15 ngm/mL), or LPD (see page 200); inadequate endometrium (see page 173); or an infection in either partner (see chapter 16). Fibroids (see page 231), scar tissue (see page 229), endometrial polyps (see page 237), genetic abnormalities (see page 272), and killer cells (see page 261) should also be considered. I (Sami) have had success with many patients using a combination of progesterone to support the luteal phase and endometrium and antibiotics to get rid of any infection.

### Chinese Medicine

Chinese medicine considers early pregnancy loss "kidney qi deficiency," in which the body is not able to resource the implanted embryo. It generally affects Dry and Tired types. See a Chinese medicine practitioner about herbs and acupuncture that may help.

*Help Yourself*

- Use your BBT chart to detect whether you are routinely conceiving but not maintaining pregnancy. The telltale pattern is a triphasic chart — three distinct temperature phases — with a sudden drop in temperature near the end of your cycle (before your period begins).
- If you experience symptoms of pregnancy, it's time to talk with your doctor about chemical pregnancy and what to do about it.

---

### Case Study: Marguerite

Marguerite took fertility drugs for more than four years but still didn't have a baby. The doctor's only suggestion was to continue taking the same drugs. But Marguerite wasn't infertile, so the fertility drugs were never going to solve her problem.

When she flew across the Atlantic to see me (Sami), she described a particular pattern of breast tenderness: her breasts always hurt for the same four days out of her regular-as-clockwork twenty-eight-day cycle, except that every few months they would hurt for two weeks straight. That clued me in on what was happening: she was conceiving a few times a year but had early pregnancy loss. I prescribed a progesterone supplement to be taken at the appropriate time in her cycle, and she was pregnant within four months.

---

STUCK

### Luteinized Unruptured Follicle Syndrome (LUFS)

Luteinized unruptured follicle syndrome, more casually referred to as *trapped egg syndrome,* is a rare condition in which a follicle develops to mature an egg, but the follicle never breaks open to release the egg. LH spikes, the usual signal to start ovulation, but there's no ovulation — and thus no pregnancy. LUFS can occur in any woman, but it is more frequent in women taking fertility drugs, women with endometriosis, and women who have had PID.

LUFS is difficult to diagnose because it seems as if ovulation has occurred: BBT rises, progesterone goes up, and other hormone levels are normal. A series of carefully timed ultrasound scans of the ovaries is required to reveal whether the follicle collapses at the expected time, and therefore whether the egg has been released. Laparoscopy can be useful in diagnosis if noninvasive approaches don't provide the necessary information.

IVF is commonly recommended for women with LUFS, because the egg is removed from the follicle with a needle. But IVF is not necessary. A well-timed injection of HCG can prompt the egg to be released. Assuming that there are no other fertility issues, once the egg is successfully released, all that remains to be done is to time intercourse (or insemination).

---

### Case Study: Lucy

Lucy, in her early 30s, had been trying to get pregnant for three years without any success. Her ob-gyn couldn't find anything wrong with her. Although I did an extensive workup when she came to see me (Sami), I also couldn't find anything to explain why Lucy wasn't conceiving. When I recommended a laparoscopy to evaluate her pelvic anatomy, she told me that she'd already had one, and her doctor had pronounced everything completely normal. She agreed to have another one, just in case her doctor had missed something.

The laparoscopy revealed that Lucy's ovaries were totally smooth — no sign of any follicles ever releasing from either one. Although she had regular menstrual cycles, I told her she had likely *never* released an egg. In all the years she'd been trying to get pregnant, she probably hadn't ovulated once. Happily, two cycles later, after two injections of HCG to stimulate the release of a mature egg, Lucy was pregnant.

---

### Chinese Medicine

Chinese medicine considers LUFS a result of stagnation. Stuck women are the type most likely to have it.

Taking an herbal formula containing Zao Jiao Ci (gleditsia spine) for about five days during the follicular phase is very effective in helping the follicle rupture. In my (Jill's) experience, this herb is nearly miraculous in getting follicles to pop (and in reducing ovarian cysts, a process that amounts to much the same thing). Conventional medicine doesn't have anything like it. Acupuncture is also useful in prompting ovulation.

### Help Yourself
- Try false unicorn root (see page 295).
- See a Chinese medicine practitioner for an herbal formula containing Zao Jiao Ci.
- See an acupuncturist to help prompt ovulation.

# MEN

TIRED

WATERLOGGED

STUCK

DRY

## Sexual Function Problems

Erectile problems, premature ejaculation, and failure to ejaculate present some of the more obvious fertility challenges for men. They are also among the most common: about 5 percent of couples struggling with infertility have one or more of these as their central concern. What you do about them will depend on the source of the problem.

Sexual function can be compromised by certain general health conditions, some medications, and congenital defects. Age is a factor. Injury to the reproductive system, including injury as a result of surgery, can also be a cause, as can injury to the spinal cord. Low testosterone or high prolactin can interfere with sexual function. Alcoholism, or even just regular intake of alcohol, can be to blame. So can fatigue, stress, anxiety, or low self-esteem. When faced with fertility issues, even people not usually prone to being stressed-out may be exceptionally anxious or low in self-esteem. "Performance anxiety" can strike for any number of reasons; struggling with fertility is certainly a big one.

You may be facing sexual function problems if you have diabetes, high blood pressure, multiple sclerosis or another neurological disorder, kidney disease, stroke, or heart disease. In these cases, you should talk to your doctor about how to manage any of those conditions better to curb this side effect. If you're having sexual function problems but don't know why, you may want to be screened for some of these conditions.

Blood pressure and heart disease medications can cause erectile dysfunction (ED). So can tranquilizers and antidepressants, which can also seriously decrease libido. If you suspect that medication is a source of your problem, talk to your doctor about cutting back your dosage or changing your prescription to reduce this side effect.

Anatomical conditions that can impair male fertility include hypospadias (an abnormally placed opening of the urethra, which in some cases hampers fertility) and Peyronie's disease (scar tissue causing abnormal curvature of the erect penis and possibly ED). Discuss conception options with your doctor; artificial insemination may be your best bet.

Radical prostate and bladder surgery can injure nerves and compromise the blood supply to the penis, which can cause ED. Drugs such as

Viagra, Levitra, and Cialis can increase blood flow to the penis. You'll also benefit from losing weight, becoming more active, and quitting smoking.

You probably don't need anyone to tell you that you have a sexual function problem, although a physical exam can detect or confirm the problem, and relevant screening tests can determine the underlying cause(s) and therefore the appropriate course of action. The most important screenings for sexual function problems are a good medical history, including a list of all medications; a physical exam; and a blood test for hormone levels.

---

### Case Study: Burt and Sarah

Burt and Sarah were significantly younger than most couples who wind up in my (Sami's) office, and medical histories and physical exams showed no clear reason why they were having trouble getting pregnant. A postcoital test revealed an important clue: no sperm.

It was a difficult conversation for Burt to have, but he confided that he was ejaculating prematurely. The sperm were released just as they entered the vagina, which wasn't giving them enough of a head start; they really needed to be dropped off right outside the cervix.

Sometimes this kind of issue is best addressed by a sex counselor. Burt and Sarah successfully used a more direct solution: pinching the scrotum just before penetration gave the couple the extra bit of time they needed to reach full penetration before ejaculation. Within a couple of months, Sarah was pregnant.

---

*Chinese Medicine*

Chinese medicine offers three main diagnoses for variations on ED: yang deficiency (Tired), damp heat (Waterlogged), or qi and blood stagnation (Stuck). Herbs and acupuncture can be very helpful in treating ED, except when the culprit is medications.

Premature ejaculation is considered qi deficiency (Tired), yin deficiency (Dry), or qi stagnation with heat (Stuck). Herbs and acupuncture may help.

*Help Yourself*
- Limit alcohol intake or avoid alcohol altogether.
- Exercise regularly.
- Reduce stress.
- Get enough sleep.
- Deal with anxiety or depression.

- Stop smoking.
- See a Chinese medicine practitioner for herbs and acupuncture. Note that Chinese treatment focuses on the cause of the problem; pharmaceuticals such as Viagra work on the symptoms. Beware of pills and potions sold on the Internet as "herbal Viagra" or some such. Like their namesake, they too treat the symptoms — though not very well. They are not strong enough or specific enough to be of much use in treating the root cause of the problem.

## WOMEN AND MEN

### Follicle-Stimulating Hormone (FSH)

DRY

PALE

#### *Women and High FSH*

The common fertility problem here is not with elevated levels of the hormone itself, but with the way most doctors use the information. If you've seen a doctor for fertility problems, FSH level is the one test you're most likely to have had.

As the name suggests, FSH spurs the ovaries to grow and mature the follicles that will release the eggs. When the ovaries have lots of eggs, they don't need to work very hard to release them, so FSH levels are low. (FSH can also be too low — more about that in a moment.) As the supply of eggs dwindles, however, the pituitary gland generally has to work harder to stimulate the ovaries to develop the eggs, and FSH levels go up to help push the ovaries along. This is why older women generally have higher FSH levels than younger women. "Normal" FSH levels, on day 2 or 3 of the menstrual cycle, should be under 12 mIU/mL.

Low ovarian reserve isn't the only reason FSH rises, however, so automatically treating every elevated result as a sign that a woman doesn't have enough eggs or has only "bad" eggs is a mistake. And high FSH should never be considered a definitive sign that pregnancy is impossible.

For one thing, "bad eggs" is a catchall diagnosis applied when the doctor doesn't know what else is wrong. Almost no one has eggs that are all "bad" anyway, although as women get older, they do have more eggs that are less viable. That does not mean, however, that there are no good, viable eggs available.

Several things other than a diminished egg supply can cause high FSH. Although they are less common, they must be investigated before you accept a conclusion of low ovarian reserve. FSH may be elevated because of certain autoimmune disorders, some genetic conditions, surgical removal of one ovary, smoking, or recovery from amenorrhea (lack of a menstrual period) due to hormone imbalance. High FSH can also be due to premature ovarian failure (POF; see page 208), or early menopause.

Commonly, FSH can run amok due to stress. As with all of its processes, the body has to work much harder to produce an egg when it is stressed-out and rundown. I (Jill) have seen my patients' FSH go up when they were stressed to the max, then come back down when relative calm returned. Many have then gone on to get pregnant. FSH can also rise for no discernible reason and then return to normal. FSH levels can vary from cycle to cycle. In any case, high FSH does not mean you can't or won't ovulate or conceive. It may be harder to get pregnant with high FSH, but it certainly doesn't rule out pregnancy altogether.

Even if high FSH does turn out to be linked to a lower number of eggs in the ovaries, it's the quality of ovulation that's important, not the quantity of eggs. As long as you are ovulating, it doesn't matter whether the one released egg came from a supply of a hundred or a thousand or a million. If you have high FSH *and* ovulation issues, you may have a problem, but high FSH alone shouldn't be the end of the story.

---

### Case Study: Imani

Imani's doctors had told her that she'd never have a baby of her own after discovering she had FSH levels ranging from 15 to 25 mIU/mL. She was only 34. When she came to my (Sami's) office, I performed a more thorough workup than she had received before being given that terrible diagnosis, including HSG (see page 198) and, ultimately, laparoscopy. That was how I discovered the true cause of her fertility problem: scar tissue on her ovaries and surrounding her fallopian tubes. After I performed surgery to remove the scar tissue, Imani conceived four months later, with no further treatment (and no change in FSH).

---

FSH is tested on day 2 or 3 of the menstrual cycle. FSH is somewhat complicated to measure, and results can vary from lab to lab. Make sure to get tested by whatever lab your doctor usually uses so that results are consistent. Most doctors have a cutoff for FSH levels above which they won't treat a patient for infertility. Different doctors use different limits, but most are set around 12 to 14 mIU/mL.

If you get elevated results, you should definitely have the test repeated. One high result should not be a cause for concern. (After menopause, FSH levels stay high. As long as they vary, you're not there yet.) Many doctors, however, take the highest result recorded as the definitive one, essentially disregarding any lower values.

High FSH does mean that fertility drugs won't help you. These drugs work by stimulating the production of more FSH (or, in the case of injectables, providing more). If your levels are already high, your ovaries can become resistant to FSH. So before you begin taking fertility drugs, make sure you have your FSH level tested.

IVF will not increase the likelihood that women with high FSH will get pregnant. Such women will do just as well, or better, by trying to conceive naturally. So the IVF docs may be right to dissuade such women from doing IVF with high-dose fertility drugs, but they are not right to offer no options other than donor egg IVF. I (Sami) give some of my patients estrogen to lower their FSH. Once FSH comes down, their ovaries may respond to the FSH in high-dose drugs.

---

### Case Study: Priti

Priti had had an FSH level of 100 mIU/mL for two years by the time she came to see me, and she hadn't menstruated in that time. Her doctors diagnosed her with POF and offered no hope for conceiving her own child. She was 33 years old.

I prescribed estrogen to suppress her FSH, then monitored her hormones to pinpoint ovulation. She developed a single egg, had an insemination, and nine months later delivered a healthy baby boy. After that, she began having regular periods again. Hers was a case of *temporary* POF.

---

TIRED

STUCK

*Women and Low FSH*

Low FSH can also present a fertility problem. This typically happens as part of a stress pattern. Stress hormones can suppress FSH. In these circumstances, a woman may ovulate, although it may happen as part of an elongated cycle. And as long as there's ovulation, there shouldn't really be a problem getting pregnant (assuming she can identify when ovulation occurs and time intercourse accordingly). If FSH drops low enough to stop ovulation, fertility drugs can help. So can stress reduction! The effect on FSH is just one of many reasons managing stress is so important to fertility.

### Men and FSH

FSH stimulates sperm production in men. Men's FSH levels rise natu-rally with age (sort of a male menopause), but they may also be forced up by testicular trauma or torsion, or when an infection destroys cells in the testicles. If a man's FSH rises too high and stays up, he'll stop making sperm. The rise usually can't be prevented, and once the level is up, there's not much to be done about it. High FSH is a symptom of testicular failure. High FSH and low sperm count combined results in a diagnosis of testicular failure.

DRY

TIRED

STUCK

Excessively low FSH levels in men probably have the same cause as they do in women: stress. If that's the case, the prescription might be the same: clomiphene, in very low doses, plus stress-reduction techniques. Low FSH due to stress is likely to be accompanied by weak sperm — low count, poor motility or morphology, or any combination thereof.

A man with either low or high FSH should see a specialist in male infertility.

### Chinese Medicine

High FSH in women or men is considered to be related to yin deficiency, which is why Dry types are especially susceptible. Pale women are the next most likely to have high FSH. In Dry and Pale women, high FSH leads to poor endometrial or follicle development and possibly to less fertile cervical mucus. Acupuncture and herbs can be useful in lowering FSH and thereby increasing fertility.

Low FSH is more related to yang deficiency, and so is more prevalent in Tired or Stuck types, male or female.

### Help Yourself

- If your FSH is high, establish whether you are ovulating and, if so, keep trying for natural conception accordingly.
- Insist on a complete workup, not just an FSH result — for your partner as well as yourself. Demand that your doctor provide the same evaluation he or she would give any patient, regardless of age or FSH levels.
- Consult an acupuncturist or herbalist for help in lowering your FSH.
- Use visualization techniques to reduce stress (see page 90) and help normalize FSH.

STUCK

### Elevated Prolactin

Prolactin is a hormone secreted by the pituitary gland. Its main function is to stimulate breast development and milk production in women. Men have it, too, at lower levels, but even the scientific experts don't really know why.

An elevated level of prolactin in the blood is known as hyperprolactinemia. It's an uncommon condition, but it can account for a good number of cases of amenorrhea (absence of period) or other menstrual cycle dysfunction and infertility. High prolactin levels can stop ovulation—not surprising since elevated prolactin is what keeps nursing mothers from having a period and getting pregnant (though it's not foolproof). Men can experience fertility problems as a result of elevated prolactin, too.

The most common cause of elevated prolactin is stress. An underactive thyroid can cause this, too, as can a benign pituitary tumor, though that's much rarer. Several types of drugs can raise prolactin levels, including alcohol, opiates, and some tranquilizers, antidepressants, blood pressure medications, and antinausea drugs. You should review all drugs you are taking with your doctor in case any of them could be responsible for your elevated prolactin.

---

### Case Study: Jess

Jess was a veteran of several failed IVFs. Since she was approaching 40, all the doctors were telling her that her eggs must be of poor quality and were advising her to do donor egg IVF. In a last-ditch effort to find another way, Jess flew to New York to see me (Sami). A basic blood test showed that she had mildly elevated prolactin, and a follow-up MRI revealed a small pituitary tumor. The tumor was otherwise benign, but it was responsible for pumping out excess prolactin. I prescribed bromocriptine (Parlodel) to suppress secretion of prolactin. It also shrank the tumor, which required no additional treatment. Jess's husband also tested positive for E. coli, so they both took antibiotics to eradicate the infection.

With her prolactin levels back to normal and the infection cleared up, Jess tried one more round of IVF with her own eggs. She told me that she had to beg her doctors to do so, since they were convinced her eggs were no good. She conceived and went on to have a healthy baby boy. A year later, she conceived again, this time with no medical intervention.

In women, high prolactin levels lead to decreased estrogen levels, interfere with regular ovulation, can cause low libido, and may lead to metabolic imbalances and infertility. A mild case may mean low progesterone and a short luteal phase, which is enough to impair fertility, even with an apparently regular menstrual cycle. A more moderate case can cause infrequent, light, or irregular periods and the associated fertility problems. Fertility remains an issue in the most severe cases, where menstruation and ovulation may stop altogether. High prolactin can cause hypogonadism — abnormally low levels of sex hormones — which in women means low estrogen and the menopause-like consequences of that. More rarely, high prolactin can cause galactorrhea — breast milk production not connected to pregnancy or childbirth.

In men, elevated prolactin levels cause fertility problems ranging from low testosterone (hypogonadism), metabolic imbalances, and low libido to interference with normal sperm production and ED.

If you are experiencing any of these symptoms, ask your doctor to check your prolactin levels along with your other hormones.

### Chinese Medicine
Stuck women are the most likely fertility type to have high prolactin. I (Jill) have found that herbs that move qi can help bring down prolactin levels.

### Help Yourself
- Get plenty of B vitamins, magnesium, and zinc in your diet.
- Find ways to ease the physical effects of stress in your life: have regular massages, learn to meditate, or discover other stress reducers that work for you.
- Get regular *gentle* exercise. (*Excessive* exercise can raise prolactin levels.)
- Avoid alcohol altogether.
- Chaste tree berry can help rebalance hormones, including taming too-high prolactin levels.
- See an herbalist for herbs that can move qi.

### Case Study: Bruce and Justine

Bruce and Justine had trouble getting pregnant, but with the help of a fertility specialist, they finally conceived. Sadly, Justine had a miscarriage the day after routine amniocentesis, and both she and Bruce spiraled into depression. They also had problems conceiving again. Bruce experienced ED, and his sperm count was low, though neither of these problems had been an issue during their original fertility treatments. Bruce's urologist wrote off both as a result of his depression.

In my (Sami's) office, further tests revealed that Bruce's prolactin levels were over 100 ng/mL (normal is under 20) and that he had a pituitary tumor. I prescribed bromocriptine (Parlodel) to inhibit production of prolactin and shrink the otherwise benign tumor, and soon thereafter Bruce's sperm count improved and his ED disappeared. The couple conceived again just three months after beginning treatment with me and had a healthy baby.

## Other Hormonal Issues

There are a range of uncommon hormonal causes of fertility problems. We don't have room to go into detail about them here, but if none of the common explanations apply to your situation, make sure your doctor rules these out before you accept a diagnosis of unexplained infertility.

### Women:

Adrenal disorders
Ovarian, pituitary, or adrenal tumors
Pituitary disease, dysfunction, or failure
Hyperandrogenism
Galactorrhea-amenorrhea syndrome
Hypothalamic-pituitary amenorrhea (usually associated with extreme stress and weight loss or bulimia)
Hyperinsulinemia
Resistant ovary syndrome

### Men:

Pituitary disease, dysfunction, or failure
Adrenal disorders
Endocrine disturbances

# Making Babies Action Plan

The following action plans summarize the testing needed to establish whether your fertility problems stem from any of these hormonal issues. They will guide you through your potential testing program as efficiently as possible. For women, we've organized them roughly the way they need to be timed to your cycle, so that you can schedule the tests appropriately and get them all completed in as short a time as possible. (Timing is not usually an issue for men.) Not everyone will need all these tests, and these may not be all the tests you need. Your doctor will guide you as to which tests you need, of course, but you should make sure that your understanding, gleaned from the descriptions in this chapter, lines up with your doctor's plans.

## TESTS FOR WOMEN

| TEST | CONDITION | TYPES MOST LIKELY TO NEED IT | TIMING |
|------|-----------|------------------------------|--------|
| Pregnancy blood test | Early pregnancy loss | TIRED / DRY | When period is a day or two late or 10 to 11 days after ovulation |
| Blood test for estrogen and FSH | Premature ovarian failure (POF); ovarian reserve (egg supply); stress | DRY | Day 2 or 3 of cycle (to test ovarian reserve) |
| Blood test for LH | Polycystic ovarian syndrome (PCOS); ovarian reserve (egg supply); stress | TIRED / WATERLOGGED / STUCK | Day 2 or 3 of cycle |

# TESTS FOR WOMEN

| TEST | CONDITION | TYPES MOST LIKELY TO NEED IT | TIMING |
|------|-----------|------------------------------|--------|
| Ultrasound of ovaries | Polycystic ovarian syndrome (PCOS); ovarian cysts | TIRED / WATERLOGGED / STUCK | Just after period ends (day 4, 5, or 6 of typical cycle) |
| Ultrasound of ovaries | To assess eggs in ovaries and development of follicles; to monitor effects of fertility drugs and track follicle development | DRY / TIRED | Just after period ends (day 4, 5, or 6 of typical cycle) |
| Cervical mucus culture (postcoital test) | Infection causing early pregnancy loss | WATERLOGGED | 1 to 3 days before ovulation is expected |
| Blood test for estrogen | To monitor effects of fertility drugs and track follicle development | DRY / PALE | Before ovulation; frequently while monitoring fertility drugs |
| Laparoscopy | Endometriosis; scar tissue; blocked tubes | STUCK / WATERLOGGED | After period ends but before ovulation (day 7, 8, or 9 of typical cycle) |

## TESTS FOR WOMEN

| TEST | CONDITION | TYPES MOST LIKELY TO NEED IT | TIMING |
|---|---|---|---|
| Transvaginal ultrasound | Luteal phase defect (LPD); thin uterine lining; early pregnancy loss | PALE, DRY, STUCK, TIRED | Just before ovulation |
| Ultrasound of ovaries | Luteinized unruptured follicle syndrome (LUFS) | STUCK | Before and after presumed ovulation |
| Serial progesterone blood test | Luteal phase defect (LPD); early pregnancy loss | TIRED, DRY | 7, 9, and 11 days after ovulation (between days 21 and 25 of typical cycle) |
| Endometrial biopsy | Luteal phase defect (LPD); early pregnancy loss | PALE, STUCK, TIRED | 8 to 10 days after ovulation (and after blood pregnancy test) |

### TESTS FOR WOMEN

| TEST | CONDITION | TYPES MOST LIKELY TO NEED IT | TIMING |
| --- | --- | --- | --- |
| Blood test for prolactin | Elevated prolactin; luteal phase defect (LPD) | STUCK | Anytime |
| Blood test for TSH | Thyroid imbalance (over- or underactive) | TIRED | Anytime |
| Blood test for testosterone and DHEA (androgens) | Polycystic ovarian syndrome (PCOS) | TIRED  WATERLOGGED  STUCK | Anytime |
| Blood test for fasting glucose and insulin levels | Polycystic ovarian syndrome (PCOS) | TIRED  WATERLOGGED  STUCK | Any morning (after fasting) |

## TESTS FOR MEN

| TEST | CONDITION | TYPES MOST LIKELY TO NEED IT |
|------|-----------|------------------------------|
| Physical exam and medical history (including medications) | Sexual function problems | Anyone experiencing sexual function problems |
| Blood test for male hormone levels (FSH, LH, testosterone, TSH) | Hormone imbalance; sexual function problems |  **TIRED** Also, anyone experiencing sexual function problems should ask his doctor about these tests. |
| Blood test for male prolactin levels | Hormone imbalance; sexual function problems | **STUCK** Also, anyone experiencing sexual function problems should ask his doctor about these tests. |

# CHAPTER FIFTEEN

# Structural or Anatomical Issues

**B**oth men and women may experience a range of structural or anatomical issues affecting fertility, and we address them in this chapter roughly in the order of their prevalence. We've covered the surgical solutions here, but in some cases there are also strategies you can implement on your own to improve fertility. You'll find these in the Help Yourself sections.

## WOMEN

STUCK

WATERLOGGED

### Blocked Fallopian Tubes

Eggs travel through the fallopian tubes to the uterus. The tubes are lined with tiny hairlike cilia, which help move an egg along, and mucus-producing cells maintain a slippery environment to ease it on its journey.

If the tubes become blocked, the egg can't get picked up and transported toward the uterus, the sperm can't get to the egg, and you can't get pregnant. The tubes can also be partially obstructed, so that sperm are able to reach the egg but the fertilized egg can't get through to the uterus. An ectopic pregnancy results.

Fallopian tube blockages are relatively common, accounting for about 20 percent of female infertility. There are four main ways the fallopian tubes can become blocked.

1. **Excess thick mucus.** Normally, there's just enough mucus generated in the tubes to coat the walls and keep them slippery enough to ensure that an egg can scoot by without

getting stuck. Mucus thickens a bit at the ends of the tubes connecting to the uterus, to delay a fertilized egg for a couple of days during its first cell divisions. If there's too much mucus, however, it can completely obstruct the tube. It also can coat the opening at the ovary end, which can prevent the egg from being swept down in the first place. Because the tubes are so narrow, it really doesn't take much to plug them up. These problems are particularly common in Waterlogged women.

2. **Infection and inflammation.** The tubes are prone to attack from bacteria coming up from the cervix. The resulting inflammation can cause the inner walls of the tubes to stick together, creating a blockage. This is often referred to as pelvic inflammatory disease (PID), although the results of PID can appear in a variety of locations. Inflammation specifically of the fallopian tubes is called salpingitis. Salpingitis (like PID generally) can result from a variety of microbes, many but not all of which are sexually transmitted, and often involves more than one. These kinds of infections are most common in Waterlogged women.

3. **Liquid.** Chronic salpingitis may result in the tubes filling with fluid (hydrosalpinx) or pus (pyosalpinx), which blocks an egg from moving along. These liquids may also leak back into the uterus, where they can create an implantation problem or be toxic to an embryo.

4. **Thickening.** If scarlike tissue called adhesions develop on the outer surface of the tubes, these adhesions can immobilize the tubes and ovaries, preventing an otherwise healthy and open tube from picking up an egg. Scar tissue resulting from pelvic surgery or previous pregnancies (traumatic vaginal deliveries, C-sections, or other complications) can block the tubes internally.

## Case Study: Virginia

Virginia had been trying to get pregnant for three years without success. Her doctors had told her that her eggs were all "bad" due to high FSH, although she was only 32 years old and healthy. When she came to see me (Sami), she'd had a reasonably thorough workup, including an HSG, which showed that her tubes were open. But there was one last test that had never been done: exploratory surgery. Not the kind of thing you want to rush into, naturally, but since all other avenues had been explored and nothing could yet explain her trouble getting pregnant, it was the path I recommended.

With outpatient laparoscopic surgery, I found and removed adhesions around Virginia's fallopian tubes, as well as around her ovaries. It was as if her ovaries were in a cellophane bag—no eggs could get out. The adhesions around her tubes immobilized them to the point that they would have been unable to pick up any eggs anyway. Removing the adhesions (caused by an earlier pelvic infection) allowed eggs to be released and the tubes to become mobile again. Less than four months after her surgery, Virginia was pregnant.

Blocked tubes generally come with no symptoms—aside from not getting pregnant—except in cases where pelvic infections, a ruptured cyst, or a ruptured appendix cause both the blockage and pain.

Your doctor can check to see if your tubes are blocked using an HSG or laparoscopy (see page 198). Sometimes these procedures can be curative as well as diagnostic. Obstructions created by mucus can be easily cleared by having the tubes "flushed" during HSG, for example. Studies have shown that pregnancy rates increase after HSG, presumably because minor blockages are broken up in the process of getting a clear picture.

A total blockage can be surgically removed using laparoscopy, an outpatient procedure. You may be able to get pregnant with no other help after laparoscopy, depending on your age, your partner, and all the other variables that contribute to fertility.

IVF may be an option, since it bypasses the need for the egg to travel through the fallopian tubes. A total blockage may still need to be repaired or removed first, however, because the fluid trapped inside the tubes can impair implantation or harm the embryo if it leaks back into the uterus.

### Chinese Medicine

Chinese medicine views blocked tubes as stagnation of blood (Stuck) or phlegm (Waterlogged). Herbs may be useful in Waterlogged women.

Acupuncture may be as well, though in a more limited way. Most Stuck women with blocked tubes will need Western intervention.

### Help Yourself

Most women with fully blocked tubes will need surgery to correct the condition, but women whose tubes are partially blocked can try the following:

- Stop smoking. Smoking impedes the action of the cilia, and this can interfere with the movement of fertilized eggs.
- If your tubes are just a bit gummed up with mucus, see an herbalist for Chinese formulas that move blood and phlegm, which can be very helpful in clearing them.
- Consult a massage therapist specifically trained in the techniques of deep abdominal massage, such as Arvigo Maya Abdominal Massage. Or practice self-massage. The techniques in chapter 4 may not clear a completely blocked tube, but they can help prevent a blockage.
- Use castor oil packs if you have scar tissue or adhesions (see page 234).

### Fibroids

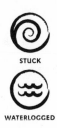

STUCK

WATERLOGGED

Fibroids are benign growths in the wall of the uterus, made of smooth muscle and fibrous tissue. They grow in response to excess estrogen in the body. Fibroids can range in size from as small as a pea to as large as a melon, although most of them fall within the orange-to-grapefruit range. An estimated 20 to 30 percent of women between 35 and 50 have fibroids, although some may never know it, because they don't necessarily cause any problems or symptoms.

But fibroids certainly *can* cause trouble, depending on their size, number, and exact location. They may change normal pelvic anatomy, alter the blood supply to the uterus, prevent the egg from being picked up, or interfere with implantation. They can also cause painful intercourse. Common symptoms include long (more than five days), heavy, clotted periods (sometimes so heavy they can cause anemia); periods that stop and start; bleeding between periods; a sensation of pressure on the bladder or elsewhere in the pelvic area; or enough swelling of the abdomen to be noticeable. Sometimes the first sign of fibroids is having trouble conceiving.

If you have these symptoms, discuss them with your doctor. A regular pelvic exam will be the first step toward diagnosis: your doctor will be able to feel if the uterus is enlarged or irregularly shaped. Further tests may be warranted to detect and measure fibroids: ultrasound, hysteroscopy (outpatient exploratory surgery in which a small camera is inserted through the cervix to give the doctor a good view of what's going on in the uterus), HSG, or laparoscopy. With a read on whether you have fibroids, where in the uterus they are, how many there are, how big they are, and whether they can prevent implantation, your doctor can advise you on whether you should have surgery. Generally, that's necessary only if any one fibroid is larger than 5 cm or if there are multiple fibroids of at least 3 cm each. A fibroid of any size *within* the uterine cavity (submucous fibroid) should be removed.

### Chinese Medicine

Chinese medicine views fibroids as related to blood or phlegm stagnation. Stuck or Waterlogged women are most prone to them.

Herbs and acupuncture can be used in conjunction with Western medical treatment to reduce the size of fibroids and their unpleasant side effects, but they are unlikely to make fibroids disappear altogether on their own. In my (Jill's) practice, I have had much success in reducing small fibroids but have not been able to resolve large ones. Blood-moving herbs may be useful for fibroids, but they must be used only under expert guidance for a safe and effective approach. Many herbs are contraindicated in pregnancy because they can cause early miscarriage.

### Help Yourself

Most of the things you can do to help combat fibroids are aimed at reducing your exposure to excess estrogen, supporting your liver (which is active in breaking down estrogen), promoting circulation of blood in the pelvic area, and checking in with yourself emotionally.

- Consult with your gynecologist about fibroids, and use herbs and acupuncture as an adjunct.

- If you are overweight, lose a few pounds. Extra fat cells increase the amount of estrogen in your system.
- Choose a low-fat, high-fiber, mostly vegetarian diet.
- Go easy on dairy products, although you don't have to avoid them altogether.
- Choose meat and dairy from animals that haven't been treated with hormones.
- Avoid soy. Many "alternative" practitioners recommend soy and other sources of phytoestrogens (plant estrogens) for fibroids, on the theory that the gentle phytoestrogens attach to receptor sites in the body that might otherwise latch onto more harmful xenoestrogens (synthetic or chemical estrogens). Over the years, however, I (Jill) have seen enough women whose fibroids have gotten worse under the influence of phytoestrogens in herbs and foods to suggest otherwise. Processed soy products seem to be the most detrimental.
- Choose organic produce, thereby avoiding exposure to estrogenic pesticides.
- Eat plenty of cruciferous vegetables, such as broccoli, cabbage, cauliflower, kale, and Brussels sprouts. They contain a phytonutrient called di-indolylmethane (DIM), which supports efficient estrogen metabolism.
- Avoid refined and hydrogenated oils.
- Limit sugar, chocolate, caffeine, and alcohol.
- Get plenty of B vitamins in whole foods such as lentils, rice bran, and blackstrap molasses or in supplements. Vitamin $B_6$, in particular, enhances the breakdown of estrogen and its removal from the body.
- Eat artichokes.
- Stimulate the liver by using lemon juice and including bitter greens such as dandelion, endive, and radicchio in your salads.
- Use liver-supporting herbs, including dandelion root, milk thistle, burdock, and turmeric.
- Follow a detoxification program. At the YinOva Center, we sell a monthlong herbal detox made by Blessed Herbs (see Resources).
- Get regular moderate exercise to help improve circulation.

- Take regular baths with Epsom salts. Dissolve 6 cups of salts in a warm bath and lie in it for 20 minutes. Get out, dry off, and lie quietly for 20 minutes more. Or try a warm bath with essential oils such as frankincense and lavender.
- Include omega-3 fatty acids in your diet; they help prevent abnormal blood clotting. Eat fatty fish, use flaxseed oil, and/or take supplements.
- Apply a castor oil pack to your lower abdomen twice a day during your period (and *only* during your period). It will invigorate the blood and help the lymphatic system move debris. Lie down, rub castor oil over your abdomen, cover the area with plastic wrap, and place a heating pad or hot-water bottle on top (warm but not scalding; if it is too hot, place a towel between the heat source and the plastic wrap). Relax for 20 minutes.
- Look within to see if you are harboring suppressed emotions that could be exacerbating your physical issues. Over the years, I (Jill) have noticed that women with certain emotional issues are more prone to fibroids. These women often feel overwhelmed or unable to cope, overworked, or sometimes creatively stifled. They might be in conflicted relationships — with their spouses or other important people in their lives, with their work, or with their feelings about motherhood. See a therapist or life coach, particularly to explore ways in which you feel blocked.
- Try meditation.
- Do yoga.
- Learn to say no!

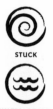

STUCK

WATERLOGGED

### Endometriosis

Endometriosis is one of the most common causes of infertility. It is estimated that about 10 to 20 percent of all women have it (with or without symptoms) and that between 20 and 50 percent of women seeking medical evaluations for infertility have it.

In endometriosis, islands of endometrial tissue — the lining of the uterus — grow *outside* the uterus. They can crop up pretty much anywhere in the pelvic area, including on the outer wall of the uterus, the ovaries, the fallopian tubes, and the pelvic wall. This misplaced tissue responds to hormones, particularly estrogen, just as it does when inside the uterus, growing and shrinking cyclically. But unlike the actual endometrium, which sloughs off each month, endometriosis tissue has no way to get out of the body when it breaks down, and it can become inflamed. In some cases, it causes scar tissue or blocked fallopian tubes. Even if it doesn't advance that far, it can cause fertility problems. Women with endometriosis may have poorer results with IVF, usually because of implantation problems.

Endometriosis symptoms may include painful periods or cramps, heavy periods, pain at ovulation, and spotting before the period begins. It can also cause pain during or after intercourse with deep penetration, painful bowel movements during menstruation, and ovarian cysts. A hallmark is chronic pelvic pain, which can be, but isn't necessarily, severe and which can include back pain. Some women have endometriosis — even over large areas or with scarring — with little or no pain. Some have severe pain but relatively mild and contained cases of endometriosis. Some women just think painful periods are normal, so endometriosis can go undiagnosed for quite a while. Not infrequently, fertility problems are the first sign of endometriosis.

No one really knows what causes endometriosis. Current best guesses include excess estrogen, immune system weakness, and retrograde menstruation (blood and tissue flowing back into the fallopian tubes). Having your first period early and having your first pregnancy later both increase the risk of endometriosis.

Whatever the underlying cause, endometriosis interferes with fertility in several ways.

- The endometrial tissue itself can block the fallopian tubes or coat the ovaries. This accounts for about 5 percent of cases of infertility in women with endometriosis.
- Endometriosis can attract or activate an increased number of macrophages. Macrophages are large cells that clean up debris and bacteria, which is a good thing as long as they stick to getting rid of misplaced endometrial tissue. Macrophages also get rid of sperm that have swum through the tubes and into the abdominal cavity. Again, that's a good thing — until,

in women with endometriosis, overactivated macrophages enter the fallopian tubes, picking off sperm there before the sperm have a chance to reach their target. Macrophages also produce cytokines, chemicals that are toxic to both sperm and embryos.

- The scattered endometrial tissue has glands similar to those in the endometrium itself, and these glands secrete mucus that can clog up the ovaries or the fringelike fimbriae, located at the ovary end of the fallopian tubes to guide the eggs into the tubes.

- Endometriosis is associated with increased levels of prostaglandins, which make the fallopian tubes less flexible, and so more likely to get blocked and less likely to be able to sweep an egg along.

- Women with endometriosis are at increased risk of luteinized unruptured follicle syndrome (LUFS; see page 212) and luteal phase defect (LPD; see page 200).

- Many cases of endometriosis are the result of an inappropriate immune response. The body detects endometrial cells in the wrong place and mounts an inflammatory reaction to protect itself, attacking *all* endometrial tissue and thus creating a hostile environment for implantation.

Sometimes endometriosis symptoms are treated with birth control pills or other hormonal contraceptives, but that's obviously not an option when you want to conceive. Your doctor may suggest other hormone therapy or outpatient laparoscopic surgery. Laparoscopy is also used to diagnose endometriosis — the doctor has to get in there and have a look around to find it. Often diagnosis and treatment are done at the same time through laparoscopic surgery. After confirming that there is endometriosis, the surgeon will cauterize or laser the misplaced endometrial tissue.

### Chinese Medicine

Chinese medicine attributes endometriosis to blood stagnation. Stuck women are prone to it, though it may affect Waterlogged women as well.

Acupuncture can clear inflammation and improve blood flow in the pelvic area. Some herbs can help, but the herbs that help the most are not safe in pregnancy. I (Jill) usually have my patients take the herbs during their periods, when we can be sure they aren't pregnant. Sometimes I use very sensitive pregnancy tests to establish as early as we can whether there's a pregnancy, and so whether it is safe to take the herbs premenstrually, too. There are over-the-counter formulas to treat endometriosis, but you should not use them on your own if you are trying to conceive.

### Help Yourself

Much of what you can do to tame endometriosis is aimed at reducing exposure to excess estrogen, supporting the liver (as it breaks down estrogen), and improving circulation, in all the same ways you would for fibroids (see page 231). There is one difference, however. I (Jill) have not seen the same pattern of suppressed emotions with endometriosis that I have with fibroids.

You also can try the following:

- See an acupuncturist to clear inflammation and improve blood flow in the pelvic area.
- See an herbalist for beneficial Chinese formulas. Be aware that the herbs that help the most are not safe if you are pregnant.
- Include omega-3 fatty acids in your diet to fight inflammation and improve blood flow.
- Take evening primrose oil, eat fruits rich in vitamin C and bioflavonoids, and avoid hydrogenated fats to combat inflammation.
- Improve blood flow by avoiding strenuous exercise during your period (gentle or moderate exercise is good), avoiding inversions (such as yoga headstands) while you have your period, and using pads instead of tampons, which can interfere with the free flow of blood.

### Endometrial Polyps

Endometrial polyps are fleshy outgrowths of the lining of the uterus. These polyps can create an environment hostile to implantation (not unlike the action of an IUD). If they develop near the fallopian tubes,

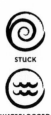

STUCK

WATERLOGGED

they can create a blockage. Polyps increase the risk of miscarriage and infertility.

Polyps are usually benign. Up to 10 percent of women have polyps, but many of them experience no symptoms at all. Signs of polyps can include long periods (more than five days), periods that start and stop, and heavy and clotted periods. Polyps can cause abnormal bleeding at any time during the menstrual cycle.

Your doctor may use a saline infusion sonogram (SIS; saline solution is used to distend the uterine cavity) or hysterosalpingogram (see page 198) to get a good look at your polyps. They may need to be surgically removed through a procedure called operative hysteroscopy. This is an outpatient procedure performed under general anesthesia or an epidural, with a camera guiding the surgeon in removing the polyp.

### Chinese Medicine

Chinese medicine views polyps essentially in the same way it does fibroids — as related to blood (Stuck) or phlegm (Waterlogged) stagnation. Herbs and acupuncture can be useful.

### Help Yourself

The advice here is the same as for fibroids (see page 232).

## Ovarian Cysts

STUCK

WATERLOGGED

An ovarian cyst is a fluid-filled sac in the ovary. These cysts are almost always benign, and most shrink away over a few cycles. But they can cause pelvic pain, back pain, or painful periods. And they can alter normal anatomy enough to prevent eggs from being picked up by the fallopian tubes, making conception impossible.

Many cysts cause no symptoms and are discovered during a routine pelvic exam (or an exam as part of a fertility workup), when the doctor feels a lump. A sonogram on day 4, 5, or 6 of your cycle can confirm the diagnosis and assess the size and appearance of the cyst.

Because most cysts go away on their own within a few cycles, one approach is to just watch and wait for two or three months. If the cyst has not resolved, your doctor may order an MRI or other 3-D ultrasound imaging.

Sometimes birth control pills are given for a few months to prevent ovulation so that no new cysts can form and any existing cysts can shrink away. But if time is critical, laparoscopic surgery might be the best course. (It might also be recommended if the cyst doesn't go away on its own, even after you've had several periods, if it gets larger, or if it looks in any way suspicious to your doctor.) Cysts can be removed through small incisions during an operative laparoscopy.

---

### Case Study: Lara

Lara, age 32, had a large ovarian cyst as a result of failed fertility treatment with FSH. (Cysts are a potential side effect of all fertility drugs.) She and her husband were still keen to conceive but couldn't because of the cyst. I (Jill) prescribed herbs, which Lara bought but never took because her doctor recommended against them.

After several months, the cyst remained the same size. Finally, Lara decided to schedule surgery, and the date was set for about a month later. Figuring that she had nothing to lose at this point, she decided to give the herbs a try. She took them for two weeks, then stopped them two weeks before the surgery. The first thing the doctor did in the operating room was to perform a sonogram of the cyst—and it was no longer there. The surgery was called off.

---

### Chinese Medicine

In Chinese medicine, ovarian cysts are usually attributed to a combination of damp stagnation (Waterlogged) and blood stagnation (Stuck).

To treat ovarian cysts, I (Jill) prescribe an herbal formula that strikes me as so effective it is practically miraculous. It reliably makes ovarian cysts go away in just one cycle. Nothing in Western medicine can do anything like it. It is not available over the counter, so an herbalist has to prescribe it. The formula contains Huang Qi (astragalus root), Zao Jiao Ci (gleditsia spine), Kun Bu (laminaria), Xia Ku Cao (prunella spica flower), San Leng (scirpus), E Zhu (zedoaria), Zao Jiao (gleditsia fruit), and Shui Zhi (leech).

### Help Yourself
- See an herbalist.

### Stenotic Cervix

DRY

Stenotic cervix is an uncommon condition in which the opening in the cervix leading to the uterus is very narrow (you might be told it is "closed"). This makes it hard for sperm to get in, and fewer of them will.

You are unlikely to have any symptoms from a stenotic cervix, although you may have bad cramps during your period as clots try to navigate the narrow opening on their way out of the uterus. Doctors diagnose stenotic cervix by direct observation—they can see and feel it during a pelvic exam.

There's no treatment for stenotic cervix, but if you need to, you can circumvent the problem with intrauterine insemination (IUI) to get pregnant (see page 325). Fortunately, a stenotic cervix usually softens and dilates normally during labor.

STUCK

### Asherman's Syndrome

Asherman's syndrome is a rare condition in which scar tissue forms in the uterus, usually after uterine surgery, including D & C. Any pelvic surgery can create scar tissue that could result in fertility problems. The scarring can cause decreased menstrual flow or amenorrhea (no period), infertility, early pregnancy loss, and/or repeated miscarriages. Scar tissue can also result from previous pregnancies with traumatic vaginal deliveries, C-sections, or other complications.

Asherman's is usually not detectable from a regular pelvic exam. It may not be detected until fertility problems occur. A vaginal saline ultrasound or HSG (see page 198) might pick it up. Hysteroscopy (see page 232) may be necessary to make the diagnosis and may also be used as a treatment, with the camera guiding the surgeon to remove problematic tissue. Such surgery resolves most cases of Asherman's syndrome, and the vast majority of women whose fertility problems are caused by the syndrome go on to have successful pregnancies after treatment.

#### *Chinese Medicine*
Asherman's is caused by blood stagnation due to trauma (such as surgery).

## MEN

NONSPECIFIC

### Sperm Problems

Men tend not to consider that a couple's fertility problems might be due to them. I (Sami) once had a man call me up and ask me to prescribe his wife fertility drugs, even though he had never been to see a doctor.

(I declined.) If sexual performance is okay, the thinking goes, there's no problem with the man.

Too many doctors are more than willing to go along with this. Sometimes those planning to wield powerful technologies to force a solution to the problem just don't care whether there's a low sperm count or the sperm are poor swimmers or somehow misshapen and ineffective. Before the advent of assisted reproductive technologies (ARTs), and especially intracytoplasmic sperm injection (ICSI; see page 334), men weren't so often ignored. But now the attitude seems to be, *I need only one good sperm. How hard can that be?* And they are right, as far as this logic goes. "Low sperm count" might still mean 10 million sperm. "Poor motility" (movement) might mean that more than half aren't swimming well. "Weak morphology" (structure) could knock out another couple of million curled, crooked, two-tailed, or otherwise ineffective sperm. A doctor armed with a good microscope is still going to have his or her choice of 2 million or so sperm for every milliliter of semen sample he or she has to work with. Pick a good-looking one, inject it straight into the egg (who cares if it has the ability to get in there itself?), and the woman is good to go — at least about a third of the time.

### Get Tested

We can't help but ask: why not just get a semen analysis? Maybe there's a problem and maybe there isn't, but at least you'll know for sure. If there *is* a problem, ICSI and IVF, or IUI, may still be the right approach. But maybe a far less invasive solution could be used instead. You will never know unless you get over the reluctance to collect a sample and bring it in to be examined under the microscope. Most "male factor" infertility is invisible, so this is the only way you're going to find out what you're dealing with. (Just make sure your doctor chooses an excellent lab specializing in semen analysis to minimize the possibility of poor lab work skewing your results.)

A semen analysis evaluates the number, movement, and shape of the sperm — officially known as count, motility, and morphology. Advanced techniques can specify structural and biochemical abnormalities within individual sperm. Problems in any one of these areas can make it difficult to conceive. Maybe not enough sperm reach the cervix — or not enough live ones, anyway. Or the ones that make it alive can't attach to or penetrate the egg effectively due to structural abnormalities. Remember the man who asked me (Sami) to prescribe fertility drugs for his wife? I convinced him to be checked out by a specialist, who determined that his sperm were abnormally shaped, so they couldn't penetrate an egg. No matter how many eggs his wife produced, his sperm weren't going to be able to fertilize any of them. Eventually, he agreed to be treated by a urologist specializing in male fertility, after which the couple successfully conceived.

There's also the possibility of low semen volume, which again results in not enough sperm heading toward the egg. Volume can be low because of anatomical issues or poor production of seminal fluid from the prostate and seminal vesicles. It can also be caused by dehydration, in which case drinking more water will fix the problem right away.

### Low on Sperm; Now What?

When a reliable semen analysis turns up any unfavorable numbers, you may want to consult a urologist who specializes in male fertility about your options. While you're waiting for that appointment, you can start improving the situation on your own: eat right, get proper sleep, and avoid alcohol, cigarettes, steroids, excessive heat, and stress. As we discussed in chapter 3, avoid hot tubs, saunas, electric blankets, tight underwear, hot baths, heated car seats, and a laptop placed on your lap. In addition, consider having more sex or otherwise ejaculating more often; prolonged abstinence can decrease sperm quality.

It makes sense to have another semen analysis after a few months to monitor the progress of any strategies you are implementing and to double-check the original results. Men make all new sperm every three months, so different behaviors can result in a different outcome on a second analysis. In addition, you can get different results depending on when you take the sample. If you are very stressed at the time, for example, volume may be low and the sperm may not be ejected from the vasa deferentia into the semen very well, leading to poor results. Under less stressful circumstances, results may well be normal. Also, other situations can cause temporary problems with sperm — for example, if you had a fever or had gone on a bit of a bender — and a repeat test once the sperm have had a chance to regenerate will come back normal.

### *Declining Sperm Counts*

Across the population at large, sperm counts have been declining steeply for decades. Pretty much all men today would have been considered infertile just two generations ago. In 1940, the average man had 113 million sperm per milliliter of semen. By 1960, he had only 66 million (a 45 percent drop), and the number has continued to go down ever since.

Average semen volume has decreased, too, as has the percentage of men with normal sperm morphology. A recent study showed that more than 40 percent of the sperm donors tracked since 1990 had abnormal sperm, versus only 5 percent of those tested before 1980.

The decline in average sperm count has been so emphatic that doctors have had to redefine "normal." Twenty years ago, men were expected to have about 40 million sperm per milliliter of semen to be considered fertile. Today 20 million is considered normal. Whatever the ideal benchmark, the number of men with sperm counts under 20 million has tripled, according to a *British Medical Journal* study. That study also found that a 30-year-old man in 2005 had, on average, just one-quarter of the sperm of a 30-year-old in 1955.

It may be that the experts have gone just a bit too far in redefining male fertility and that what is considered normal now is just too low. Twenty million sperm may be the average, but calling it "normal" can't obscure the fact that it's often not enough to conceive a child easily. A *New England Journal of Medicine* study showed that men who successfully conceived with their partners averaged more than 48 million sperm per milliliter of semen.

What's "normal" for motility is a closer match to reality. A semen analysis will come back as A-OK if about 60 percent of the sperm show good forward movement. The *New England Journal of Medicine* study found that successful spontaneous conceptions occurred with men with about 63 percent motility.

### *Causes*

The cause of the overall decline in sperm quantity and quality remains something of a mystery, but a number of factors are clearly at play, including rising rates of prescription drug use; more exposure to alcohol, cigarettes, and recreational drugs; and increasing exposure to environmental toxins such as pesticides and other pollutants (including exposure in the womb) that interfere with crucial hormones. Genetic disorders (which account for somewhere between 2 and 5 percent of men diagnosed with infertility), kidney disease, diabetes, and cancer and cancer treatments can also negatively affect sperm count and quality. We've already mentioned stress as a cause, and that goes for physical as well as psychological stress.

### Chinese Medicine

Chinese medicine relates sperm production to kidney qi. Most sperm problems can be attributed to yang deficiency (Tired) or yin deficiency (Dry), although some may be due to damp stagnation (Waterlogged). Stuck or Pale could be affected as well.

Acupuncture and Chinese herbs can help increase sperm count and motility, and to a lesser degree morphology (see the box on pages 158–59). The herbs that work vary widely according to type and specifics of the problem.

### Help Yourself

- Consult an acupuncturist and/or an herbalist for help with sperm problems.

STUCK

### Varicoceles

Varicoceles are one of the most common conditions affecting men's fertility. Up to about 20 percent of all men have varicoceles, but among men with fertility problems, up to 40 percent have them. This rate is even higher among men who have already fathered children and are now having fertility problems ("secondary infertility").

A varicocele is a cluster of enlarged veins (more or less the same thing as varicose veins) in the testicles. The blood that collects in the area of a varicocele heats up the testicle to 98.6°F; the ideal testicular temperature is 96°F to 97°F. The extra heat can damage or destroy existing sperm, change sperm shape, and impair the production of new sperm, which can impair fertility or contribute to miscarriage. Varicoceles can also cause low testosterone levels.

Most men with varicoceles have no symptoms; a fertility problem may be the first sign of this condition. But varicoceles may cause discomfort, a kind of pulling pain. You or your doctor, on routine exam, may discover a varicocele by noting that one of your testicles feels like "a bag of worms."

If you do feel a varicocele, or wonder whether you have one because you haven't found another explanation for your fertility issues, see a urologist or other specialist in male fertility for diagnosis and discussion of your options. Microsurgery can eliminate a varicocele and restore fertility. You may still need a bit of patience, however. Only about 35 percent of couples get pregnant within a year after surgical correction of a varicocele, but up to 80 percent are pregnant within two years.

---

### Case Study: Khalid and Fatima

Khalid and Fatima had been trying for more than a year to conceive, and I (Sami) had seen them several times already for inseminations. I had been urging Khalid to see a specialist in male fertility as well, and when he finally took my suggestion, his doctor discovered a varicocele and suggested surgery to correct it. Just a couple days after the surgery, I had good news for them: Fatima was pregnant.

Khalid called me to give me a piece of his mind. He was none too pleased to have had surgery he "didn't need" since the latest insemination had worked. But sadly, Fatima had a miscarriage a few weeks later, presumably because of abnormal DNA in the sperm.

I never had another appointment with them because they went on to have two children with no further inseminations or any other intervention or assistance. Once the varicocele was gone, Khalid's sperm were healthy enough to do the job on their own.

---

### *Chinese Medicine*

It's easy to understand the Chinese view of varicoceles: blood stagnation. This is a common problem among Stuck men.

There is some evidence that Chinese herbs can help improve circulation, shrink varicoceles, and improve sperm count and motility in patients with varicoceles. There is no doubt, however, that surgery is even more effective and, of course, faster and more permanent.

### *Help Yourself*
- See an herbalist.

NONSPECIFIC

### Testicular Trauma

Injury of the testicles can compromise the blood supply, and this can damage the sperm production mechanism. A severe blow from playing sports or from a fight may be all it takes. Be especially concerned if there's swelling of the testicles or bleeding in or around them. The particular injury known as testicular torsion (twisting) can create a similar problem unless it is quickly treated surgically.

#### *Chinese Medicine*

Chinese medicine looks at testicular trauma as blood stagnation due to trauma. Herbs and acupuncture may be useful.

#### *Help Yourself*
- Keep swelling down after a blow to the testicles with cold compresses and anti-inflammatories.

STUCK

WATERLOGGED

### Blockage of the Vas Deferens

An obstruction of the vas deferens (the tube that transports sperm from the testicle to the urethra) can prevent sperm from getting where they need to go and from becoming fully or properly formed. Following are the most common causes of blockage.

**Surgery.** Hernia repair, correction of an undescended testicle, prostate surgery, surgery for testicular cancer, surgery to correct a hydrocele (a fluid-filled sac surrounding a testicle that results in swelling of the scrotum) — any surgery in the groin, in fact — can create an obstruction of the vas deferens.

**Vasectomy.** The whole point of a vasectomy is to obstruct the vasa deferentia. Keep in mind that men who have had a vasectomy "reversed" may still run into trouble with blockages if scar tissue remains.

**Congenital absence of vas deferens.** Some males are born with no vas deferens on one or both sides. The seminal vesicles, which make other components of semen, may be missing as well.

**Undescended testicle.** This must be corrected surgically

(most often in infancy or childhood) to protect fertility. But even when caught early, surgery is not a guarantee of future fertility.

**Infection.** Any infection can cause a blockage of the vas deferens. Chlamydia, gonorrhea, and tuberculosis are particularly troublesome in this way.

**Orchitis.** Viral infections can cause testicular inflammation, known as orchitis, which can in turn cause sperm production to fail.

**Mumps orchitis.** This is a common side effect of mumps, occurring several days after the virus first appears and affecting about a third of male mumps patients who are past puberty. Mumps orchitis can destroy sperm-producing cells in the testicles, resulting in a permanently low, or even absent, sperm count. Fortunately, most cases of mumps orchitis affect only one testicle, so most men who have had it after puberty do make sperm, although the count may be low. They can get their partners pregnant, but they may need assistance from IUI or IVF. Mumps orchitis can cause testicular atrophy, but again usually only on one side.

### Chinese Medicine

Chinese medicine attributes vas deferens blockages to stagnation of blood (Stuck) or phlegm (Waterlogged).

## OTHER STRUCTURAL OR ANATOMICAL ISSUES

A range of uncommon structural or anatomical issues can cause fertility problems. They are rare, but if none of the common explanations apply, be sure that your doctor has ruled out these issues before you accept a diagnosis of unexplained infertility.

**Women:**
Endometrial hyperplasia
Adenomyosis (endometriosis inside the muscle of the uterus)
Pelvic adhesions or scarring
Dysfunctional uterine bleeding

Septated uterus

Bicornate uterus

Vaginismus

Vulvitis

Vulva vestibulitis

Congenital defect causing sexual malfunction

Painful intercourse or other sexual malfunction

**Men:**

Hydrocele

Blocked ejaculatory duct

Genetic or congenital disorder

## Making Babies Action Plan

The following action plans summarize the testing needed to establish whether your fertility problems stem from any of these structural or anatomical issues. They will guide you through your potential testing program as efficiently as possible. For women, we've organized them roughly the way they need to be timed to your cycle, so that you can schedule the tests appropriately and get them all completed in as short a time as possible. (Timing is not usually an issue for men.) Not everyone will need all these tests, and these may not be all the tests you need. Your doctor will guide you as to which tests you need, of course, but you should make sure that your understanding, gleaned from the descriptions in this chapter, lines up with your doctor's plans.

## TESTS FOR WOMEN

| TEST | CONDITION | TYPES MOST LIKELY TO NEED IT | TIMING |
|------|-----------|------------------------------|--------|
| Ultrasound of ovaries and uterus | Fibroids; ovarian cysts; adenomyosis | STUCK / WATERLOGGED | Just after period ends (day 4, 5, or 6 of typical cycle); for fibroids, anytime |
| HSG | Blocked fallopian tubes; fibroids; endometrial polyps | STUCK / WATERLOGGED | After period ends but before ovulation (day 7, 8, or 9 of typical cycle) |
| | Asherman's syndrome; repeated miscarriages; to check shape of uterus | NONSPECIFIC | After period ends but before ovulation (day 7, 8, or 9 of typical cycle) |
| Laparoscopy | Blocked fallopian tubes; fibroids; endometriosis; pelvic adhesions (scar tissue) | STUCK / WATERLOGGED | After period ends but before ovulation (day 7, 8, or 9 of typical cycle) |
| Pelvic exam | Stenotic cervix | DRY | Best before ovulation |

| TEST | CONDITION | TYPES MOST LIKELY TO NEED IT | TIMING |
|---|---|---|---|
| Saline infusion ultrasound | Asherman's syndrome; endometrial polyps; sub-mucous fibroids | STUCK; WATERLOGGED | After period ends |
| Hysteroscopy | Fibroids; endometrial polyps | STUCK; WATERLOGGED | After period ends |
| | Asherman's syndrome; endometrial polyps; abnormal endometrial pathology | STUCK | After period ends |
| MRI or other 3-D imaging | Fibroids; ovarian cysts; endometrial polyps | STUCK; WATERLOGGED | After period ends |
| Pelvic exam | Fibroids; ovarian cysts | STUCK; WATERLOGGED | After ovulation |

## TESTS FOR MEN

| TEST | CONDITION | TYPES MOST LIKELY TO NEED IT |
|---|---|---|
| Semen analysis | Sperm count, motility, or morphology problems; infection | NONSPECIFIC |
| | Blockage of vas deferens (no sperm) | STUCK |
| Physical exam | Varicocele | STUCK |
| | Testicular trauma | NONSPECIFIC |
| Scrotal sonogram | Varicocele; testicular tumor | STUCK |
| | Testicular trauma | NONSPECIFIC |
| Testicular biopsy | Azoospermia (no sperm) | STUCK |
| Semen cultures | Prostatitis; urethritis | WATERLOGGED   Also, anyone with these conditions should talk with his doctor about a semen culture. |
| FSH, LH, testosterone levels | Hormone imbalance; testicular failure | NONSPECIFIC |

# CHAPTER SIXTEEN

# Infections

nfections can affect anyone, of course, and they can also affect fertility. In fact, undetected and untreated infections are the most commonly overlooked cause of infertility. About 15 percent of infertility cases can be traced back to an infection, and infections account for an even higher percentage of early pregnancy loss. An infection is so often the answer to the puzzle of unexplained infertility that we joke that antibiotics are Sami's favorite fertility drugs. Infections are also a common cause of IVF failure. Waterlogged types are especially prone to fertility problems stemming from infections.

Any woman undergoing IVF will get antibiotics as part of her treatment. That's because of the concern that any bacteria lingering in her reproductive tract — even if it doesn't cause signs of an infection — could interfere with pregnancy. The docs are right to worry: one study showed that E. coli found in the cervical mucus greatly diminished success rates of IVF. So it's absolutely a legitimate concern, but it's addressed in a completely backward manner. If bacteria can prevent pregnancy, why not just treat the couple with antibiotics, let them do their work, and then see if nature is able to take its course before jumping to IVF?

According to the Centers for Disease Control (CDC), the rate of sexually transmitted diseases (STDs) in this country is at an all-time high, and the rate continues to rise for many types of infections. Between 5 and 10 percent of people carry chlamydia bacteria, for instance, and that's more than twice the level of a decade ago. By far the majority of these people have no symptoms whatsoever.

Silent infections like these are so widespread that we think they are probably a major cause of unexplained infertility. But we want to emphasize that not all of the infections causing infertility are sexually transmitted, or *only* sexually transmitted. Ureaplasma, mycoplasma, E. coli, klebsiella, and others are not spread solely by sexual relations, and they often linger without causing symptoms — apart from infertility or early pregnancy loss. So don't make the mistake of thinking that just because you are in a monogamous relationship, you can ignore these infections.

Every couple struggling with unexplained infertility ought to be screened for bacteria and infections so mild that they're flying under the radar. (In fact, it would probably be a good idea for anyone preparing for pregnancy to be screened.) And couples ought to do it long before they sign up for IVF or any other major intervention. As mentioned previously, Waterlogged people are especially prone to infections that hamper fertility, but all fertility types can experience this. So Waterlogged types might want to get tested for infections right away, while other types probably don't need to rush into testing unless they have an unexplained fertility problem.

A strong immune system, bolstered by a good diet and good sleeping habits, can eradicate infections on its own. This may take a long time, however — time you may not feel you have, especially since you can't know for sure in advance if your immune system can beat the infection. It's also possible that you've already had the infection for a long time and haven't been able to clear it. So we recommend attacking bacteria with antibiotics *and* a healthy lifestyle to support the immune system. And in all cases, both partners should be treated at the same time.

Infections may look different or act differently in men and women, as described in the next two sections.

## WOMEN

NONSPECIFIC

Untreated chlamydia has long been known as a cause of female infertility. Chronic chlamydia infection can develop into pelvic inflammatory disease (PID), which can cause scarring in the fallopian tubes and an increased risk of ectopic pregnancy or infertility. Once it's gotten that far, the problem is no longer treatable with antibiotics. Chlamydia infection is often without symptoms, however, so it often goes undetected.

Chlamydia is just one bacteria that can interfere with fertility. Other common culprits include E. coli, enterococcus, staphylococcus, ureaplasma, mycoplasma, and gonorrhea. Yeast infections (*Candida albicans*) can be problematic as well. Studies have shown that about 25 to 30 percent of women seeking treatment for infertility carry microorganisms that can impair fertility.

In addition to causing problems in the female reproductive tract, these infections can damage, inhibit, or kill sperm. They can cause the sperm to stick together (agglutinate) so they can't function properly, impair the sperm's ability to move, or affect the sperm's ability to penetrate an egg. Bacteria in the cervical mucus (cervicitis) can also attach to sperm swimming through and eventually attach to the egg, thereby infecting the embryo. Sperm can also carry bacteria they pick up as they pass through a catheter for IUI or IVF.

These infections can be very subtle, causing essentially no symptoms, so the only way to know you have one may be for your doctor to order a lab test of your cervical mucus (see page 269). They can also cause odor or burning, pain and fever, and in severe cases, as with chlamydia and gonorrhea, pelvic scarring and infertility that is much harder to treat than by simply taking a course of antibiotics.

Both partners must be treated with antibiotics if one is diagnosed with an infection. They likely have already shared the bacteria, and if one partner is left untreated, he or she could easily reinfect the other.

---

### Case Study: Evelyn

Evelyn, whom we mentioned in chapter 1, had been battling infertility since before she was 30. Over the course of ten years, she'd been in the care of four different doctors, been pumped up with incredibly strong fertility drugs fifty times, and never been pregnant. Evelyn was literally risking her life and health by taking so many drugs, and no one ever stopped to investigate why she wasn't getting pregnant.

In the end, all it took was a course of standard antibiotics. On her first visit to my (Sami's) office, I cultured her cervix for bacteria, a routine check (at least in my office) when there's no obvious cause for failure to get pregnant. The lab found a mycoplasma infection, which can indeed cause infertility or early pregnancy loss. After the antibiotics cleared that up, Evelyn was pregnant with her daughter within a month. Two years later, when she was 42, she had a son, conceived without any medical intervention at all.

## MEN

NONSPECIFIC

The same bacteria that cause fertility problems in women also cause fertility problems when they take up residence in the male reproductive tract. Infections can cause low sperm count, impaired motility, low sperm quality, and genetic damage to sperm. Men may experience fertility problems even if their sperm look normal and no problems show up on basic semen analysis. Furthermore, with infection in the prostate (prostatitis) or urethra (urethritis), bacteria may attach to the sperm at the time of ejaculation, and the sperm can transport that bacteria all the way to the egg.

Just as with women, most of the time these bacteria cause low-grade (mild) infections without any symptoms, and they go undetected and untreated, sometimes for years. To find out if you have a silent infection, your doctor has to order lab tests of your semen. Even if the semen culture shows no bacteria, if white blood cells show up on standard semen analysis, indicating that an immune response is under way, that's reason enough to presume that there's an infection and both partners need to take antibiotics. In some cases, bacterial infections can cause severe symptoms in men. Untreated chlamydia, for example, can lead to swelling of the testicles or epididymis, scarring, and sterility. These cases are almost always treated, however, because of the painful symptoms and so, ironically, are of less concern than silent infections.

If a man tests positive for an infection, it is easily treated with a course of antibiotics. Antibiotic treatment will not only clear the infection but also reverse the negative effects of the infection on sperm—and in so doing, dramatically increase pregnancy rates. Immediately after treatment, the body will produce far fewer abnormal sperm and keep making new healthy sperm, so sperm quality will quickly be back to normal. A study in Mexico underlined this point: Of 193 men seeking fertility treatment with their partners, about three-quarters were infected with both chlamydia and mycoplasma. After taking antibiotics, the vast majority of those couples got pregnant with no other treatment.

By the way, any infection, anywhere in the body—a viral flu with a high fever, for example, or even just a bad cold—can have a negative impact on sperm for as long as two months afterward. Pretty much anything causing a fever can hamper a man's reproductive efforts until the natural turnover of sperm replaces damaged sperm with healthy new ones.

---

### Case Study: Ang Suk and Myung

Ang Suk and Myung live halfway around the world but heard about me (Sami) from a doctor friend in New York. They had two lovely daughters, but after the second was born, they had experienced two miscarriages, then two years of what but after the doctors labeled "unexplained secondary infertility." They had spent more than $100,000 on IVF and other medical interventions to help them get pregnant, but nothing had worked.

After one visit with them, I ordered lab tests, which found ureaplasma in Ang Suk's cervical mucus. Ureaplasma can cause miscarriage and infertility. It also produces inflammation that can harm an embryo. His-and-hers doses of tetracycline got rid of the bacteria, and Ang Suk was pregnant two months later, with no other help from me or their previous doctors. She went on to have a healthy baby boy.

---

## CHINESE MEDICINE

Chinese medicine, like Western medicine, considers infections to be the result of pathogens, but also the result of an environment inside the body that makes the presence of pathogens more likely. The infection itself is seen as dampness combined with heat and toxicity. Waterlogged people are more susceptible to infections than others, but infections can strike in all fertility types. An infection can't take hold unless the defensive qi (the immune system) is weak and the conditions are right for the growth of the pathogen.

Chinese herbs and acupuncture can be helpful in fighting reproductive system infections. They should always be used with antibiotics to help stop a recurrence.

## HELP YOURSELF

- Boost your immune system by eating a nutrient-rich diet, especially foods rich in beta-carotene and vitamins C and E. Zinc boosts immunity and has been shown to prevent the recurrence of infections, so be sure to include that in your diet as well.
- Eat garlic, which has strong antibacterial properties, to help fight infections.
- If you take antibiotics, take a probiotic such as *Lactobacillus acidophilus* to restore the "good" bacteria in your gut once

treatment is complete. Half a cup of yogurt twice a day is a good alternative, if not quite as effective. At YinOva, we use probiotic capsules from Metagenics (see Resources), which contain no dairy. Take according to package instructions.

- See an herbalist and/or an acupuncturist to help fight infections. Some infections are very stubborn, however, and recurrence is a major issue. Always use herbs or acupuncture in conjunction with antibiotics to prevent a recurrence.

## Making Babies Action Plan

The following action plans summarize the testing needed to establivsh whether your fertility problems stem from an infection. Infections that interfere with fertility can strike in all fertility types. Waterlogged types are particularly prone to infections, including bacterial infections, so people who are Waterlogged should consider being tested for infections early in the process of getting worked up for infertility. Other types should be tested if there is no other explanation found for their fertility troubles. Not everyone will need all these tests, and these may not be all the tests you need. Your doctor will guide you as to which tests you need, of course, but you should make sure that your understanding, gleaned from the descriptions in this chapter, lines up with your doctor's plans.

### TESTS FOR WOMEN

| TEST | CONDITION | TYPES MOST LIKELY TO NEED IT | TIMING |
|---|---|---|---|
| Cervical mucus culture (postcoital test) | Infection | WATERLOGGED | 1 to 3 days before ovulation is expected |

| | TESTS FOR MEN | |
|---|---|---|
| TEST | CONDITION | TYPES MOST LIKELY TO NEED IT |
| Semen culture | Infection |  WATERLOGGED |
| White blood cell count (in semen) | Immune response (sign of infection) | WATERLOGGED |

# CHAPTER SEVENTEEN

# Immune System Issues

Immunological fertility issues occur in all fertility types, particularly among women. The first part of this chapter covers autoimmune reactions that can cause pregnancy loss or IVF failure (primarily because of their effects on women); the second part covers antisperm antibodies, which cause immune infertility.

## AUTOIMMUNE REACTIONS

NONSPECIFIC

Over the past five years or so, we've seen more women with autoimmune problems of one kind or another (allergies, lupus, Crohn's disease, rheumatoid arthritis, chronic fatigue, thyroid problems) affecting their fertility. Endometriosis, recurrent miscarriages, and IVF failure are common among these women. Unfortunately, not all doctors recognize how these issues affect reproduction. We believe that immunity issues are the third most commonly overlooked cause of infertility (after infections and endometriosis).

If you are suffering from repeated miscarriages, your immune system may be to blame. Experts estimate that up to 20 percent of miscarriages are related to autoimmune reactions. It's as if the woman's body has an allergic reaction to the embryo. In addition, "unexplained infertility" is often not infertility at all, but rather early and recurrent miscarriages due to inappropriate immune reactions.

Miscarriage may not technically be a fertility problem (conception and implantation *do* take place), but we're including it here for two reasons. The first is that the end result is the same — your desire for parenthood is frustrated — and solving the problem will help you become a parent. The second is that the same immune system issues that result in miscarriage also cause fertility problems (no conception and implantation). There are four main markers of immune problems in women with recurrent pregnancy loss: antithyroid antibodies, antiphospholipid antibodies (thrombophilias), natural killer cells, and antinuclear antibodies. This section looks at each in turn.

### Antithyroid Antibodies

Hypothyroidism (low thyroid hormone levels) is most commonly caused by high levels of antibodies directed against the thyroid gland. It is also possible to have notable levels of these antibodies and a thyroid gland that's working just fine, at least for now. The antibodies increase the risk of hypothyroidism, however, so your doctor should keep tabs on them. Just as hypothyroid women are at greater risk for miscarriage (see page 272), so too are women with high antibodies but normal thyroid levels. That holds true for women undergoing IVF as well. Keep in mind that thyroid function can change during pregnancy, and your doctor should be monitoring this, especially during the first trimester. Closer attention must be paid to women with known thyroid problems, but all pregnant women should be tested once during the first trimester, as should anyone having problems getting pregnant. A blood test can determine whether you have high antithyroid antibodies.

Scientists are as yet unsure exactly why the antithyroid antibodies–miscarriage link exists. It may be that antithyroid antibodies come along with other immune system problems that are the real troublemakers. Or it could be that the antibodies just get a bit confused and "cross-react" against the placenta or the embryo. In any case, taking supplemental thyroid hormone can reduce the risk of miscarriage.

### Antiphospholipid Antibodies (APAs)

Antiphospholipid antibodies (APAs) mistakenly attack normal cells as if they were invaders. When APAs attach to the phospholipids (the fat molecules that help make up cell membranes), it makes them sticky, and they clump together, leading to poor blood flow and clots. This can cause several health problems, including stroke or heart attack, later in life. Improper blood flow to the endometrium or placenta means that not enough nutrients and oxygen are supplied, and this can prevent implantation or cause early miscarriage.

If you are experiencing unexplained infertility, recurrent miscarriages, or chemical pregnancies but don't know why, talk with your doctor about getting a blood test for APAs. APAs show up in about 15 percent of women with recurrent miscarriages.

If you have APAs, your doctor will probably prescribe daily low-dose aspirin (formerly "baby aspirin") and/or an injectable anticoagulant such as heparin or Lovenox in more severe cases, to counter their effects. This regimen will thin out the blood, reducing the risk of blood clots and miscarriage.

I (Sami) recommend daily low-dose aspirin to almost all my patients. Aspirin is a blood thinner, and low doses can improve blood flow to the uterus and placenta and prevent clotting that can interfere with implantation. Chinese medicine uses a similar pathway when acupuncture is given to increase blood flow to the uterus. (Be sure to consult with a professional before taking aspirin in combination with herbs or anything else.)

Many women have problems with implantation that are hard to detect or pin down, and aspirin can help. It is not likely to hurt the mother or fetus (with the possible exception of people with a history of stomach ulcers or bleeding or gastritis, or people with clotting disorders, who should not take aspirin). Just as low-dose aspirin is widely used to help prevent heart attack and stroke, a daily dose is useful for a broad range of women who are trying to get pregnant.

Women who have had repeated miscarriages, early pregnancy losses, or failed IVF cycles should be evaluated for more serious clotting disorders, including thrombophilia (overactive clotting). They may need to see a hematologist, who specializes in this kind of thing. In some cases, injectable blood thinners may be called for. Although most women should stop taking low-dose aspirin after the first trimester, in some cases it should be taken throughout pregnancy. For example, a woman with the marker for MTHFR, a genetic abnormality that increases clotting and with it the risk of heart attack, stroke, and miscarriage, may be able to carry a baby to term with low-dose aspirin throughout pregnancy, given along with high doses of folic acid.

## Natural Killer Cells

Natural killer (NK) cells are a normal and, despite the fearsome name, helpful part of your immune system. Your body makes these particularly aggressive white blood cells specifically to seek out rapidly growing and dividing cells—such as bacterial and viral infections and cancer—and destroy them. They are also normally present in the uterine lining in the luteal phase, where they help promote implantation.

NK cells may also be a cause of recurrent miscarriages, however. In some women, these cells go into overdrive and overreact to a pregnancy, attacking the embryo the same way they attack cancer cells. All it takes is a simple blood test to determine whether your NK cells are working too hard.

The treatment I (Sami) recommend is intravenous gamma globulins, steroids, or intralipid infusions to suppress the immune system just long enough to get pregnancy established (usually through the first three months), though not all fertility specialists take this approach or even test for NK cells.

### Antinuclear Antibodies

Antinuclear antibodies exist to attack the nuclei of cells invading your body. If the fertilized egg is mistaken for an invader, they can sometimes attack its nucleus, too. Small amounts of antinuclear antibodies in the blood are normal—about 5 percent of healthy people have them. People with autoimmune diseases such as lupus and rheumatoid arthritis tend to have high levels of these antibodies, which can lead to inflammation in the uterus and placenta and then to implantation failure, recurrent miscarriages, or unexplained infertility. Women with high levels of antinuclear antibodies face lower chances of success with IVF and ICSI, too.

If you are having trouble getting pregnant, discuss with your doctor having the simple blood test that measures your level of antinuclear antibodies. Standard treatment is a steroid such as prednisone to suppress inflammatory and immune response, lowering the level of antibodies. If your level is very high, above 1:160, you should also see a rheumatologist.

### Chinese Medicine

You might think the best way to handle immune issues is to boost the immune system—just what you'd want to do if you caught colds all the time or had some other sign of immune deficiency. But simply making the immune system stronger, when it is already rather hyperactive, is a mistake—and a commonly made one. What you really want to do is bring your immune system back into balance, not turbocharge it. Substantially improving these conditions requires a certain amount of finesse on the part of an herbalist.

In the Chinese medicine view, no one fertility type is more likely than others to have immune system issues. They are rooted in weak qi and yang (Tired), leading to poor fluid metabolism (Waterlogged), leading to stagnation of qi and blood (Stuck), leading to heat and thus causing deficiency in yin (Dry) and blood (Pale).

Clotting disorders such as APAs and MTHFR are considered to be about blood stagnation. From the Chinese medical perspective, blood stagnation refers to any kind of poor blood circulation, in this case in the uterus. Stuck types are particularly prone to such stagnation.

When applied correctly, Chinese medicine can be very effective in treating a misbehaving immune system. Treatment should focus on your particular fertility type, as well as any other condition you might have. The goal is to achieve a balanced system, not simply to boost qi.

### Help Yourself

- See a Chinese medicine practitioner for herbs and acupuncture tailored to your specific situation — to clear heat, move qi and damp, and/or support qi and yin.
- Adopt a daily stress management routine, such as yoga, meditation, or going for a walk after work to unwind. Stress increases the production and release of cortisol, which ultimately suppresses your immune system.
- Avoid alcohol and smoking altogether, and keep refined sugar and caffeine to a minimum, as they all put extra stress on your immune system.
- Load up on antioxidants such as vitamin C (in reasonable amounts), vitamin E, and beta-carotene, which are beneficial to the immune system. Include them in your diet and also consider supplements.
- Consider taking a zinc supplement, as zinc is helpful to the immune system.
- Ask your doctor about taking a para-aminobenzoic acid (PABA) supplement to improve some autoimmune conditions.
- Eat more alkaline-producing foods, such as whole grains and

vegetables, and fewer acid-producing ones, such as meat, alcohol, and coffee.

- Make sure you're getting enough folic acid — 2 to 3 mg (2,000 to 3,000 mcg) a day.

### *Antiphospholipid Antibodies*

- After consulting with a professional if you take herbs or other medications or supplements, take one low-dose (81 mg) aspirin daily. This is especially important for Stuck types. You can buy a bottle of low-dose aspirin, formerly known as "baby aspirin," at any drugstore. It's the equivalent of about one-quarter of one regular strength tablet. Aspirin should be taken after a full meal to prevent irritation of the stomach. You can take low-dose aspirin for as long as you like while trying to get pregnant, but you should stop at the end of your first trimester unless your doctor advises otherwise. Using aspirin this way has been shown to improve the uterine lining, and this improves implantation. A study published in 2000 demonstrated that treatment with baby aspirin increased the thickness of the uterine lining, thanks to improved blood flow, which in turn increased pregnancy rates in women struggling with infertility. An Israeli study demonstrated that women who were diagnosed with autoimmune problems and had repeated IVF failures achieved an amazing 37 percent pregnancy rate when they used low-dose aspirin along with IVF.
- See a licensed herbalist for blood-moving herbs (herbs with anticoagulant effects). This is not a condition to treat herbally on your own; you need the supervision of an herbalist. This is doubly important if you want to combine herbs with aspirin therapy.
- Try acupuncture to increase blood flow to the uterus.

### *Natural Killer Cells*

- Take a fish oil supplement to moderate NK cell activity.
- Use a liquid chlorophyll supplement to move NK cells from the blood into tissues. Fewer NK cells floating in the bloodstream means fewer NK cells available to overreact to sperm or embryos.

*Antinuclear Antibodies*

- See an herbalist for damp- and heat-clearing herbs. This is not a condition to treat herbally on your own; you need the supervision of an herbalist.

## ANTISPERM ANTIBODIES

NONSPECIFIC

The most common immune system issue affecting fertility is what is essentially an allergy to sperm. In many cases of unexplained infertility, the mystery can be solved by a test for antisperm antibodies.

As mentioned earlier, antibodies are proteins the immune system uses to identify and protect itself against foreign intruders. That's good when it means combating a cold virus but bad when the body mistakenly attacks innocents abroad, such as tree pollen (as in seasonal allergies) or, more directly to the point here, sperm.

A woman's body may make antibodies to her partner's sperm, killing or disabling them as soon as they get into the cervical mucus. Or a man might make antibodies against his own sperm, putting them out of commission one way or another well before they ever get near an egg. If the sperm aren't killed outright, the antibodies may inactivate their ability to attach to and penetrate an egg. Antisperm antibodies can also cause sperm to stick together (agglutination), rendering them ineffective. In men, antisperm antibodies are usually made after an obstruction (including blockage of the vas deferens; see page 246) or injury of some kind, especially vasectomy reversal. In women, the cause is unknown.

The submicroscopic antibodies can't be seen in the mucus or semen or on the sperm, and they cause no symptoms. The simplest way to find out if antisperm antibodies might be your problem is to have a postcoital test (see page 197). If it shows fertile cervical mucus of appropriate stretchiness and a neutral pH (not acidic), but the sperm are dead or shaking in place rather than swimming heartily around, antisperm antibodies could be the problem.

The only definitive way to know whether you or your partner have antisperm antibodies, however, is to have an immunobead binding test. This test examines the man's semen to see if it contains antibodies, which appear as telltale beads on the sperm, and it looks at the sperm mixed with the man's blood and with the woman's blood to see if antibodies form.

Antibodies may attach to the head or tail of the sperm. If they attach to the head, the proteins coat the head like a layer of plastic wrap, so the enzymes that help it bind to and penetrate the egg can't get out to do their thing. If the antibodies are directed at the tail, the sperm can't swim. Either way, the sperm will be nonfunctional but alive, so a post-coital test may not raise a red flag. If you have had a good postcoital test, with live sperm, but are experiencing unexplained infertility, you should get tested for antisperm antibodies. Likewise, if you've had IVF where there's been "good sperm" and a "good egg" but no fertilization, you and your partner should have this checked out.

---

### Case Study: Sherry and Tom

Sherry, age 38, had struggled with infertility for sixteen years, through three marriages. She had sought help from infertility specialists and had three "full" infertility workups, but the results had always been the same: she was normal. Her husbands each tested normal as well. The doctors found absolutely nothing in their evaluations to explain why Sherry wasn't getting pregnant, so she was given the diagnosis of "unexplained infertility."

But none of them had ever been tested for antisperm antibodies. I (Sami) ordered an immuno-bead binding test on Sherry's and Tom's blood and on his sperm, and this showed that her body was having an allergic reaction to sperm, killing them off as if they were hostile invaders. Next time she ovulated, Sherry took a moderate-dose steroid for seven days to block her immune system's overreaction. She was then inseminated with her husband's sperm via IUI, to get the sperm as close as possible, as quickly as possible, to the fallopian tubes so that her body had less time to react. It took a few tries, but within four months Sherry was pregnant.

---

The typical response to this problem (as it is to most fertility problems) is to try IVF with ICSI. That can work, but so can the less invasive IUI. In either case, a low-dose steroid such as prednisone should be taken for a few days before ovulation to suppress the inappropriate immune reaction. This greatly improves the chances for pregnancy. (It's also possible to get pregnant through intercourse, but that won't work as well as IUI.) If three or four ovulatory cycles with IUI don't do the trick, IVF is the next logical step.

### Chinese Medicine

Women or men making antibodies to sperm are considered to be exhibiting a subtle form of blood stagnation which could be seen in any type.

A yin-nourishing herbal formula with blood-moving herbs added can reduce the antibody load for men and women.

### Help Yourself

- See an herbalist for a formula that's appropriately tailored to your situation.
- Try the over-the-counter Chinese herbal formula Zhi Bai Di Huang Wan (anemarrhena, philodendron, rehmannia). According to research done at Shanghai Medical University in 1995, this formula reduced antisperm antibodies in more than 80 percent of infertile couples with the antibodies. You should be able to find it in your health food store. Take it according to package directions.

## Making Babies Action Plan

The following action plan summarizes the testing needed to establish whether your fertility problems stem from any of these immunological issues. It will guide you through your potential testing program as efficiently as possible. These tests are the same for men and women, except the postcoital test, which is performed only on women. Not everyone will need all these tests, and these may not be all the tests you need. Your doctor will guide you as to which tests you need, of course, but you should make sure that your understanding, gleaned from the descriptions in this chapter, lines up with your doctor's plans.

| TEST | CONDITION | TYPES MOST LIKELY TO NEED IT | TIMING |
|---|---|---|---|
| Postcoital test | Antisperm antibodies | NONSPECIFIC | 1 to 3 days before ovulation is expected |
| Antithyroid antibodies blood test | Antithyroid antibodies | NONSPECIFIC | Anytime |

| TEST | CONDITION | TYPES MOST LIKELY TO NEED IT | TIMING |
|---|---|---|---|
| Antiphospholipid antibodies blood test | Antiphospholipid antibodies | NONSPECIFIC | Anytime |
| Natural killer cells blood test | Natural killer cells | NONSPECIFIC | Anytime |
| Antinuclear antibodies blood test | Antinuclear antibodies | NONSPECIFIC | Anytime |
| Immunobead binding test | Antisperm antibodies | NONSPECIFIC | Anytime |
| Blood test for thrombophilia and other clotting disorders | Clotting | NONSPECIFIC | Anytime |

# CHAPTER EIGHTEEN

# General Health Issues

Several general health concerns have a negative impact on fertility, across all fertility types and in both men and women. This chapter looks at the most common—and the most commonly overlooked. They are covered roughly in the order in which we see them, from most to least often.

## CERVICAL MUCUS

To conceive (naturally) you must have enough fertile ("egg-white") mucus at ovulation. It allows the sperm to swim easily and provides them with nourishment. If you don't have enough cervical mucus, or if your cervical mucus is too thick or too acidic, the sperm aren't going to thrive and may not be able to swim well enough or live long enough to reach the egg. You probably won't have any symptoms other than fertility problems.

Your doctor can check your cervical mucus as part of a postcoital test (see page 197) by grabbing a bit of mucus and pulling it out of the cervix with long forceps (through a speculum). This is done during the one to three days before ovulation is expected—that is, when your mucus should be most fertile. The doctor will stretch the mucus between the jaws of the forceps, testing its spinnbarkeit (stretchiness), and measure the pH (acidity or alkalinity) with a small strip of litmus paper. The best pH for sperm is 7 or 8. This is done right in the doctor's office.

Some of the mucus can also be sent off to a lab to be cultured for bacteria—that is, to check to see if you have an infection. A bacterial infection can cause "hostile" cervical mucus, and if that's the case, a course of antibiotics is in order—for you and your partner (see page 254). If there's no infection, try the simple strategies in the Help Yourself

DRY

STUCK

WATERLOGGED

section to improve the quality of your mucus. You may need IUI (see page 325) to bypass hostile mucus. With IUI, sperm live a much shorter time in the uterus, only about twelve hours, precisely because they don't have mucus to sustain them.

---

## Case Study: Elisheva

Elisheva had been taking Clomid as her doctor prescribed, one pill a day, for a few months, but she still wasn't pregnant. So her doctor doubled the dose of the fertility drug. Still no luck. She was only in her mid-twenties and generally healthy, so there was no obvious explanation for why she wasn't getting pregnant.

When she came to see me (Sami), I was surprised to find that she'd never had a sonogram to see how many eggs she was forming with the Clo-mid and that she'd never had a postcoital test. So no one knew why she wasn't getting pregnant. I prescribed a lower dose of Clomid — half a pill each day, which was half as much as she had started with and just a quarter of her current dose. When I did a sonogram, it showed two eggs, so ovulation was not the problem. I also performed a postcoital test, which showed that her cervical mucus was too thick, a side effect of Clomid. So I told her to take Mucinex for a few days before her next ovulation. She did — and got pregnant that same cycle.

---

### Chinese Medicine

Chinese medicine connects lack of mucus to yin deficiency (Dry), and acidic or thick mucus to internal heat from qi stagnation (Stuck or Waterlogged).

Acupuncture can increase fertile cervical mucus. My (Jill's) patients often tell me they notice an increase in the amount of fertile cervical mucus after starting a course of acupuncture treatment (even when that wasn't the main goal of treatment).

### Help Yourself

- See an acupuncturist to help increase fertile cervical mucus. Herbs may be useful as well.
- If your cervical mucus has been tested and is too acidic (the pH is too low), use a baking soda douche before having sex around ovulation. (This is the only situation in which we recommend douching of any kind. Douching with water or vinegar will kill sperm — though not reliably enough to act as birth control, of course.) Baking soda is alkaline. The pH of mucus changes rapidly, so the brief exposure to the alkaline douche is enough to get the pH back up to where it should be. The douche will not wash out the cervical mucus — like oil and water, they

don't mix. Use only when having intercourse at mid-cycle, during the two to three days ending with ovulation. Here's how you do it.

1. Thoroughly dissolve 1 tablespoon fresh baking soda in 1 cup hot water.
2. Allow the solution to cool to room temperature.
3. Fill a simple handheld douche with the mixture.
4. Lie down flat in the tub. To keep warm, line the tub with a towel or fill it with two inches of warm water.
5. Gently douche for 1 minute. You do not need to use all of the mixture.
6. Stand up in the tub.
7. Remove the remaining water in your vagina by placing a finger in your vagina and coughing.
8. Wait at least 1 hour (but no more than 12 hours) before having intercourse.

- If your cervical mucus is too acidic, avoid acid-producing foods such as coffee, alcohol, and red meat. Eat alkaline-promoting foods such as vegetables and whole grains.
- If your cervical mucus is too thick, use the over-the-counter decongestant guaifenesin (Mucinex or Humibid) to thin it out. (This is the stuff used to thin out mucus in your lungs so you don't feel congested.) Take 600 mg twice a day for the five days ending with ovulation.
- Drink more fluids. Keeping yourself well hydrated will help prevent too-thick cervical mucus.
- If your cervical mucus is both thick and acidic, use both the guaifenesin and the baking soda douche.

---

### Case Study: Clara

Clara was turned down by two different IVF doctors who told her that she'd never get pregnant because of her age (41) and the fact that her FSH was too high. I (Sami) don't consider either of those factors to be good indicators of the ability to conceive. What I did find was that her cervical mucus was very acidic. Sperm can die in acidic environments in as little as twenty minutes, so in Clara's body, they simply weren't getting a chance to complete their all-important swim. I advised Clara to use a baking soda douche (see Help Yourself) one to two hours before intercourse, to make the vagina and mucus as alkaline as possible. Once was all it took, and Clara got pregnant and had identical twins.

NONSPECIFIC

## GENETIC AND CONGENITAL DISORDERS

Small additions, omissions, or coding mistakes in the chromosomes can cause all kinds of problems, including infertility. Repeated miscarriages (or failed IVF treatments), sexual malfunction, anatomical problems, and low or no sperm count can in rare cases be traced back to the genes. This happens, for example, in Klinefelter's syndrome (an extra X—female—chromosome in males) and Turner's syndrome (only one X chromosome in females). Sometimes the problem is identified by signs and symptoms such as ambiguous genitalia, the absence of sperm, multiple miscarriages, or no menstruation (ever). Sometimes the investigation into fertility problems is the first time these disorders pop up. One patient I (Jill) saw turned out to have two uteruses. (Happily, she could get pregnant in either one.)

Genetic disorders like these can occur in all fertility types, and there's not usually much you can do about them on your own. The key is to make sure genetic causes have been considered if your infertility is unexplained. Should one turn out to be at the heart of the matter, your doctor will advise you on the best treatment, including hormone supplements, surgical correction, or fertility treatments that work around the problem.

TIRED

## HYPOTHYROID

Having an underactive thyroid—hypothyroidism—increases your chances of having trouble conceiving and of miscarrying. Low levels of thyroid hormone affect metabolism, slowing it down, and meddling with metabolism can affect the production of hormones. If your thyroid is sluggish, the effect can be significant enough to stop ovulation (even with a regular period) or cause early pregnancy loss. Or it can cause irregularities in your menstrual cycle, enough to complicate conception. In addition, some underlying causes of hypothyroidism—some autoimmune and pituitary disorders—can also impair fertility. It's not uncommon, for example, to find polycystic ovarian syndrome (PCOS) underlying low thyroid, and PCOS brings its own fertility problems (see page 202). Some women with an underactive thyroid have luteal phase

defect (LPD; see page 200), which can cause infertility or early pregnancy loss (see page 210). A low level of thyroid hormone can cause an
increase in the hormone prolactin (see page 220), which can impede fertility by causing irregular menstrual cycles, anovulatory cycles (no egg is
released), or the lack of any period at all.

Low thyroid is ten times more common in women, but it can affect
men, too. One percent of infertile men have hypothyroidism, which can
cause poor semen quality, low testosterone levels, and decreased sex drive.

The classic symptoms of low thyroid for men and women are fatigue,
weight gain, sensitivity to cold, loss of libido, constipation, joint stiffness,
depression, hair loss or thin hair, dry skin and hair, brittle nails, and skin
problems. For women, the menstrual cycle may also offer some clues.
Hypothyroidism often comes along with a short cycle, a heavy period, a
long period, and PMS. A severely underactive thyroid can cause anovulation, amenorrhea (no period), or irregular cycles.

Your thyroid levels may be low for one of three reasons: failure of
the thyroid gland, failure of the feedback mechanism that prompts the
gland to secrete thyroid hormone, or failure of the body to use thyroid
hormone effectively. Whichever is in play, the treatment options are the
same: prescription thyroid-stimulating hormone (TSH).

Your doctor can test your blood to determine your thyroid hormone
level. Experts sometimes disagree on the optimum levels, but your TSH
should be between 1.0 and 2.5 mIU/L. Correcting the levels by taking prescription TSH should take care of the symptoms of hypothyroidism, including fertility problems. You'll need to continue having your
thyroid levels monitored regularly so that the dosage of medication can
be adjusted to accommodate the changes your body will naturally go
through over time.

### Chinese Medicine

Chinese medicine considers hypothyroidism weak yang (Tired).

Yang tonifying herbs can help the body to produce more TSH on
its own. Because they contain no thyroid hormone, you can take Chinese herbs with your pharmaceutical TSH, as long as a clinical herbalist
monitors you and has your thyroid levels checked regularly. As the herbs
improve the function of your own thyroid, you may need less medication. Acupuncture also may help strengthen thyroid function.

### Help Yourself

- See an herbalist for a tonic to help your body produce more TSH. It is not a good idea to tackle hypothyroidism with "alternative" methods alone, however. The best results come from combining Western diagnostics and treatment with complementary strategies.
- See an acupuncturist to help strengthen thyroid function. Again, acupuncture should not substitute for prescription drugs.
- Do not take supplements within three hours of taking thyroid medication, to make sure they won't interfere with absorption.
- Steer clear of fluoride. Fluoride displaces iodine in the thyroid gland and interferes with proper thyroid function by preventing the formation of thyroxine (the thyroid hormone commonly abbreviated as T4).
- Eat seaweed. It's a good source of iodine, which is essential for proper thyroid function.
- Take 500 mg daily of the amino acid tyrosine, which the body uses to build TSH.
- Take supplemental coenzyme Q10, magnesium, and B vitamins, which are especially important in people with low thyroid levels.
- Make a point of cooking broccoli, cabbage, collard greens, kale, Brussels sprouts, bok choy, cauliflower, turnips, kohlrabi, and rutabagas. These vegetables inhibit the thyroid if eaten raw.
- Avoid sugar and refined carbohydrates.
- Avoid soy, which can make a thyroid condition worse.
- Get regular gentle exercise.

NONSPECIFIC

## REPEATED MISCARRIAGES

Repeated miscarriages are not technically a form of infertility, but we're addressing the problem in this book, just as we do early pregnancy loss (see page 210), because it is a major impediment to having a healthy baby. Furthermore, a miscarriage that ends with incomplete passage of the placenta can cause fertility problems by interfering with ovulation or implantation. Miscarriage can also create scar tissue that can result in infertility. And miscarriage is one of the common causes of failure in IVF.

We've categorized it as a general health issue because it's impossible to pin down one underlying cause. Here we look at miscarriages that occur at seven weeks of pregnancy or later. Before that, a miscarriage is considered early pregnancy loss.

The key to treating repeated miscarriages is to figure out the cause. After seven weeks, low progesterone would not be the prime suspect. Most doctors focus mainly on hormones, anatomy (especially of the uterus), genetics (abnormal chromosomes in either partner or the fetus), and thrombophilia (overactive clotting). Those are likely causes, but you're not getting a complete picture if you don't also investigate environmental, immunological, and infectious causes. In our experience, immunological problems and infections are the most commonly overlooked causes of repeated miscarriages. And it's important to consider what's going on in both partners, not just the woman.

Miscarriages are not uncommon, and sometimes there are good reasons for them biologically speaking. But a second miscarriage bears thorough investigation with your doctor, and if you are age 38 or over, that evaluation should begin after just one.

Your doctor may use a variety of tests, as well as a medical history and physical exam, to home in on the cause of a miscarriage. Blood tests for hormone levels, including thyroid, prolactin, and progesterone, may be useful. A blood pregnancy test may be used to check for a retained placenta. HSG (see page 198) can be used to check for scarring of the uterus and to check its structure. Hysteroscopy (see page 232) can be used to identify and remove scar tissue or retained products of conception. Genetic testing may be recommended.

Once the cause of a miscarriage has been identified, corrective steps can be taken. You may need supplemental hormones, antibiotics, or treatment for an overactive immune system. You might need to track down and remove an exposure to toxins. You may need surgery to correct scarring or anatomical issues such as a septate uterus (when the uterus is internally divided by a wall, leaving insufficient room for a baby to grow). This is why pinpointing the cause is crucial: if you skip any step, you can't know what the most effective solution would be.

### Chinese Medicine

Chinese medicine attributes miscarriages to central qi dropping (Tired), while early pregnancy loss is related to kidney deficiency (Dry). Tired and Dry types are the most likely to have these problems, but they may occur in any type.

Acupuncture and herbs can help prevent miscarriages due to hormone or immune system issues. They are not effective in preventing miscarriages due to chromosomal abnormalities in the fetus or structural abnormalities in a woman's anatomy.

### Help Yourself

- Continue or adopt healthy lifestyle choices. Pay particular attention to appropriate exercise, good nutrition, healthy weight, and stress management.
- See a doctor specializing in miscarriage.
- See a Chinese medicine practitioner for help preventing miscarriages due to hormone or immune system issues.

TIRED

STUCK

WATERLOGGED

## INTESTINAL DISORDERS

Celiac disease, Crohn's disease (or ulcerative colitis), candidiasis, and similar chronic intestinal disorders can all interfere with the absorption of nutrients from food, sometimes enough to make you undernourished. This can impair ovulation or otherwise compromise fertility. Candidiasis has also been implicated in miscarriage and premature birth. The drugs used to treat these conditions can sometimes hamper fertility as well, by suppressing the immune system or damaging DNA. Women who have had intestinal surgery for Crohn's are most likely to have fertility problems. (That's *not* a recommendation not to have surgery. It may well be the best treatment.) Celiac disease seems more related to hormone abnormalities than to other intestinal problems, in men as well as in women. Many men with celiac disease have smaller than average testicles and low fertility; their partners have an elevated rate of miscarriage.

Talk to your doctor about possible digestive disorders if you have chronic diarrhea and fatigue, abdominal pain, occasionally bloody diarrhea, recurrent constipation, or frequent vomiting. You may need a referral to a gastroenterologist.

## Chinese Medicine

Different intestinal disorders have different diagnoses in Chinese medicine, but in general they are related to qi deficiency leading to damp (Waterlogged), or qi stagnation leading to qi deficiency (Tired or Stuck). Acupuncture and herbs may be useful.

### Help Yourself

- Chew your food well.
- Take time to eat. Don't eat on the run or when you are angry or upset.
- Limit carbs in the evenings. Digestion slows down at night, and any carbs left standing in the intestines can ferment, giving off alcohols that can weaken digestion.
- Limit cold raw foods in the evenings, when your digestion is slowing down.
- Cut out refined sugars.
- Limit wheat. You probably don't need to cut it out altogether (unless you have celiac disease), but Americans in general eat too much.
- Eat only until full. Do not overeat.
- Limit stimulants such as tea, coffee, and alcohol.
- Eat a diet comprising whole foods—focusing on whole grains, beans, legumes, a wide range of vegetables, free-range eggs, and fish—with only small amounts of lean meat and poultry.
- Take a probiotic supplement and include natural yogurt with live cultures in your diet.
- Eat lots of garlic.
- Sprinkle ground flaxseeds on your breakfast grains or salads.
- Test your tolerance for dairy. Try cutting out all dairy products for two weeks, replacing cow's milk with almond, oat, or rice milk, and see whether you feel better. (Soy milk makes matters worse for many women because of the hormonal effects.) If it seems to be helping, you can figure out your own limits with dairy products by gradually reintroducing them in small amounts. Many people seem to

have fewer problems with organic milk and do better with hard cheeses (such as Parmesan) rather than soft ones.

- To help identify problematic foods, keep a diary for one month, recording everything you eat and any digestive symptoms.
- See a gastroenterologist if digestive symptoms are severe.

# ANEMIA

PALE

If you are a woman with anemia, you might not be producing enough oxygen from red blood cells to support a pregnancy. Anemia can be caused by too little iron in the diet or by factors that limit iron absorption, such as high zinc intake, insufficient B vitamins, too much coffee, or overuse of antacids. Women with heavy periods are also susceptible, as are vegetarians and strict dieters. You may want to talk with your doctor about being tested for anemia if you are pale and lethargic or have fatigue, shortness of breath, dizziness, or palpitations.

## Chinese Medicine

In Chinese medicine, anemia is seen as blood deficiency. This is typical of the Pale type.

Acupuncture can help build blood and help with iron absorption.

## Help Yourself

- See an acupuncturist for help with anemia.
- Take supplemental iron. For mild cases of anemia, look for Floradix at your health food store; it does not seem to cause constipation, as other iron supplements tend to do. Or talk to your doctor about a supplement that's right for you, especially if you have a more serious case of anemia.
- Eat iron-rich foods, such as red meat, kidney beans, spinach, cherries, leafy green vegetables, apricots, and sunflower seeds.
- Drink nettle leaf tea, which is naturally rich in minerals, including iron. This is an ancient remedy for anemia. You can buy it in tea bags at your health food store.
- Include plenty of good sources of vitamin C in your diet, such as citrus fruits, bell peppers, broccoli, cantaloupe, and strawberries. Vitamin C improves iron absorption.

## HYPERTHYROID

DRY

STUCK

An overactive thyroid—known as hyperthyroidism, or Graves' disease—can disrupt your metabolism and hormone balance just as surely as an underactive thyroid can, potentially causing the same lack of ovulation (even with a seemingly normal cycle) or early pregnancy loss.

You may want to have your thyroid level tested if you have unexplained or unintended weight loss, heat intolerance, insomnia, loose or frequent bowel movements, nervousness or agitation, and palpitations. Your TSH should be between 1.0 and 2.5 mIU/L, and the more tightly controlled it is in that range, the better ovulation will be. Long-term untreated hyperthyroidism causes the characteristic "pop eyes." Women who are hyperthyroid often have light periods. Their BBT tends to be too high during phase 1 (menstruation) and phase 2 (pre-ovulation).

Talk with your doctor about medications to tame a hyperactive thyroid. Another option is to have your thyroid gland surgically removed, which is just what one of my (Sami's) patients did. She was in too much of a hurry to get pregnant to take the time to sort out proper medication dosages when there was no guarantee that medication would immediately restore her fertility. Without a thyroid gland, however, you'll be *hypo*thyroid, and you'll need medication to deal with that.

### Chinese Medicine

Chinese medicine attributes hyperthyroidism to heat from yin deficiency (Dry) or qi stagnation (Stuck).

### Help Yourself

- Add calories and protein to your diet if you've lost a great deal of weight or experienced muscle wasting.
- Make sure you get enough calcium to counter thinning bones, which can be exacerbated by hyperthyroidism.

## DIABETES

Both men and women with diabetes (type 1 or type 2) are at increased risk of infertility. Women with diabetes have a higher risk of miscarriage, fetal abnormalities, and bigger babies, although if your diabetes

TIRED

DRY

WATERLOGGED

is well managed, you are unlikely to have a problem. Like the insulin resistance that can be a precursor of the disease, diabetes itself directly affects hormone production and metabolism, and the resulting hormone imbalance and weight issues can compromise fertility.

If you have diabetes, proper monitoring and management is essential for conception and a healthy pregnancy. Blood sugar needs to be stable at ovulation; when it is not, there is an increased risk of chromosomal abnormalities in the fetus. In men, poorly controlled blood sugar can affect cell division in the testicles, leading to abnormal sperm. It can also cause erectile dysfunction (ED) and retrograde ejaculation (where sperm ends up in the bladder).

With proper care and attention, type 2 diabetes can be controlled with diet and exercise. (The Making Babies plan for your type will probably do the trick.) Medications such as metformin (Glucophage) can help in some cases; other cases require treatment with insulin.

### Chinese Medicine

Diabetes is considered a wasting and thirsting disorder in Chinese medicine. It can be either a yin deficiency (Dry type) or a yang deficiency (Tired type). Roughly speaking, these correspond to type 1 and type 2 diabetes, although some people with the Tired type move into the Dry type over a long period of time.

Some herbs can be helpful, but treatment should always be supervised by an herbalist and coordinated with Western medical care.

### Help Yourself

- Consult an herbalist for help with diabetes.
- Eat a low-fat, low-carb diet.
- Control your weight.

## OTHER GENERAL HEALTH ISSUES

Women with amenorrhea (lack of periods), oligomenorrhea (infrequent periods), or dysmenorrhea (severe uterine pain with periods) should work to find the cause—and cure—before settling for a diagnosis of unexplained infertility.

Men can experience fertility problems in the wake of cancer, liver disease, kidney disease, or chronic renal failure.

# Making Babies Action Plan

The following action plans summarize the testing needed to establish whether your fertility problems stem from any of these general health issues. They will guide you through your potential testing program as efficiently as possible. Not everyone will need all these tests, and these may not be all the tests you need. Your doctor will guide you as to which tests you need, of course, but you should make sure that your understanding, gleaned from the descriptions in this chapter, lines up with your doctor's plans.

| | TESTS FOR MEN AND WOMEN | | |
|---|---|---|---|
| TEST | CONDITION | TYPES MOST LIKELY TO NEED IT | TIMING |
| Genetic tests | Genetic and congenital disorders, such as cystic fibrosis and Tay-Sachs disease | NONSPECIFIC | Anytime |
| Blood test for TSH | Hypothyroid | TIRED | Anytime |
| Chromosome tests (karyotypes) | Repeated miscarriages | TIRED | Anytime |
| History of environmental and toxic exposures | Repeated miscarriages | DRY | Anytime |
| Medical history and physical exam | Intestinal disorders | TIRED WATERLOGGED | Anytime |

## TESTS FOR MEN AND WOMEN

| TEST | CONDITION | TYPES MOST LIKELY TO NEED IT | TIMING |
|---|---|---|---|
| Test for celiac disease | Celiac disease | TIRED / WATERLOGGED | Anytime |
| Blood tests for fasting glucose and 2 hours post-breakfast | Diabetes | TIRED / WATERLOGGED | Anytime |

## TESTS FOR WOMEN

| TEST | CONDITION | TYPES MOST LIKELY TO NEED IT | TIMING |
|---|---|---|---|
| Postcoital test | Cervical mucus acidity/thickness/ "hostility" | DRY / STUCK | 1 to 3 days before ovulation is expected |
| Blood test for TSH | Hyperthyroidism and hypothyroidism | DRY | Anytime |
| Thrombophilia workup | Repeated miscarriages | NONSPECIFIC | Anytime |
| Blood test for anemia | Anemia | PALE | Anytime |

# PART FIVE

# Pre-mester:
# The 3-Month Making
# Babies Program

# CHAPTER NINETEEN

# Pre-mester: How to Use the Making Babies Program for Your Fertility Type

Think of the next three months as a sort of pre-trimester — a "pre-mester," if you will. What you do during this time is just as important to a healthy pregnancy as what you do after conception — maybe even more so, because taking care of your body properly now just may be what allows you to get pregnant in the first place.

You learned earlier in this book how food, exercise, supplements, and other lifestyle choices can bolster (or harm) fertility. In the following chapters, you'll learn how that general knowledge applies to your specific fertility type. Exactly what constitutes eating right, how and how much you should exercise, and which supplements will benefit you the most depends on your type. Each chapter also provides similarly tailored advice about your mind and emotions, do-it-yourself fertility boosts, medical interventions to consider, and Chinese medicine strategies. It's all designed to get you into the best possible shape for conception by bringing your body into balance, optimizing your overall health, and circumventing any specific roadblocks to conception. That will increase your odds of getting pregnant and lay the groundwork for an all-around healthy pregnancy. That's why we think everyone should have a Making Babies pre-mester, even people who have had no fertility problems and have no reason to expect they will. And it definitely behooves men as well as women to follow the program for their type.

## THINGS YOU SHOULD KNOW

The principles of diet, exercise, supplements, and lifestyle choices laid out in earlier chapters form the foundation of the Making Babies program for every fertility type. The recommendations that follow, type by type, are to be layered on top of those basics. Here are a few things to keep in mind about following the Making Babies program for your type.

- When general advice from the earlier chapters reappears in the program for a particular type, that means it is especially important for that type. If at any point information appears to conflict with the guidelines from earlier chapters, you should follow what's given for your particular type.
- Some fertility strategies are especially helpful at a particular point in a woman's cycle, and those are recommended for certain phases, although they are generally good anytime (unless specifically noted). If you find that you can't fit in everything every day, focus your efforts on the key phases.
- Each type begins with diet recommendations, including the percentages of macronutrients for that type. Please don't treat these as exact figures; they are meant to serve as rough guidelines to help you balance your meals. We don't want anyone weighing or otherwise measuring their food precisely. Instead, think of these percentages as approximately how much real estate each food group should have on your plate. Tired types, for example, do best on about 50 percent complex carbs, 30 percent fruits and veggies, and 20 percent high-quality protein. If this is you, you'll want to cover about half your plate with complex carbs, then divide the other half in two again, with a slightly bigger portion given over to fruits and veggies and a slighter smaller portion devoted to protein. A big sweet potato, a heap of garlicky broccoli, and a small serving of salmon would fit the bill.
- Unless otherwise specified, you should take supplements according to package directions.

## CHINESE MEDICINE

You can successfully use the Making Babies program without ever consulting a Chinese medicine practitioner. But if you do choose to try herbs or acupuncture, you will maximize your plan's effectiveness.

### Chinese Practitioners

If you decide to use Chinese medicine, your first task is to find a reputable practitioner. Most likely you are looking for a licensed acupuncturist (LAc), a specialist formally trained in Chinese medical theory and basic biosciences as well as acupuncture, who may also have studied herbal medicine and/or bodywork. Licensing rules vary from state to state. Most states require a three- to five-year master's degree in Oriental medicine from an accredited acupuncture school and written and practical state board exams. In some states, licensed practitioners specializing in acupuncture carry titles other than LAc, including DOM (doctor of Oriental medicine), DAc (doctor of acupuncture), and AP (acupuncture physician).

Check with the board of the professions in your state to find a licensed acupuncturist in your area. The National Certification Commission for Acupuncture and Oriental Medicine (NCCAOM) has a "find a practitioner" section on its Web site. The organization tests practitioners to ensure they are knowledgeable about Chinese medicine and appropriate sterile technique. Many, but not all, states require this test for licensing. Some states do not license acupuncturists; in this case, look for someone who is NCCAOM certified. He or she will have a degree in Oriental medicine from an accredited school or will have worked as an apprentice acupuncturist for at least four years and will have passed a written and a practical exam.

Some other health care providers, such as physicians, dentists, and chiropractors, also practice acupuncture. They may have had less training than an LAc, so it may be best to find an MD or DO (doctor of osteopathy) who is also an LAc. Or look for a Western doctor who is a member of the American Academy of Medical Acupuncture (AAMA), which requires a minimum of two hundred hours of training for membership.

Besides establishing the credentials of a practitioner and the details of his or her training (where and for how long), you should also be sure to ask how long he or she has been in practice and what experience he or she has in treating infertility and your specific issues.

If you know people who have used Chinese medicine, ask about their experiences and for their recommendations. Make sure the person you select is someone you like and feel you can trust. Just as with a medical doctor, this is an important relationship, and if something doesn't feel right to you, you should find a different practitioner.

A good practitioner will pinpoint and then correct any subtle imbalances in your body to improve your ability to conceive. You should get a specific diagnosis and specific recommendations for regular acupuncture and herbal formulas. You don't need to fully understand everything the practitioner tells you in terms of Chinese medicine, but you should have a general idea of what you are being treated for, how, and why. (For example, your practitioner might say, "Your qi is stuck. Qi needs to flow smoothly to allow for conception, and acupuncture at certain points can free up qi." Of course, this is a simplification of what should be a detailed analysis.) You should also receive an explanation of how progress will be monitored ("We'll be looking for your period to become more regular within a few months").

Make sure both your medical doctor and your Chinese medicine practitioner are aware of what other treatment you may be receiving. If you are lucky, you'll find a practitioner who will give your doctor a call to discuss your case. If your practitioner doesn't work that way, you'll need to take responsibility for accurately conveying information from one to the other and satisfying yourself that it is being taken into account on both ends. Your medical doctor is unlikely to know much about Chinese treatments, but your Chinese medicine practitioner should have a basic facility with Western treatments and how Chinese approaches may interact with them. Generally, Chinese herbs and acupuncture can be used right alongside Western treatments, but there are some instances in which the effects might overlap too much, and one side or the other should be curbed. In some cases, as with using herbs that boost hormones at the same time you are using fertility drugs, careful and knowledgeable coordination will be required. In others, the two approaches just shouldn't be combined. For instance, ovulation-stimulating herbs might cause the body to develop a single primary follicle. That would be the body's normal route, but it's not desirable in an IVF cycle when fertility drugs are being used to get lots of eggs to start at the same time.

### Chinese Herbs

In prescribing an herbal formula for you, an herbalist should be taking into account both your underlying condition or constitution (your fertility type) and your current symptoms or medical condition. A typical formula will contain about ten to fifteen herbs, combined just for you.

Exactly how you obtain your formula will vary by practitioner. I (Jill) use an Internet pharmacy. I send in my prescription for a patient, the pharmacy makes up the formula, and my patient gets an e-mail saying that it is ready and can be "picked up" online. I use a lab that makes freeze-dried granules from the herbs, to be mixed with water and taken as a tea. Other practitioners use dried herbs in a packet that must be brewed into a tea. Others use pills or tinctures that you receive right in the office. Some provide prescriptions to take to a Chinese herb store.

Over-the-counter Chinese herbal formulas are also available. Your practitioner may sell them, some health food stores carry them, and you can order them on the Internet. (The one place you shouldn't buy them is from a Chinatown storefront—or do so only with specific professional advice on what to get and where. Otherwise, you run the risk of counterfeits and contamination, including contamination with Western drugs.) These formulas are one size fits all, so they can't measure up to personalized formulas. They tend to be weaker, which can mean they are less effective but also that they are less likely to cause any side effects. To achieve maximum benefit from Chinese herbs, you should consult an herbalist.

Chinese herbs are the gentlest possible first intervention if you have fertility problems that require treatment beyond the self-help strategies in this book. Herbs are much gentler than hormones, for example, but they are fully able to handle the kinds of minor hormone imbalances that are significant enough to interfere with conception. Of course, you should discuss any herbal supplements you use with your doctor. And you should stop taking herbs during the first four days of your period unless otherwise instructed, and again once you are pregnant. No responsible practitioner will prescribe herbs contraindicated in pregnancy to someone trying to get pregnant, of course, but stopping provides an extra layer of protection.

## GET YOUR PROGRAMS HERE

With these general pointers in mind, you are prepared for your personal pre-mester. You'll need to read only the one or possibly two chapters of the five that follow that pertain to your type (or combination type). Give the program at least a month. Ideally, you should follow it for three months to bring you into peak fertility fitness before you even start trying to get pregnant. That will make conceiving, as well as pregnancy, easier. And should further fertility treatment become necessary, the Making Babies program will allow you to minimize short- and long-term side effects and increase your success rate. No matter the ultimate details of the journey you are embarking on, three months is an investment that will be well worthwhile.

## Making Babies Action Plan

❑ Follow the Making Babies program for your type for at least one month, preferably three.
❑ Layer the advice for your type on top of the general advice in the preceding chapters.
❑ If you are interested in acupuncture and Chinese herbs, consult a licensed Chinese medicine practitioner.
❑ Find and purchase Chinese herbs carefully.
❑ Facilitate communication between your medical doctor and Chinese medicine practitioner.
❑ Remember, successful conception is not the end of the road. Medical monitoring of any first-trimester pregnancy is very important in fertility patients.

# CHAPTER TWENTY

# The Making Babies Rx: Tired

The Making Babies program for Tired types can improve many aspects of your health and fertility, but most of these strategies are aimed particularly at improving metabolism and digestion, especially as they affect your hormones.

## FOOD

**Choose:**

- Simple, well-cooked foods, with relatively few components at each meal. Ideally, your meals should be full of locally grown seasonal produce. Emphasize complex carbohydrates (50 percent), with the addition of vegetables and fruits (30 percent) and high-quality protein (20 percent).

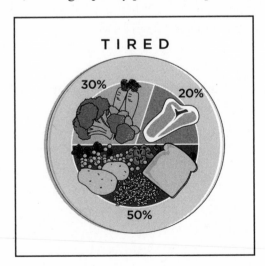

- Easy-to-digest, warming, slow-cooked foods such as soups and stews. They arrive in the stomach warm and broken down and so do not ask your digestive system to work too hard.
- Lightly cooked vegetables, for better digestibility. Corn, celery, watercress, turnip, pumpkin, alfalfa sprouts, button mushrooms, radishes, and capers are especially good choices. Buy organic as much as possible.
- Lots of legumes, especially kidney beans, adzuki beans, and lentils.
- Small amounts of lean organic meat and poultry, preferably hormone-free, and fish such as salmon. Animal protein (if you partake) has warming properties that are beneficial for this type.
- Seeds, especially sesame, pumpkin, and sunflower.
- Seaweed, such as kelp.
- Green tea, jasmine tea, red raspberry leaf tea, and Spicy Fertili-Tea (see box on next page).
- Whole grains, including brown rice, quinoa, barley, and oats. Whole grains are good for everyone, but they are particularly important for Tired types who crave the energy from carbs and tend to binge on cookies and the like. Letting your body get the sugars it needs in a slow-release form keeps blood sugar levels stable and you feeling satisfied. You may feel particularly in need of a sugar fix during phase 1 of your cycle (menstruation), but that just makes it even more important for you to get what you need from whole grains rather than simple sugars in refined and junk foods during that time.
- Regular mealtimes.
- To take your time with meals, chewing food well.
- To prepare your own food rather than eat in restaurants.
- Several small meals throughout the day, to stabilize blood sugar levels. Don't wait until you are very hungry to eat.
- Spicy foods—foods seasoned with chiles and warming spices such as ginger, cinnamon, cloves, cumin, cardamom, cayenne, rosemary, nutmeg, turmeric, and fennel.
- Foods that Chinese medicine considers warming, such as rice, oatmeal, parsnips, onions, leeks, lamb, beef, chicken, and stewed fruit.

## SPICY FERTILI-TEA
## FOR TIRED TYPES

**1 cup black tea leaves**        **2 tablespoons ground cardamom**

**2 tablespoons ground allspice**    **Fresh ginger slices**

Combine all the ingredients except the ginger in a small resealable container. Place 2 teaspoons of the mixture in a teacup. Add two slices of fresh ginger, pour boiling water over the tea and ginger, and let steep for 10 minutes. Strain and serve.

### Avoid:

- Dairy products.
- Wheat.
- Fruit juice, since it concentrates the sugar and loses most of the fiber. Try vegetable juice instead, or water or tea.
- The junk foods and refined sugars and carbohydrates you're liable to crave. That goes for artificial sweeteners, too. Scratch the itch with whole grains instead. This is particularly important during phase 4 of your cycle (potential implantation).
- Eating on the run.
- Overeating.
- Raw foods and cold or frozen foods. (Your digestion is not working as well as it should and does not have enough energy to warm foods up to a temperature at which they can be easily digested.) Don't put ice in your drinks, and avoid ice cream. Steering clear of cold foods and drinks is especially important during phase 3 of your cycle (ovulation). When you do have, say, a salad, accompany it with something warm, such as a cup of soup or a baked potato.
- Fried foods. They are not really good for anybody, but Tired types really don't metabolize the fat well, and it's likely to compound whatever their digestive issues are.
- Tofu and processed soy products.
- Stimulants such as caffeine, coffee, or energy drinks, even when you feel sluggish. The boost they provide is only false energy and over time will make you feel even more rundown.
- Excess salt.

- Alcohol. None of it will do you any good, with beer being your very worst choice from the bar.
- Indigestion—or at least the foods and situations that you know give you indigestion.

## EXERCISE

- Get regular, moderate exercise that leaves you energized, not exhausted. Don't exercise in short, intense bursts or start a high-energy program. Be careful not to overexercise. About thirty minutes three times a week is good. You can do up to thirty minutes a day as long as you are not exercising until you are exhausted. Tired men can exercise a bit longer—about forty minutes three times a week (or daily, as long as it stays moderate). Avoiding heavy exercise is especially important for Tired women during phase 1 of their cycle (menstruation). Being active is okay, but you want to avoid really getting your blood pumping during this time. You also want to be sure to exercise only moderately during phase 4 (potential implantation).
- Build up endurance gradually. Pace yourself so that you don't overexert.
- Daily gentle exercise is better than sporadic intense activity and will boost your metabolism better. It can be as simple as walking around the block every evening.

## LIFESTYLE

- Do all that you can to conserve your energy. Women should keep their energy up in whatever ways they can, especially during phase 1 (menstruation) and phase 4 (potential implantation) of their cycle.
- Be careful not to overdo it with work.
- Limit stress. Learn and use stress-reduction techniques that work for you.
- Get enough rest and enough sleep.
- Keep warm. Dress appropriately for the weather. Take warm baths. Keep your feet warm with slippers or socks.
- Keep a regular schedule. Establish a regular bedtime and a regular bedtime routine.

- Write down your goals and devise a plan for how you will achieve them.
- Make space in your life for fun and laughter.
- Consciously set limits with the people in your life. Practice saying no.
- Protect your back — it's your weak point. Use your knees when lifting heavy items, for example.
- Try the visualization exercises beginning on page 90.
- Try the self-massages beginning on page 92.

## SUPPLEMENTS

- Royal jelly.
- Wheatgrass.
- Chromium boosts metabolism by enhancing the action of insulin.
- L-arginine.
- For women only: Chaste tree berry (*Vitex agnus-castus;* in Chinese medicine, Man Jing Zi) works to restore hormone balance, thereby improving fertility. It helps increase LH and inhibit the release of FSH, which can improve progesterone levels. It can also improve the ratio of progesterone to estrogen by curbing excess estrogen. It can help sustain progesterone in phases 3 and 4 of your cycle (ovulation and potential implantation), especially when ovulation is delayed. It can be used to regulate periods, restart periods that have stopped, and moderate heavy menstrual flow. *Men should not take Chaste tree berry when their partners are trying to conceive,* as it can decrease sperm count.
- False unicorn root can strengthen the uterine wall and promote the growth of follicles, which explains why it has been used for centuries as a fertility tonic.
- Avoid black cohosh (Sheng Ma). Black cohosh is one of the most common gynecologic herbs in Western herbalism, and if you seek advice at a health food store, this may well be what the clerk recommends. It is properly used to relieve menopausal symptoms and to bring on a period. Precisely because it is good at doing the latter (it can inhibit ovulation), this is not an herb we recommend on its own. (You are, after

all, essentially trying to stop your period temporarily.) Black cohosh is also not to be taken during pregnancy. There are some cases, however, in which an herbalist may rightly use it as part of a formula for women trying to conceive.

## HELP YOURSELF FERTILITY STRATEGIES

- **Women.** Warm your lower abdomen (and/or your lower back) with a hot-water bottle or a heating pad set on low or medium for twenty minutes each evening during the first half of your cycle. (This kind of warmth is good for you in general, so feel free to use it at any other time you please.) It is key for relieving menstrual cramps and improving ovulation.
- **Men.** Don't masturbate; focus on sexual experiences that reinforce connection.

## MEDICAL ASSISTANCE

- If your doctor advises a serial progesterone test, do it during phase 4 of your cycle (potential implantation)—the luteal phase. This test will help determine whether you should take supplemental progesterone during this phase to improve implantation.
- Consult with your doctor about potential hypothyroidism and anemia if you have lethargy, weight gain, sensitivity to cold, and low BBT in phase 2 of your cycle (pre-ovulation).

## CHINESE MEDICINE

- Acupuncture can help boost your qi, especially if you feel tired and washed-out during your period.
- Acupuncture can help speed up follicle development in Tired women who have a long follicular phase (not enough FSH to produce a follicle in a timely manner).
- Acupuncture and Chinese herbs can help stimulate your metabolism and warm you up a bit, bringing you back into balance. Consult a Chinese medicine practitioner. This is especially beneficial for Tired women who are hypothyroid or anemic or who have low BBT, lethargy, weight gain, and sensitivity to cold in phase 2 (pre-ovulation).

# CHAPTER TWENTY-ONE

# The Making Babies Rx: Dry

The Making Babies program for Dry types can improve many aspects of your health and fertility, but most of these strategies are aimed particularly at helping your body build follicles and a healthy endometrium.

## FOOD

**Choose:**

- A diet that prioritizes vegetables and fruits, combined with complex carbohydrates and a small amount of protein and healthy fats, for concentrated nutrition that nourishes tissue and increases moisture levels. Aim to fill your plate with roughly 10 percent animal protein (if you eat it), 10 percent vegetable protein (e.g., soy products and beans; increase to 20 percent if you are vegetarian), 40 percent vegetables, and 40 percent complex carbohydrates.

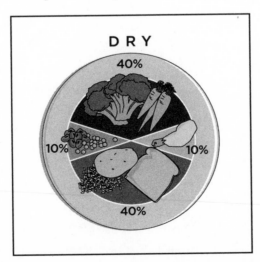

- Five small meals and one larger one at regular times during the day.
- Small portions of protein throughout the day, including meat, dairy products, beans, and legumes. Protein is especially important during phase 2 of your cycle (pre-ovulation) because it helps to build good follicles.
- Flax and soy products for their phytoestrogens, protein, and healthy fats. Try ground flaxseeds on your breakfast cereal or flaxseed oil in your salad dressing (whole flaxseeds are not easily digested, so you reap less benefit). Flax and soy are especially useful during phase 2 of your cycle (pre-ovulation). If you are Stuck as well as Dry, however, limit yourself to two portions a week.
- Lightly cooked foods (go for steamed or stir-fried rather than roasted or deep-fried), salads, and some cold raw foods.
- Dairy products, including eggs.
- Seaweed and concentrated green juice, such as spirulina.
- Foods rich in vitamins B and E, such as eggs and wheat germ, especially during phases 2 and 3 of your cycle (pre-ovulation and ovulation).
- To hydrate with at least eight 8-ounce glasses of water or other healthy fluids, such as green or chamomile tea or Anise-Chrysanthemum Fertili-Tea (see box), at regular intervals throughout the day. Proper hydration is important for everyone but crucial for fertility in Dry types, especially during phase 2 of your cycle (pre-ovulation) so that you are hydrated enough to produce fertile cervical mucus.
- Foods Chinese medicine considers moistening and lubricating, cooling, or yin nourishing. These include seeds, beans (especially mung beans), nuts, sardines, bone marrow, wheat, oats, rice, millet, celery, spinach, Swiss chard, cucumbers, lettuce, radishes, asparagus, eggplant, cabbage, tomatoes, broccoli, cauliflower, zucchini, alfalfa sprouts, squash, sweet potatoes, green beans, beets, mushrooms, apples, pears, bananas, watermelon, blueberries, and blackberries.

### Avoid:

- Alcohol, which is dehydrating and will make your symptoms worse. It is also a stimulant. Chinese medicine says it generates heat. Avoiding alcohol is good advice for everyone, but it is crucial for Dry types, particularly during phase 1 of your cycle (menstruation), and especially if your period is heavy, since it can make bleeding heavier.

- Rich or fatty foods, such as dishes that are deep-fried or have heavy cream sauces.
- Coffee, black tea, caffeine, energy drinks (including herbal ones), weight-loss formulas, and other stimulants.
- Sugar.
- Eating late at night.
- Low-calorie diets; extreme, imbalanced diets; being too controlling about what you eat.
- Spicy foods and spices Chinese medicine considers to be warming, such as chiles, curry, ginger, cinnamon, garlic, and wasabi. This is especially important during phase 1 of your cycle (menstruation) and particularly if your period is heavy.

---

### ANISE-CHRYSANTHEMUM FERTILI-TEA FOR DRY TYPES

All these ingredients should be available at your health food store. Check the herb, spice, supplement, and tea sections.

**1 cup chrysanthemum tea leaves**          **¼ cup stinging nettle tea leaves**
**2 tablespoons marshmallow root**          **2 teaspoons anise**

Combine all the ingredients in a small resealable container. Place 2 teaspoons of the mixture in a teacup. Pour boiling water over the tea and let steep for 10 minutes. Strain and serve. This is good hot or cold.

---

### EXERCISE

- Choose energizing, revitalizing exercise that is replenishing and meditative — activities that will help quiet the mind as well as work the body, such as yoga, tai chi, qi gong, swimming, or simply walking in nature.
- Avoid exercise that is intensely aerobic or exhausting, such as running or using a stair-climber. Limit your aerobic exercise to about thirty minutes at a pop, three times a week.

This is especially important during phase 1 of your cycle (menstruation). Additional exercise that is more meditative or that focuses more on stretching is fine.

- Balance exercise that builds bulk, such as weightlifting, with exercise that encourages movement and flexibility. (Dry men, we are especially talking to you!)
- Avoid sports drinks, especially the ones with caffeine. They are too yang. Instead, try water or nourishing fruit nectars diluted with water.
- Avoid saunas and bikram ("hot") yoga.

## LIFESTYLE

- Get enough good-quality sleep.
- Avoid smoking and recreational drugs. This is especially important for Dry types because cigarettes and drugs are yin depleting and particularly likely to throw you severely out of balance. This can have harmful effects on fertility even in the short term.
- Don't use weight-loss pills; they are stimulants.
- Limit your time in the stale air of sealed, climate-controlled buildings as much as possible. Spend time in natural environments (forests, lakes, and beaches) to balance yourself out.
- Limit the time you spend near electrical machinery. This includes the time you spend sitting in front of a computer.
- As much as is humanly possible, avoid toxic fumes, such as those emitted by paints, construction materials, and dry cleaners.
- Don't cause yourself to get overheated. Avoid saunas, steam rooms, hot tubs, and hot baths.
- Moisturize your skin.
- Reduce your stress level. Learn and use stress-reduction strategies that work for you.
- Lead a sensibly paced life, allow yourself downtime, and cut down on partying. Cultivate pastimes that serve as an antidote to the hectic pace of modern life. Try reading a book

or exercising. Relaxing and resting are especially important during phase 1 of your cycle (menstruation), when your energy is naturally low, and during phase 2 (pre-ovulation).

- Establish a regular routine. Besides eating meals at consistent times, aim for regular bedtimes and exercise sessions.
- Avoid overstimulation. Stay away from loud environments (e.g., big parties and rock concerts), scary movies, and the like.
- Be patient, especially if you are over 35. You've gotten out of balance over time, and it's going to take time to restore your balance. It might take six to twelve months of eating well, exercising regularly, and getting good-quality sleep before you see fertility results.
- Try the visualization exercises beginning on page 90.
- Try the self-massages beginning on page 92.

## SUPPLEMENTS

- Essential fatty acids (EFAs), which are good for everyone but particularly important for Dry types.
- L-carnitine.
- Royal jelly.
- Liquid chlorophyll. This is especially useful in phase 2 of your cycle (pre-ovulation) because it supports follicle building.
- Floradix herbal iron supplement is beneficial during phase 1 of your cycle (menstruation), when you are losing blood and iron. Iron also supports follicle building, among other things, and so is particularly beneficial during phase 2 (pre-ovulation).

## MEDICAL ASSISTANCE

- Dry women are prone to problems in phases 1 and 2 of their cycle (menstruation and pre-ovulation). Without sufficient FSH and estrogen, they don't have sufficient resources for optimally developing follicles or the endometrium. They may also have less fertile cervical mucus.
- Check with your doctor if your BBT is too high in phase

2 of your cycle (pre-ovulation) or if you have insomnia, unintended weight loss, or feelings of agitation. You might have hyperthyroidism or excessive sex hormone activity. Dry men are also prone to these conditions.

- Consider your options very carefully with your health care practitioner before you take fertility drugs. Your ovaries are less likely to respond well to those drugs, and some of them can deplete cervical mucus and thin the endometrium, two issues you may already be struggling with.

- If you decide to use fertility drugs in an attempt to boost ovulation, carefully prepare your body for them before you begin. We recommend at least three months on the Making Babies program before starting treatment. Wait to try fertility drugs until your main symptoms have subsided (until you're no longer having hot flashes or night sweats, your period is strong, and you have good cervical mucus, for example).

## CHINESE MEDICINE

- If you decide to try fertility drugs or assisted reproductive technologies (ARTs), acupuncture and herbs can help prepare your body for them and increase your odds of responding — or at least dampen important side effects, such as depleted fertile cervical mucus and a thinner endometrium. Consult a Chinese medicine practitioner for the right formulas for you.

- Herbs and acupuncture can nourish yin and clear heat. Acupuncture can bring blood to the follicles, where growth might be impeded by low estrogen; increase fertile cervical mucus; and help regulate hormones.

- If your follicular phase is too long (there is not enough FSH to produce a follicle in a timely manner), acupuncture can help normalize the process.

- A Chinese herbal formula can thin too-thick cervical mucus.

# CHAPTER TWENTY-TWO

# The Making Babies Rx: Stuck

The Making Babies program for Stuck types can improve many aspects of your health and fertility, but most of these strategies are aimed particularly at easing hormonal transitions, especially premenstrually; improving blood flow; and minimizing the impact of fibroids and endometriosis.

## FOOD

**Choose:**

- A diet that won't stress your liver with too many synthetic compounds. The whole, unprocessed foods we recommend to everyone are even more important for this type. Aim for 60 percent vegetables and fruits, 30 percent complex carbohydrates, and 10 percent protein (lean meat, oily fish, low-fat cheese, nuts, and seeds).

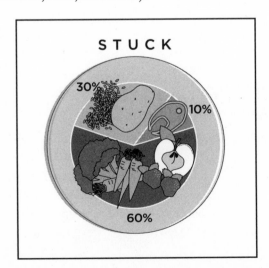

- Plenty of fiber, especially for women in phase 4 of their cycle (potential implantation).
- Cruciferous vegetables such as broccoli, which will help metabolize and eliminate excessive estrogen efficiently, taming PMS. They are particularly helpful for Stuck women in phase 4 of their cycle (potential implantation).
- Essential fatty acids (EFAs) found in plants, such as evening primrose oil, which is chock-a-block with omega-6 fatty acids. EFAs are especially good for Stuck women during phase 4 of their cycle (potential implantation).
- Calcium-rich foods to offset the way calcium levels drop in times of stress. This is particularly important for women, especially before their periods, because low calcium ultimately leads to reduced blood supply to the uterus.
- A daily glass of fruit or vegetable juice to make sure you get all the vitamins A and C you need to allow your body to absorb calcium efficiently. Get a little sun every day to take care of the vitamin D that works alongside them.
- Small amounts of foods that are naturally sour, such as citrus, vinegar, and pickles, to support liver function. (Monitor how much of these you eat. Too much sour food can stagnate the liver.) Try hot water with a little lemon in it first thing in the morning.
- Spices that move qi, including turmeric, thyme, rosemary, basil, mint, and garlic.
- To sit down and eat your meals slowly, chewing your food thoroughly.

## MINT-ORANGE FERTILI-TEA FOR STUCK TYPES

All these ingredients should be available at your health food store. Check the herb, spice, supplement, and tea sections.

**1 cup mint leaves**

**¼ cup oat straw tea leaves**

**½ cup red raspberry leaf tea leaves**

**2 teaspoons dried orange peel**

Combine all the ingredients in a small resealable container. Place 2 teaspoons of the mixture in a teacup. Pour boiling water over the tea and let steep for 10 minutes. Strain and serve.

## Avoid:

- Overeating or eating too frequently (eating again before the last meal has been digested).
- Eating on the run or eating when angry or upset.
- Food with preservatives or other added chemicals.
- Large or frequent servings of red meat.
- Animal products treated with hormones, especially red meat. The synthetic estrogens you'll be exposed to can worsen endometriosis and fibroids.
- Caffeine. Cut it out or at least limit it.
- Coffee (regular and decaf). Stuck types will benefit from eliminating coffee across the board, but Stuck women will see an immediate benefit by avoiding it during phase 4 of their cycle (potential implantation); PMS symptoms such as breast tenderness will subside.
- Salty foods and hard cheeses, if you tend to bloat.
- Excessively sour foods and drinks, or excessive quantities of sour foods. In small quantities, sour is good for the liver, but a little goes a long way.
- Fried or fatty foods.
- Dairy products.
- Flaxseeds and soy products such as tofu and edamame. Their phytoestrogens can make endometriosis and fibroids worse.
- Alcohol. Drinking may be tempting as a way to relieve tension, but it is a stimulant and will just worsen hormone imbalances and the symptoms that go with them.

## EXERCISE

- Get regular exercise. Do something aerobic, but don't let it get too intense. Half an hour of jogging every day would be a good choice. Besides the direct physical benefits, including improving circulation, it's a healthy way to let off steam. Regular moderate exercise is particularly beneficial to Stuck women during phase 4 of their cycle (potential implantation), supporting a good blood supply to the uterus.
- Stop jogging and all high-impact exercise during phase 1 of

your cycle (menstruation). That kind of exercise will just make heavy periods even heavier. But do get in motion to keep things flowing smoothly (moving blood and qi) and to ease cramps. Light exercise, such as walking, is a good choice. Daily but gentle exercise also is important during phase 3 of your cycle (ovulation).

- Engage in regular exercise with a meditative component, such as qi gong, yoga, tai chi, or even just walking outdoors. Exercise that is repetitive by nature, such as swimming or jogging, tends to quiet the mind while it occupies the body.
- Do not swim in cold water.

## LIFESTYLE

- Reduce stress. Develop an arsenal of relaxation techniques (meditation, deep breathing, meditative exercises, or whatever works for you) and put them into regular practice to relieve physical and mental tension. This is especially important for Stuck women during phases 3 and 4 of their cycle (ovulation and potential implantation). If you have a long follicular phase, stress may be getting in the way of ovulation.
- Take a look at how you handle your emotions, particularly whether you tend to bottle up your feelings, and find healthy ways of expressing your needs.
- Laugh.
- Avoid people or situations that you find frustrating.
- Practice breathing deeply so that you fill your abdomen with each breath.
- Focus on achieving balance in your life.
- Try the visualization exercises beginning on page 90.
- Try the self-massages beginning on page 92.
- Do not have intercourse during menstruation.
- Use pads instead of tampons, which impede blood flow.

## SUPPLEMENTS

- Zinc (especially premenstrually).
- Vitamin B complex.

- Magnesium.
- Calcium.
- Evening primrose oil, an omega-6 fatty acid usually available in capsule form, can increase and improve the quality of cervical mucus. It also can enhance fertility by smoothing hormonal transitions (including easing PMS and painful periods). It is useful throughout the cycle for Stuck types, but combination types may instead want to switch to flaxseed oil after ovulation to avoid possible cramps.
- Red raspberry leaf, usually in a tincture or tea, can improve blood flow, toning the uterus and helping to make it ready for pregnancy. Although it has been given to women during pregnancy for centuries, modern research suggests that red raspberry leaf may increase the risk of preterm labor, so if you use it to boost fertility, you should discontinue it once you become pregnant.
- Low-dose aspirin (see page 261) once a day. This is good for most people having trouble getting pregnant, but it is especially important for Stuck types.

## MEDICAL ASSISTANCE

- Ask your doctor about having a blood test to determine your prolactin level.
- Talk to your doctor about having a sonogram to detect or evaluate fibroids or endometriosis.

## CHINESE MEDICINE

- Acupuncture can smooth the flow of qi and blood, ease cramps, prevent clots, and stimulate even menstrual flow (especially in women whose periods stop and start or who have spotting). This may ultimately improve your ability to conceive, since any obstruction to the menstrual flow can have negative implications for fertility.
- Acupuncture can offset the effects of stress. It is particularly helpful to Stuck women who have BBT spikes in phase

2 of their cycle (pre-ovulation) not due to fever, alcohol consumption, or disturbed sleep, because stress is most likely the cause. It's also good for women with a long follicular phase, which can signal that stress is interfering with ovulation.

- For Stuck women with pain at ovulation, a long follicular phase, or PMS, herbs to move qi and blood can help alleviate symptoms, including pain, bloating, or sore breasts at ovulation, as well as breast tenderness, mood swings, irritability, weepiness, food cravings, skin breakouts, and bloating before your period. By correcting the imbalance in your reproductive system that is creating those symptoms, herbs can also improve your fertility. A licensed Chinese herbalist can prescribe a customized formula.

# CHAPTER TWENTY-THREE

# The Making Babies Rx: Pale

**T**he Making Babies program for Pale types can improve many aspects of your health and fertility, but most of these strategies are aimed particularly at being well nourished; ensuring good blood flow, especially in the pelvic area; and building a good uterine lining.

## FOOD

**Choose:**

- A diet that averages out to be around 30 percent protein (animal protein is especially beneficial), 30 percent complex carbohydrates (grains and starchy vegetables), and 40 percent vegetables and fruits.

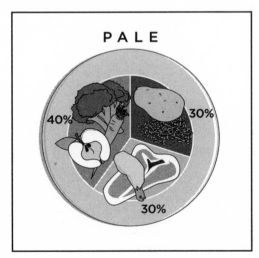

- Plenty of protein. We recommend at least one serving a day of meat (hormone-free, if possible), poultry, fish, eggs (specifically the yolk), or legumes. Meat that has been well marinated before cooking or has been slow-cooked for a long time is especially beneficial. If you are a committed vegetarian, make sure you eat a broad range of protein from different plant sources (nuts, seeds, beans, high-protein sprouts, and grains such as quinoa) in order to get the essential amino acids you need. Also consider supplementing with whey protein powder. Protein is doubly important for Pale women during phases 1 and 2 of their cycle (menstruation and pre-ovulation), while they are losing blood, and to help the body regenerate the endometrium and build follicles.

- Regular meals.
- Foods with phytoestrogens, such as flaxseeds and soy, to help build follicles. This is key during phases 1 and 2 of your cycle (menstruation and pre-ovulation), but good for you anytime. Pale/Stuck combination types should *avoid* phytoestrogens, however.
- Iron-rich foods, including blackstrap molasses, eggs, lentils, watercress, lean meat, liver and kidneys, and black currants. Vitamin C helps with the absorption of iron, so be sure to get plenty of that, too, from sources such as black currants, leafy dark green vegetables, oranges, broccoli, and kiwifruit.
- Soups with stock made from bones, such as chicken stock. This is particularly beneficial during phase 2 of your cycle (pre-ovulation). See the Chinese Medicine section for suggested ingredients for making a soup.

## PALE GREEN FERTILI-TEA FOR PALE TYPES

All these ingredients should be available at your health food store. Check the herb, spice, supplement, and tea sections.

**1 cup green tea leaves**                    **½ cup stinging nettle tea leaves**
**¼ cup dried wolfberries (Goji berries)**

Combine all the ingredients in a small resealable container. Place 2 teaspoons of the mixture in a small pot containing a cup of cold water. Bring to a boil and let boil for five minutes. Strain and serve.

**Avoid:**

- Caffeine, which inhibits the absorption of iron. It also promotes poor blood sugar regulation and cravings for simple sugars, which lead to reduced blood quality.
- Having liquids with meals, which decreases the absorption of nutrients. Try doing most of your drinking between meals.
- Eating dairy products to excess. Having milk with your cereal and in your tea and a daily yogurt are fine, just don't overdo it.
- Cold raw foods such as salads, ice cream, and drinks straight from the fridge. If you do eat cold foods, combine them with something warm. Have soup or a baked potato with your salad, for example.
- Eating on the run or while standing up, and eating while stressed.
- Dieting.
- Phytoestrogens, such as flaxseeds and soy, if you are a Pale/Stuck type.

## EXERCISE

- Limit aerobic exercise to thirty minutes three times a week.
- Engage in regular exercise with a meditative component, such as yoga, qi gong, or tai chi, and feel free to add whatever you like in terms of stretching or flexibility work.

## LIFESTYLE

- Be sure to get enough rest. This is particularly important during phase 1 of your cycle (menstruation).
- Develop your time management skills and work or study habits.
- Try not to worry about things you can't do anything about.
- Try the visualization exercises beginning on page 90.
- Try the self-massages beginning on page 92.

## SUPPLEMENTS

- Floradix (iron with herbs) is especially useful during phase 1 of your cycle (menstruation), when you are losing blood and iron.
- Liquid chlorophyll.
- L-carnitine.

## MEDICAL ASSISTANCE

- Ask your doctor about a blood test for anemia.

## CHINESE MEDICINE

- Acupuncture can help bring blood to the endometrium.
- Herbal formulas can help you build a thick endometrium. See an herbalist.
- A blood-nourishing soup can be especially beneficial in phase 2 of your cycle (pre-ovulation). One simple recipe is to boil a whole chicken with a selection of vegetables (such as carrots, mushrooms, onions, and sweet potatoes) and herbs available in any Chinese herb store. For herbs, try Shan Yao (wild yam), Goji (wolfberries), Sheng Jiang (fresh ginger), Da Zao (red dates), and Long Yan Rou (longan).

# CHAPTER TWENTY-FOUR

# The Making Babies Rx: Waterlogged

The Making Babies program for Waterlogged types can improve many aspects of your health and fertility, but most of these strategies are aimed particularly at preventing the accumulation of mucus and minimizing the impact of fibroids and endometriosis.

## FOOD

**Choose:**

- A diet relatively high in protein (30 percent) and low in complex carbohydrates (20 percent), with lots of vegetables and fruits (50 percent).

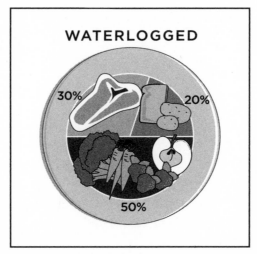

- Nutrient-rich foods, especially "living" foods such as green vegetables.
- Whole grains and other slow-releasing carbs to avoid

fluctuations in blood sugar levels as much as possible. Replace refined sugars with natural sugars such as agave nectar.

- Barley, which is a natural diuretic.
- Green tea, which, in addition to all its other beneficial properties, is a natural diuretic. (See box for a green tea mixture that's particularly good for Waterlogged people.)
- A diet relatively low in carbohydrates. When you do eat carbs, partner them with protein to hold your blood sugar steady.
- Yogurt, although you should otherwise avoid dairy products. In our experience, the body reacts differently to yogurt than to other dairy.
- Sheep's and goat's milk and milk products. Many people tolerate them better than dairy products made from cow's milk.
- To hydrate, hydrate, hydrate. Ironically, a lot of Waterlogged people are actually dehydrated. Drinking water helps flush out retained fluids.

## SPICY GREEN FERTILI-TEA FOR WATERLOGGED TYPES

All these ingredients should be available at your health food store. Check the herb, spice, supplement, and tea sections.

**1 cup roasted barley tea**                    **½ cup green tea leaves**

**2 tablespoons ground cardamom**

Combine all the ingredients in a small resealable container. Place 2 teaspoons of the mixture in a teacup. Pour boiling water over the tea and let steep for 10 minutes. Strain and serve.

### Avoid:

- Overeating.
- Raw or cold foods.
- Heavy, hard-to-digest meals and rich or greasy foods, such as cream sauces and anything deep-fried.
- Spicy foods.
- Alcohol.
- Dairy products made from cow's milk (with the exception of yogurt), which can lead to excess mucus.

- Processed foods. Waterlogged types are especially likely to react badly to them.
- Sugars and artificial sweeteners, especially high-fructose corn syrup.
- An overabundance of refined wheat products.
- Yeast, fungi, molds, and anything fermented, because Waterlogged types are prone to candida (yeast infections). Beer, bread, soy sauce, wine, vinegar, mushrooms, and blue cheeses are out.
- Excessive salt. (Another reason to avoid processed foods: they tend to be very salty, even the ones that don't taste salty.)
- Pork and rich, fatty meat, including many cuts of beef.
- Saturated fats.
- Fatty or oily foods, especially deep-fried foods.
- Soy, flaxseeds, and other sources of phytoestrogens, especially if you have endometriosis or fibroids.
- Yams, if you've been diagnosed with polycystic ovarian syndrome (PCOS; see page 202). Although yams are often touted as fertility boosters, they have too many carbs for PCOS bodies.

### EXERCISE

- Keep moving. Keeping your body in motion helps keep the fluids in your body moving as they should.
- Get regular aerobic exercise; about thirty minutes a day is fine. Avoid exercise that is too intense. Get your blood pumping, but don't exhaust yourself.
- Set exercise goals and make a plan for achieving them.

### LIFESTYLE

- Keep your environment mold-free. Be vigilant about damp areas in your home where mold might appear (especially basements and bathrooms). Autumn leaves are another common source of mold. Make sure they are cleaned up promptly and properly, but let someone else do the raking.

- Try an herbal digestive such as hawthorn flakes or fennel seeds after a rich meal, as many Asian people do. (See Resources.)
- Keep a BBT chart if you have trouble tracking ovulation by observing your cervical mucus. Waterlogged women may produce mucus at other times in their cycle as well, obscuring the time of ovulation.
- Try the visualization exercises beginning on page 90.
- Try the self-massages beginning on page 92.

## SUPPLEMENTS

- Chromium.
- Probiotics boost the population of beneficial bacteria in the digestive tract. They also combat candida (yeast infections or overgrowth), which Waterlogged people are particularly prone to.

## MEDICAL ASSISTANCE

- Consult with your doctor if you have PCOS. You may not be ovulating at all.

## CHINESE MEDICINE

- Acupuncture can improve ovulation in women with PCOS.
- Herbs that combat fluid metabolism problems can help thin or clear mucus secretions that are impeding flow in the fallopian tubes. The same type of herbs may also correct implantation problems due to mucus on the uterine lining or ineffective pinocytosis (the mechanism pressing together the front and back walls of the uterus). Consult an herbalist.

# PART SIX

# Getting Pregnant with a Little Help

CHAPTER TWENTY-FIVE

# Assisted Reproduction:
# When You Need the Next Step

**N**ot everyone will be able to get pregnant naturally. In some cases, there comes a time when nature needs a little help. If you've been through the Making Babies program, have had a thorough medical history and physical exam, and have received a specific fertility diagnosis and done whatever is necessary to correct the problem, that time may have arrived for you. This chapter describes the menu of assisted reproductive technologies (ARTs) available to you. As you peruse it, don't abandon the idea of sticking as close to nature as possible. Even in these high-tech realms, it still pays to be guided by the wisdom of your body.

The Centers for Disease Control (CDC) defines assisted reproductive technologies (formerly known as *artificial* reproductive technologies) as fertility treatments in which eggs and/or sperm are manipulated in the lab. For our purposes, we've expanded this definition to include all common fertility treatments. Here they are arranged from most "natural" to least. In general, an approach earlier in this chapter will be easier (and cheaper) than one later in the chapter. For each treatment, you'll also find ways to make that approach as gentle and as effective as possible. We often find that the less invasive techniques are not just less risky and easier on the body but also more successful.

### FERTILITY DRUGS

For couples struggling to get pregnant, the first treatment option is usually fertility drugs. Used judiciously to enhance ovulation, they can be very helpful for women who are not ovulating or are ovulating irregularly. Women with polycystic ovarian syndrome (PCOS; see page 202) often benefit from fertility drugs. The ovary-stimulating medicines can

319

also help with unexplained infertility. Some doctors use them to treat luteal phase defect (LPD; see page 200) when FSH is low, but I (Sami) usually use progesterone to treat LPD.

Fertility drugs are also generally used during the first part of treatment with ARTs, including IUI (see page 325) and IVF (see page 327), in an effort to produce more than the usual one egg per month.

Fertility drugs are very good at stimulating ovulation; the vast majority of women who take them will ovulate within the first three months of treatment. About half of the women who ovulate with drugs will get pregnant; results depend on all the other factors that influence pregnancy, including age and sperm quality. Oral fertility drugs are not as expensive as other medical treatments for fertility, although the costs of repeated office visits for monitoring can add up well beyond the cost of the medication.

But fertility drugs are not without risks. They can cause a range of minor side effects, including bloating and tenderness in the abdomen and/or breasts, mild swelling of the ovaries, stomach pain, nausea and vomiting, fluid retention, weight gain, headaches, insomnia, fatigue, irritability, depression, and blurred vision. Any one of these may not be so bad on its own, but layered on top of one another and repeated month after month, they can be pretty difficult to handle. In rare cases, fertility drugs can cause ovarian cysts (see page 238), which in turn can cause fertility problems as well as unpleasant symptoms. There is also the risk of ovarian hyperstimulation syndrome (OHSS; see page 323), which in a small portion of cases can be quite serious. Long-term and/or high-dose use of these powerful drugs can increase the risk of ovarian, breast, and uterine cancers. (Standard use of these drugs for a few cycles, however, does not increase the risk.)

Taking fertility drugs also increases the chances of twins (or more), which in turn increases the risks of the pregnancy for both mother and children (see page 15).

So it makes sense to use fertility drugs carefully, at sensible doses, and for a reasonable number of cycles. Most couples under age 35 should try to conceive for a year before beginning fertility drugs. (Following the Making Babies program will improve the odds.) If you decide to use fertility drugs, make sure you understand both the cause of your infertility and how the treatment the doctor suggests can address it. In general, we think that these drugs are prescribed too quickly and in doses that are too high. Sometimes doctors will go on providing them ad infinitum, despite the evidence that they are not effective for a particular patient. In addition, many doctors ignore the fact that lower doses aren't just safer and less likely to cause side effects, but they also can work better than higher doses in some patients. Using fertility drugs for up to four to six cycles is appropriate, but the odds of success don't improve after that. At that point, you should talk with your doctor about a different dose or medication or about moving on to another strategy altogether.

There are two commonly used fertility drugs, clomiphene and gonadotropins. When using either, you'll need a sonogram just before ovulation to monitor the effects on your ovaries, as well as a blood test to track estrogen and follicle development.

## Clomiphene

Clomiphene (including brand names Clomid and Serophene) essentially tricks the body into believing it has lower levels of estrogen, thereby prompting increased production of gonadotropin-releasing hormone (GnRH), which in turn stimulates release of LH and FSH and so triggers the ovaries to mature follicles and release eggs.

Clomiphene is taken orally for about five days starting three to five days into your cycle. (If your period is irregular or you aren't menstruating, your doctor may induce menstruation with another drug in order to time the clomiphene properly.) The most common dose is 50 mg a day, but I (Sami) usually prescribe 25 mg a day, at least to start with. Ovulation generally occurs between five and twelve days after the last dose. For patients with PCOS who have high or high normal levels of male hormones, I prescribe dexamethasone, too, to enhance the effectiveness of the clomiphene by suppressing the production of male hormones. Your doctor will monitor you via sonograms and blood tests to confirm your body's response to the medication and identify the timing of ovulation. It may take a couple of months before you start ovulating regularly with the drugs.

Clomiphene comes with the side effects and risks described in the previous section. The chances of conceiving twins (or more) are about 5 to 8 percent (compared with 2 percent in the general population). In addition, it can dry up cervical mucus to the point where healthy sperm have a hard time reaching the eggs efficiently. In this case, you may have lots of eggs, but they are unlikely to get fertilized. High doses of clomiphene (even the standard dose, depending on a woman's reaction to it) can also thin out the endometrium to the point where implantation may not occur.

Specialists in male fertility use clomiphene and, less frequently, gonadotropins (see the next section) to treat men. Clomiphene can improve sperm count, quality, or motility in cases where low testosterone is to blame for infertility. It is very effective as long as it is used only after other causes of low testosterone have been ruled out: varicoceles, thyroid disorders, and high prolactin. If testosterone is low because of general physical or psychological stress, however, clomiphene is an option. In men, it is used at very low doses (25 mg) daily for about twenty-five days each month, and only for a limited amount of time, usually no more than four to six months.

### Gonadotropins

Gonadotropins (including brand names Bravelle, Follistim, Gonal-f, Menopur, and Repronex) are also used to stimulate ovulation, though by a different hormonal mechanism. Because they must be injected, are much more expensive, and come with a greater chance of pregnancy with multiples compared to clomiphene, gonadotropins generally aren't used unless a patient has tried and not responded to clomiphene or for some reason can't use clomiphene. Like clomiphene, gonadotropins are useful in treating ovulation problems, PCOS, LPD, and unexplained infertility and as part of ARTs.

Gonadotropin use is a two-step process. First comes seven to twelve days of daily injections of FSH or a mixture of FSH and LH, depending on how long it takes your eggs to mature, starting on day 3 of your cycle. This coaxes the ovaries to mature and release more eggs than the usual one at a time. Then there is a shot of human chorionic gonadotropin (HCG), which triggers the release of the eggs within one to two days. (You or your partner gives the shot. You'll learn how in the doctor's office.) You'll be monitored via ultrasounds and blood tests to time the shot appropriately and to pinpoint ovulation.

Generally, the success rate of gonadotropins is about 20 percent per cycle, but this depends on several factors, including age, sperm quality, and the nature of the fertility problem. The chances of conceiving twins (or more) can be as high as 20 percent with gonadotropins.

### Ovarian Hyperstimulation Syndrome (OHSS)

Anyone considering or taking fertility drugs needs to be aware of ovarian hyperstimulation syndrome. Although it occurs in only a small percentage of treatment cycles and the effects may be mild, OHSS can be severe enough to require hospitalization and in rare instances can even be life threatening.

OHSS occurs when the ovaries are overstimulated by fertility drugs, even when used in typical doses. In effect, the ovaries respond *too* well, developing too many follicles and swelling to a few times their normal size. Symptoms typically begin within four to five days of ovulation and include nausea, abdominal bloating and a feeling of fullness, and weight gain. Abdominal distension, vomiting, diarrhea, decreased urine, darker urine, excessive thirst, dry skin and hair, a measurably larger abdomen, and rapid weight gain (2 pounds a day) would count as "moderate" symptoms and usually come layered right on top of the "mild" ones mentioned above. Some women get ovarian cysts (see page 238). Typically, all symptoms resolve on their own within a few days if you are not pregnant, although your doctor should monitor your condition.

This is the extent of the OHSS experience for most women, but some severe cases can involve any or all of the above and also lead to fullness or bloating above the waist; fluid around the lungs; difficulty breathing or painful breathing; shortness of breath; dizziness; pelvic, calf, or chest pain; overly concentrated blood cells; and blood clots. These can be serious enough to require hospitalization.

Anyone taking fertility drugs is at risk for OHSS, but certain women are more prone to it than others. These include younger women, women with PCOS (taking metformin as well as fertility drugs reduces the risk of OHSS), and women with high estrogen levels and a large number of follicles or eggs.

### A Better Way

Don't rush thoughtlessly into using fertility drugs. At the very least, you should be sure you understand the nature of your fertility problem, so that you know it is something fertility drugs can address. Despite the name, fertility drugs only make more eggs; they do not necessarily make you fertile.

The other key thing to remember is that when it comes to fertility drugs, more is not always better. Cutting back on the dosage can still prompt your ovaries into action without sapping your endometrium. And lower doses of clomiphene mean less of a drying effect on the cervical mucus.

For women with PCOS, taking metformin along with fertility drugs can reduce the risk of OHSS.

### Chinese Medicine

Yin tonifying herbs taken at the same time as fertility drugs can increase the chances of their effectiveness in women who are "poor responders." Chinese medicine considers fertility drugs to be yang tonics, and powerful ones at that. So yin-nourishing herbs, taken under the care of a Chinese medicine practitioner, can also help offset the side effects of the drugs, including a thin uterine lining and decreased fertile cervical mucus.

Combining these two treatments is a good path for many patients, but it has to be done with great care and good communication between the medical doctor and the Chinese medicine practitioner. Better still is to begin the herbs well in advance of the drugs. Six months is ideal, but even one month makes a difference. This can improve response, and consequently the number of eggs released.

Herbs can also help in cases of OHSS, particularly those that benefit the corpus luteum, as can acupuncture in conjunction with supplemental progesterone.

Dry women often don't respond well to fertility drugs, so taking yin tonifying herbs in advance is particularly beneficial for them. (Interestingly, some IVF clinics are now applying a parallel strategy called *estrogen priming,* giving patients like this estrogen the month before the IVF cycle.)

Tired women generally react better to fertility drugs than other women, both in terms of outcome and having an easier time with side effects.

---

### Case Study: Louise

Louise had irregular menstrual cycles, which were making it very difficult for her and her husband to conceive. After trying for more than a year, she decided, at her gynecologist's suggestion, to take Clomid. She took one pill (50 mg) a day for five days in two menstrual cycles but still wasn't pregnant. The doctor then doubled the dose, which Louise took for two more cycles. Still no dice, so her doctor referred her to me (Sami).

After a thorough medical history and physical exam that didn't reveal any other issues, I simply recommended a *lower* dose of Clomid. In her next cycle, Louise took just half a pill (25 mg) each day for six days and quickly conceived. Louise and her husband now have a beautiful, healthy baby.

---

## INTRAUTERINE INSEMINATION (IUI)

Once known as "artificial insemination" and, rightly or wrongly, jokingly associated with turkey basters, the process of placing sperm into the uterus (without intercourse) has gone high-tech. Today the sperm are "washed" and placed in sterile fluid, which is then concentrated to a small volume and injected, through a catheter inserted through the cervix, directly into the uterus.

To increase the chances of success, in most cases doctors prescribe fertility drugs for the week before ovulation to stimulate the ovaries to mature several eggs. There may also be a "trigger shot" to induce ovulation at a very specific time in order to coordinate the IUI procedure most effectively.

I (Sami) usually do two IUIs, two days in a row, to make sure we get the timing right. After each IUI, I place a special cap over the cervix temporarily, so that what I put in there stays in there. I also give progesterone in the luteal phase of the cycle to ensure that the uterine lining is ready for implantation.

Doctors use hormone blood tests, ultrasounds, and/or ovulation predictor kits to track ovulation and time IUI accordingly. Once the woman ovulates, her partner is called upon to produce a sperm sample an hour or two before the IUI procedure. If the timing of all this isn't right, the couple is just wasting their time and effort (and money).

Studies have shown that pregnancy rates improved significantly in men who were abstinent no more than three days before collecting sperm for IUI as compared to men who were abstinent for longer. Ideally, sperm should be collected after no more than two days of abstinence.

Experts used to recommend longer periods of abstinence before collecting sperm, as sperm counts generally go up a bit under those circumstances. But it turns out that sperm motility goes down at the same time, and sperm that sit around for a while are vulnerable to structural and functional damage.

Even though the sperm are about to get washed in the lab, getting a clean sample to begin with is important. And once you have it, you need to deliver it safely, or your efforts will be for naught. It's helpful to follow these steps when collecting sperm.

1. Shower with antibacterial soap. If applicable, pull back the foreskin to wash.
2. Masturbate to ejaculation and collect the ejaculate in a sterile container according to the doctor's instructions.
3. Keep the sample at room or body temperature (this is especially important in cold weather) and bring it to the doctor's office within one to two hours at most.

The sperm are processed right in the doctor's office, then inserted into the uterus. The entire IUI procedure takes about an hour. Two weeks later, you'll know whether the insemination was successful.

IUI is one of the first interventions couples struggling to get pregnant should try. Fertilization takes place "naturally," inside the body, and not in a laboratory dish. It's less invasive than IVF, since the eggs don't have to be retrieved. And because it's less involved, it's also much cheaper. One study calculated the relative costs of IUI and IVF per delivery of a baby and found that on average, IVF rang up a bill several times that of IUI.

In cases of male factor infertility, IUI is more effective than timed intercourse. IUI produces better results than fertility drugs alone in cases of unexplained infertility. And in a man with normal sperm count, motility, and morphology, results are as good with three to four IUI attempts as with one cycle of IVF.

Of course, IUI is most successful when it is used appropriately. It's most helpful in cases of low sperm count or poor motility. If sperm count is *really* low, IVF with intracytoplasmic sperm injection (ICSI; see page 334) may be more appropriate. And if there's no sperm at all, you might consider IUI with donor sperm or sperm extracted directly from the male partner's testicle. IUI is also beneficial when infertility is officially unexplained. And because the technique bypasses cervical mucus, it's one way to address hostile cervical mucus. (Others are described on pages 269–71.)

On average, there's about a 15 to 20 percent pregnancy rate per IUI attempt. We recommend that our patients undergo three to four cycles of IUI (when appropriate) before seriously considering IVF.

## IN VITRO FERTILIZATION (IVF)

In vitro fertilization is far and away the most common high-tech fertility treatment. It accounts for about 90 percent of ART procedures in the United States and results in about 48,000 babies born each year in this country.

Most descriptions or explanations of IVF will say that it is used in cases of ovulation problems. That's true — it *is* used for ovulation problems, but it *shouldn't* be. If the only problem is failure to ovulate or poor quality of ovulation, going straight to IVF is like hitting a nail with a sledgehammer. Many other strategies should be employed long before IVF is even considered.

When appropriately applied, however, IVF is a most valuable option for couples trying to surmount blocked (badly scarred) fallopian tubes, poor sperm quality, or unexplained infertility. These are the conditions IVF was, in fact, originally developed and used for. In the intervening decades, however, couples have developed an attitude of "We've been trying for three or four months already; let's just do IVF." I (Sami) might in fact refer a couple for IVF after a few months — but only if the woman is 38 or older or the couple has been diagnosed with one of these problems. Even then, I'd rather they try other strategies first.

Younger women, as well as couples with other fertility issues, generally have much better options than IVF open to them — options that are safer, cheaper, easier, and more effective. Younger women also have time on their side, so there's simply no need to rush into IVF without fully exploring the alternatives. (If they have had a complete medical history and evaluation and have already tried other methods — including just giving it time — IVF may indeed be a good choice.) Younger women are much more likely to be successful with IVF than older women—but they are also much more likely to be successful without it.

### What Happens in IVF?

With IVF, you need to get a lot of eggs at once. First, the woman takes injectable fertility drugs to stimulate the ovaries to develop several eggs rather than the usual one. Sometimes doctors also prescribe Lupron, a synthetic hormone, to prevent premature release of those eggs. In some cases, Lupron is prescribed for a month before the IVF cycle begins, to suppress the normal hormones before waking them up again with the ovary-stimulating drugs.

The doctor will monitor the development of the eggs via ultrasound and hormonal blood tests to detect when they are mature. When enough follicles are the right size, the woman is given an injection of HCG to complete the process of egg maturation. Thirty-six to forty hours after the HCG shot, the eggs are removed from the ovary using a needle inserted through the vaginal wall and guided by ultrasound images. (This procedure is performed under general anesthesia.)

Meanwhile, the male partner collects the sperm, as described on page 326. Donor sperm can also be used if needed. The sperm and eggs are combined in a dish in the lab, then monitored to confirm fertilization. Fertilized eggs develop for two to five days, at which point each is a small ball of cells officially known as an embryo, ready to be placed in the uterus.

Standard practice today is to place between two and four embryos at a time, depending on the age of the woman. This is done to increase the chances of one implanting, but it also increases the chances of more than one implanting. About a third of IVF pregnancies are twins (or more), and this brings increased risks to mother and children. This is why we applaud the small but growing trend toward placing one embryo at a time (discussed later in this section).

The embryos make their journey into the uterus through a thin catheter inserted through the cervix. Any embryos created but not transferred can be frozen for potential use in future cycles. If all goes well, at least one transferred embryo will implant in the uterine wall and grow into a baby. The woman has to wait about ten to twelve days after transfer to take a pregnancy test.

For any given IVF cycle, pregnancy will result an average of 35 percent of the time. At the most successful clinics, this translates into an average of about a 28 percent chance of the birth of a baby per cycle (after factoring in miscarriages). It's a bit less when using frozen embryos. Success rates can range from 15 to 50 percent, depending on age and the underlying fertility problem.

Success doesn't come without risks, starting with the risks associated with multiples pregnancies. There are also risks of using fertility drugs, including the risk of OHSS (see page 323). In addition, babies born from high-tech fertility treatments such as IVF are at mildly increased risk of birth defects and low birth weight, though no one can yet say for sure whether that's because of the underlying fertility problem or the treatment itself. IVF also leaves most couples in the uncomfortable moral position of having to decide what to do with unused embryos.

Fertilizing eggs outside the body is expensive. In the United States, one cycle of IVF costs on average $12,400 and may not be covered by insurance.

### Genetic Screening

Preimplantation genetic diagnosis (PGD), sometimes called preimplantation genetic screening (PGS), is a way of screening embryos for chromosomal defects such as Down syndrome before they are transferred in IVF. In this relatively new procedure, a single cell is extracted from a days-old embryo for screening.

This allows couples carrying genes for serious genetic disorders such as cystic fibrosis and Tay-Sachs disease to choose embryos without the disease. PGD is increasingly being used in IVF even when there's no particular genetic concern. The idea is that screening for the healthiest embryos will improve success rates. The vast majority of IVF clinics offer PGD — for an extra fee, of course.

But a recent Dutch study published in the *New England Journal of Medicine* suggests that women over age 35 — when risks of Down's and the like are at their highest — should *not* use this screening, at least not routinely. The women in the study ranged in age from 35 to 41. The group that received PGS had a substantially *decreased* chance of getting pregnant — 25 percent, as opposed to 37 percent in the group that had IVF but no screening.

Scientists don't yet know whether the removal of the one cell could be more harmful than has previously been thought to be the case, or whether there's a flaw in presuming that the one cell is representative of the whole embryo — so a cell that tests normal could actually be representing an embryo with abnormalities, or a cell that tests abnormal could actually be representing a healthy embryo. I (Sami) recently had two patients who started IVF with PGD but were told that all their embryos were genetically abnormal, and so none were implanted. Both went on to get pregnant without fertility drugs or IVF and to have healthy babies.

More research is needed to answer these crucial questions and to find other ways to improve IVF success rates. Women over age 35 need answers: they already face lower odds of IVF pregnancy than younger women, and in the Dutch study fully 60 percent of the embryos that were tested were deemed abnormal. (Other estimates put that figure at more like 40 percent, but that is still high.) Furthermore, a single screening test can cost up to $5,000.

### A Better Way: Natural Cycle, or Soft, IVF

Although the American way of using IVF has gone overboard — too much of a good thing — in Europe there is a growing trend toward a kinder, gentler application of the same technology. Natural cycle, or soft, IVF uses lower doses of fertility drugs (maturing fewer eggs), high-tech scanning to select high-quality eggs (so it isn't necessary to stimulate the ovaries to overproduce), and single embryo transfer with a more mature embryo. This approach lowers side effects and risks for mother and child, while improving success rates over single embryo transfers as they are typically performed in the United States. Natural cycle IVF can't yet compete with multi-embryo IVF cycles on the basis of pregnancy rates alone, but we believe it's getting there. In our opinion, the lower pregnancy rate is compensated for by the reduction of risks. It's not for everyone, but for many couples, especially for younger women who don't feel such time pressure to have more than one child at a time, we think this is a better way of doing IVF.

In some European countries where national health insurance programs cover IVF and regulate its application, natural cycle IVF is more common than standard IVF. IVF birthrates across the whole population are more or less the same as they are in this country, but with only

5 percent of those births being twins. Not only can natural cycle IVF be as effective as standard IVF and safer, it also costs less, societally speaking, than does IVF the way we do it here. Total costs of pregnancy and childbirth for all women seeking fertility treatments are lower in groups that use only single embryo transfers than in groups that have several embryos transferred—even factoring in the possibility of more cycles being necessary in the single embryo group. A group average like that won't make any difference to an individual American deciding about how to approach IVF, but it does speak to how we think our current system ought to be revamped.

Several early studies of soft IVF have demonstrated that it is effective and also have revealed some of the reasons why. A study of four hundred couples in the Netherlands compared patients who had standard IVF with patients who had natural cycle IVF. Over the course of one year, both groups had exactly the same rate of births, even though only one embryo at a time was transferred in the soft group, as opposed to two or three embryos in the other group.

In Spain, researchers found genetic abnormalities in fully half of all embryos after standard amounts of fertility drugs were used. But when the same couples used just half the standard dose, only a third of the embryos had such abnormalities.

A Belgian study confirmed that babies born after single embryo transfer were as healthy as babies conceived without any assistance from reproductive technology. Multiples pregnancies raise the risk of low birth weight and preterm birth, but in this study gestational age and birth weight were the same in single embryo transfer babies as they are in spontaneously conceived babies. Besides demonstrating that single embryo transfer is safer because it avoids the risks of a multiples pregnancy, this study also highlighted its effectiveness: more than 46 percent of the single embryo transfers resulted in conception.

Most natural cycle IVF transfers technically do not involve an embryo but the more mature *blastocyst*. This is an embryo that has been growing in a lab for five or six days (versus two or three days in standard IVF). Only the healthiest embryos survive to the blastocyst stage, and then the best of these can be selected for transfer into the uterus, raising pregnancy rates. This is how IVF is generally done in the UK, where increasingly only one embryo is transferred.

We'd like to see what's happening in Europe also happen here, and there are some signs that it is coming. In 2006, the American Society for Reproductive Medicine (ASRM) issued new guidelines on the appropriate number of embryos to transfer. For women age 35 and up, the recommendations range, by age, from two or three up to no more than five. But for women under age 35, the official recommendation is for one or two, and we are heartened by the inclusion of single embryo transfer as a valid option. Better still, the Institute of Medicine, part of the National Academies, issued a report calling for guidelines promoting single embryo transfer (as well as stricter guidelines for use of fertility drugs). Even when using quite an advanced ART such as IVF, we are still always in favor of the approach using as subtle an intervention as possible.

## Acupuncture

Acupuncture has been proven to significantly increase success rates in standard IVF. We've already seen various ways in which acupuncture can improve fertility in several situations, long before IVF is considered, as well as in conjunction with some medical treatments. All those benefits are important in technological intervention as well as in natural conception.

There's a growing body of work appearing in top-drawer research journals providing proof that acupuncture is effective. In 2006, for example, the preeminent fertility medicine journal *Fertility and Sterility* devoted an issue to a series of studies demonstrating the effectiveness of combining acupuncture and infertility treatments.

Several studies have demonstrated that just a few acupuncture treatments dramatically improve success rates of standard IVF. Longer-term acupuncture treatment before IVF begins can draw on all of the fertility benefits to improve IVF results (and sometimes obviate the need for IVF at all), as well as curb side effects and risks of IVF treatment. But even acupuncture treatments given before and after embryo transfer can raise pregnancy rates and birthrates by 50 percent or more.

One of the earliest studies to demonstrate this was actually comparing acupuncture and standard anesthesia during IVF egg retrieval. The data unexpectedly revealed that the group receiving acupuncture had a higher "take home baby" rate than the group that got standard anesthesia.

Since then, research looking directly at this effect began to quantify the benefit of acupuncture, and a series of studies showed that women who received acupuncture around the time of embryo transfer had pregnancy rates 50 percent higher than women who didn't. (Acupuncture was found to have similar results when compared with sham acupuncture treatments, too, ruling out the possibility that the benefit was just a placebo effect.) Even more recent work analyzing a group of studies demonstrated that IVF success rates can go up by as much as 65 percent with acupuncture.

### *How to Use Acupuncture with IVF*

I (Jill) use essentially the same procedure with my patients as researchers have used in their studies of acupuncture and IVF: one treatment one to two days before embryo transfer (three to five days after egg retrieval) and one treatment one to two days after transfer. There's no need to stress about the precise timing of acupuncture, as long as you get one treatment on either side of transfer. These sessions focus on improving blood flow. Whatever treatment I do is always designed to support what the medical doctors are doing, so I follow their lead.

I also use one treatment a day or two before egg retrieval, to soften the cervix and bring blood to the uterus. And I like to see a patient twice a week for acupuncture while she is taking the medications to stimulate her ovaries. Acupuncture can also stimulate the ovaries, so this is especially useful in patients who don't respond well to ovary-stimulating drugs (women who don't develop many follicles). A doctor may see this poor response (or nonresponse) on a sonogram, and if the patient comes to me for acupuncture that day, the next day's sonogram often shows that the follicles have grown, amazing the doctors even more than the patients.

These limited treatments can be very powerful. But if I had my way, every patient would get three months of acupuncture before IVF is even started, to get into tip-top shape for IVF. Some benefits (balancing reproductive hormones and ameliorating stress) take longer to bring about than others (getting more blood to the endometrium for implantation). Three months of treatment, possibly with herbs, too, will allow time for the benefits to accrue. (You usually need to stop using ovulation-stimulating herbs before an IVF cycle, however, because the herbs help the body develop a lead follicle, following the natural process, while fertility drugs aim to get lots of eggs started at the same time.) Combined with the Making Babies program, acupuncture is the ideal way to prepare the body for optimal success with IVF.

---

### Case Study: Althea

Althea was 38 when she came to me (Jill) and had already had three unsuccessful IVF treatments. She was herself a medical doctor and very reticent about seeking alternative care (though equally disillusioned with the medical care she had tried). But she had done her research, read the study about acupuncture increasing IVF pregnancy rates by 50 percent, and decided to give it a chance.

Althea's next IVF attempt was scheduled to begin the next month, but I suggested that she take three months to get her body in shape for pregnancy before trying again. Based on what she told me about her previous attempts, I felt that if she went ahead with the next IVF so soon, even with the addition of acupuncture, she would get the same disappointing results. She had not produced many follicles in response to the fertility drugs she'd taken to prepare for IVF. Although I'm in favor of acupuncture timed around embryo transfer, such an approach could do nothing about the difficulty in obtaining an embryo in the first place. Althea agreed, somewhat reluctantly, to delay her next IVF cycle.

Women who respond poorly to fertility drugs are usually Dry types (yin deficient), and sure enough Althea had other Dry symptoms, including night sweats, hot flashes, and very light periods. I prescribed weekly acupuncture sessions and yin tonifying herbs.

Over the next three months, Althea's Dry signs came back into balance. She was less tired, her periods got heavier, and her hot flashes and night sweats subsided, so I told her to go ahead and schedule her next IVF. She stopped taking herbs just before she began that fourth IVF treatment but continued with the acupuncture throughout the cycle.

This time, she responded to the drugs. In fact, she not only produced enough follicles to go ahead with the IVF, but she also had two spare embryos to freeze for future use. The doctors—including Althea herself—were amazed at the change. The fourth time was the charm, and Althea got pregnant during that cycle. At this writing, she is the mom of a two-year-old and pregnant again, having had one of her frozen embryos successfully transferred with IVF supported by acupuncture.

---

## INTRACYTOPLASMIC SPERM INJECTION (ICSI)

Intracytoplasmic sperm injection is a form of IVF in which instead of eggs being placed in a petri dish with up to half a million sperm swimming around them, vying for fertilization rights, a single sperm is injected directly into an individual egg with a fine glass needle.

ICSI is best for couples in which the male partner has an extremely low sperm count, poor sperm motility, or structurally damaged sperm. It can also be used when one or both of the tubes that carry sperm (the vasa deferentia) are damaged or missing, or when the man has had an irreversible vasectomy. It's also useful for couples who have had poor or no fertilization in a previous IVF cycle.

For the woman, ICSI proceeds just as standard IVF does. For most men, their part is the same, too: the usual sperm collection via masturbation. If there aren't enough sperm in the ejaculate, a minor operation under anesthesia may be required to collect sperm directly from the testicles with a needle. Frozen sperm or donor sperm may also be used.

One good sperm is then isolated in the lab and inserted into an egg. That process is then repeated to create the desired number of embryos. The rest of the process proceeds just as standard IVF does: embryos are inserted into the uterus, extra embryos are frozen, and pregnancy testing is done in two weeks.

ICSI success rates are similar to those of standard IVF: there's a 34 percent chance of conceiving per cycle, and a 28 percent chance of ultimately having a baby, which, taken together over twelve months, translates to a 45 percent pregnancy rate, although, just as with IVF, results vary according to age, the nature of the underlying fertility problem, general health, and so forth.

ICSI is more useful than IVF alone for certain couples, but it also has some drawbacks. The lab work is more involved and expensive, tacking on about $1,500 to the already high cost of IVF, and insurance may not cover this. ICSI also potentially enables fertilization by abnormal sperm. Studies have established that children born after ICSI face a slightly increased risk of birth defects, although it's unknown whether that's due to the technique itself or to abnormalities in the sperm. Infertile men are more likely than fertile men to have genetic abnormalities, usually alterations of the Y chromosome. Men with missing vasa deferentia are also more likely to carry mutations responsible for cystic fibrosis. It may be that the fertility problem itself is handed down from generation to generation, so it's a good idea to speak to a genetic counselor and have all relevant genetic tests before having ICSI.

Yet ICSI is fast becoming the preferred method of IVF. A study from the University of Illinois at Chicago published in the *New England Journal of Medicine* demonstrated that although ICSI makes a pricey procedure even more expensive, does not improve results overall, and increases risks, its use is mushrooming in couples not diagnosed with male factor infertility.

A recent analysis of government statistics showed that 58 percent of IVF attempts used ICSI, up from 11 percent a decade earlier, while the proportion of couples with male factor infertility having IVF stayed the same (about 34 percent). The same set of stats revealed that ICSI treatments were actually no better than IVF alone in terms of successful pregnancies.

Some clinics perform ICSI when only a few eggs are available, since it reduces the risk of poor fertilization. Some favor it for couples who have already failed with standard IVF. And some use it for everyone, promoting it as the best chance for success. Although it is true that ICSI has higher success rates than standard IVF in cases with severe sperm deficiency, the routine use of ICSI seems to provide no benefit to couples with normal sperm. Thus, many people are paying a lot for ICSI without any evidence that it's helping them at all.

## GAMETE INTRAFALLOPIAN TRANSFER (GIFT)

Gamete intrafallopian transfer is no longer a common intervention, having been supplanted by IVF, and we never recommend it. You'll still see it discussed as an ART option, though, and we are including it here so that you understand what it is.

In the early years of ARTs, GIFT produced higher pregnancy rates than IVF, but that has since been reversed. In GIFT, sperm and unfertilized eggs (the male and female gametes) are placed directly in the fallopian tubes, so fertilization occurs more naturally than with IVF—that is, inside the fallopian tubes rather than in the lab. This technique requires laparoscopic surgery and as a result, given the less invasive alternative of IVF, is rarely used. GIFT also is generally more expensive than IVF. GIFT currently accounts for less than 1 percent of ART procedures.

GIFT begins with drug stimulation and then monitoring of the ovaries, just as in IVF. The eggs are removed through a small incision in the abdominal wall, guided by a laparoscope. The eggs are combined on the spot with the sperm sample, which has been collected in the usual way and is ready and waiting. The sperm and eggs are inserted into the fallopian tubes through the same incision. This is day surgery, but it does entail more in the way of recovery than standard egg retrieval.

Most doctors place about four eggs, which increases the rate of multiples pregnancy to about 15 to 20 percent. Overall success rates vary, of course, with age and fertility issues, but on average there is about a 21 percent chance of producing a baby with each GIFT cycle.

Most clinics no longer perform or recommend GIFT, and it is not to be used for male factor infertility.

## ZYGOTE INTRAFALLOPIAN TRANSFER (ZIFT)

As with GIFT, zygote intrafallopian transfer is generally outmoded. We never recommend it but include it here because you might see or hear it discussed, and we want you to at least understand the basics.

ZIFT is more invasive than IVF, less "natural" than GIFT, and more expensive than both of those techniques. It may be used when it is important to be able to confirm that fertilization has occurred. About two hundred babies are born this way in the United States each year.

In ZIFT, sperm fertilize eggs outside the body. ICSI can be used for fertilization, if necessary. It takes about a day to be sure fertilization has occurred, and then it is time for surgery—the zygotes (fertilized eggs) are transferred laparoscopically into the fallopian tubes.

Most doctors place between one and four zygotes, and if all goes according to plan, the zygotes then travel through the fallopian tubes to implant in the uterus. About 25 percent of ZIFT pregnancies result in multiples. Success rates vary with age and other factors, but on average there is about a 26 percent chance of producing a baby with each ZIFT cycle.

## DONOR EGGS

For women over age 43 who are not making healthy eggs, women in premature menopause, or women who don't produce sufficient eggs even with fertility drugs, the final technological option is usually donor eggs. Eggs from a donor are fertilized with sperm from the patient's partner, and the resulting embryo is placed in the patient's uterus. (Some clinics offer donor embryos; donor sperm can be used as well.)

Once again, this process is a variation on standard IVF, except it is the donor who takes fertility drugs and has her eggs collected. The patient takes medications, too, to manipulate her estrogen levels in order to get her cycle in sync with the donor's. The patient is given progesterone as well, to prepare her uterine lining to support an embryo at the appropriate time. Sperm are collected, and then IVF proceeds as usual.

Each cycle of donor egg (or embryo) IVF provides about a 60 to 70 percent chance of having a baby (less with a frozen embryo). As always, results vary according to age, nature of the fertility problem, general health, and other factors. Donor egg IVF often has a higher success rate than standard IVF because donor eggs usually come from younger and more fertile women. The process is considerably more expensive than standard IVF, mainly due to compensation for the donor, although the additional tests and treatments can add up as well. One cycle can cost up to $30,000, and insurance may not cover it. There is also a high risk of multiples: 40 percent of donor egg pregnancies result in twins (or more).

For many couples, the biggest drawback to donor eggs is the lack of genetic connection to the child. Using a known, rather than an anonymous, donor may partially address this issue, although it comes with its own potential complications (interpersonal, not medical). For some people, donor eggs are the best option if the woman is at risk of passing a genetic disease on to her child. Some couples use donor eggs because carrying a child is more important to them than a genetic connection. These woman want to carry the child themselves so that they can maintain control over the pregnancy, keeping it as healthy as possible. And some couples decide not to tread this far down the path of technological options and choose another route to parenthood. There's no right answer; every couple has to decide what's right for them.

## WHAT THE FUTURE HOLDS

Scientists in labs around the world are already working on new ARTs that will make donor egg IVF seem positively old-school. Researchers have reported early successes with freezing eggs and tissue from ovaries for later use, treating human stem cells to a chemical and vitamin cocktail to make sperm and eggs, growing human ovaries complete with eggs in lab mice, and making sperm out of stem cells extracted from a human tooth and injected into the testes of lab mice. These examples just scratch the surface of the race for the next generation of infertility treatments.

Whenever these or other novel approaches come to fruition, we'll welcome them for our patients who need them. But our fervent hope is that by then, the medical community will have a better grasp of who needs what kind of fertility treatment and when. With the right kind of care, many more people could conceive and carry a pregnancy much more naturally, without ART. We understand why couples will go to such extraordinary lengths to have a child, but we would like to see them give ordinary measures a chance to work first.

## Making Babies Action Plan

- ❏ Follow the Making Babies program for three months before pursuing assisted reproduction.
- ❏ Before you try fertility drugs or other assisted reproduction, make sure you understand the cause of your infertility and how the treatment proposed addresses it.
- ❏ Evaluate other less invasive ARTs before using those that are more invasive.
- ❏ Weigh the negative aspects of IVF and other ARTs along with the potential benefits.
- ❏ Consider working with a Chinese medicine practitioner to support any Western fertility treatments you use. Especially consider acupuncture with IVF.
- ❏ If you are under age 35, try to conceive for a year before considering fertility drugs.
- ❏ Consider lower doses of fertility drugs and limit their use to six cycles.
- ❏ Collect sperm for IUI, ICSI, or IVF properly and after no more than two days of abstinence.
- ❏ If lack of ovulation is the only fertility problem, don't start with IVF.
- ❏ Consider IVF in cases of blocked fallopian tubes, poor sperm quality, or truly unexplained infertility.
- ❏ Move more quickly to IVF if you are age 38 or older, but even then a few months of less invasive strategies are probably appropriate.

❏ Carefully consider ICSI and PGD before signing on for the additional risks and expense they entail. Both are useful in some circumstances but are prescribed far too often.

❏ If you decide to use IVF, investigate natural cycle, or soft, IVF.

❏ Remember, there's no one right path, only the one that's best for you.

# Appendix

## THE MAKING BABIES
## BASAL BODY TEMPERATURE CHART

Age ____ Fertility Cycle No: ____ Last 12 Cycles: Shortest ____ Longest ____ Month _____ Year _____ Cycle length _____

| | 1 | 2 | 3 | 4 | 5 | 6 | 7 | 8 | 9 | 10 | 11 | 12 | 13 | 14 | 15 | 16 | 17 | 18 | 19 | 20 | 21 | 22 | 23 | 24 | 25 | 26 | 27 | 28 | 29 | 30 | 31 | 32 | 33 | 34 | 35 | 36 | 37 | 38 | 39 | 40 |
|---|---|---|---|---|---|---|---|---|---|---|---|---|---|---|---|---|---|---|---|---|---|---|---|---|---|---|---|---|---|---|---|---|---|---|---|---|---|---|---|---|
| Cycle Day | | | | | | | | | | | | | | | | | | | | | | | | | | | | | | | | | | | | | | | | |
| Date | | | | | | | | | | | | | | | | | | | | | | | | | | | | | | | | | | | | | | | | |
| Weekday | | | | | | | | | | | | | | | | | | | | | | | | | | | | | | | | | | | | | | | | |
| Time Temp Normally Taken | | | | | | | | | | | | | | | | | | | | | | | | | | | | | | | | | | | | | | | | |
| Waking Temperature | | | | | | | | | | | | | | | | | | | | | | | | | | | | | | | | | | | | | | | | |
| Period | | | | | | | | | | | | | | | | | | | | | | | | | | | | | | | | | | | | | | | | |
| Sticky | | | | | | | | | | | | | | | | | | | | | | | | | | | | | | | | | | | | | | | | |
| Creamy | | | | | | | | | | | | | | | | | | | | | | | | | | | | | | | | | | | | | | | | |
| Egg-White | | | | | | | | | | | | | | | | | | | | | | | | | | | | | | | | | | | | | | | | |
| Pregnancy Test | | | | | | | | | | | | | | | | | | | | | | | | | | | | | | | | | | | | | | | | |
| Circle Intercourse on Cycle Day | 1 | 2 | 3 | 4 | 5 | 6 | 7 | 8 | 9 | 10 | 11 | 12 | 13 | 14 | 15 | 16 | 17 | 18 | 19 | 20 | 21 | 22 | 23 | 24 | 25 | 26 | 27 | 28 | 29 | 30 | 31 | 32 | 33 | 34 | 35 | 36 | 37 | 38 | 39 | 40 |
| Ovulation (LH) Test | | | | | | | | | | | | | | | | | | | | | | | | | | | | | | | | | | | | | | | | |
| Cervical Position | | | | | | | | | | | | | | | | | | | | | | | | | | | | | | | | | | | | | | | | |
| Other Symptoms | | | | | | | | | | | | | | | | | | | | | | | | | | | | | | | | | | | | | | | | |

The Waking Temperature grid is marked with temperature scale values from 99 down to 97 (reading 99, 9, 8, 7, 6, 5, 4, 3, 2, 1, 98, 9, 8, 7, 6, 5, 4, 3, 2, 1, 97) across all 40 cycle-day columns.

# Resources

At www.makingbabiesprogram.com, you will find links to the following URLs, along with lots more helpful information and advice on conceiving as naturally as possible. And we want to remind you about one of our favorite resources: the quiz on our Web site that will help you quickly and clearly identify your fertility type.

## Finding Other Good Books

*Conceptions and Misconceptions: The Informed Consumer's Guide Through the Maze of In Vitro Fertilization and Assisted Reproduction Techniques,* 2nd ed., by Arthur L. Wisot, MD, and David R. Meldrum, MD

*Conquering Infertility: Dr. Alice Domar's Mind/Body Guide to Enhancing Fertility and Coping with Infertility* by Alice D. Domar and Alice Lesch Kelly

*Healing Mind, Healthy Woman: Using the Mind-Body Connection to Manage Stress and Take Control of Your Life* by Alice D. Domar, PhD, and Henry Dreher

*Inconceivable: A Woman's Triumph over Despair and Statistics* by Julia Indichova

*The Infertility Cure: The Ancient Chinese Wellness Program for Getting Pregnant and Having Healthy Babies* by Randine Lewis

*Preventing Miscarriage: The Good News* by Jonathan Scher, MD, and Carol Dix

*Taking Charge of Your Fertility: The Definitive Guide to Natural Birth Control, Pregnancy Achievement, and Reproductive Health,* 10th ed., by Toni Weschler

*The Unofficial Guide to Getting Pregnant* by Joan Liebmann-Smith, PhD, Jacqueline Nardi Egan, and John J. Stangel, MD

## Finding Physicians and Other Practitioners

www.americanpregnancy.org/infertility/index.htm

American Pregnancy Association, Irving, Texas. Directories of infertility specialists, genetic counselors, acupuncturists, chiropractors, and massage therapists searchable by city and state or ZIP code.

www.arvigomassage.com

The Arvigo Institute, Antrim, New Hampshire. Click "Practitioner Listings" to find someone trained in Arvigo techniques, by state or country.

www.fertilegardenmassage.com

Fertile Garden Massage, Nicole Kruck, LMT, New York, New York. A licensed massage therapist certified in the Arvigo Mayan Massage technique and a fertility massage specialist, Nicole Kruck provided the massage information for *Making Babies*.

www.ihr.com/infertility/ ·

Internet Health Resources. Directories of all kinds of service providers, including natural and "alternative" health care providers, IVF clinics, egg donor programs, tubal and vasectomy reversal doctors, sperm banks, male infertility specialists, pharmacies, surrogacy programs, counselors, PGD programs, adoption agencies, and lawyers.

www.nccaom.org

National Certification Commission for Acupuncture and Oriental Medicine (NCCAOM), Jacksonville, Florida. Click the search button under "Are you looking for an acupuncturist or an Oriental medicine practitioner?" to search the database by name, state, or ZIP code.

www.nine-infertility.org

National Infertility Network Exchange (NINE), East Meadow, New York. Professional referrals available to members.

www.nlm.nih.gov/medlineplus/infertility

Medline Plus by the National Library of Medicine and the National Institutes of Health. Provides links to directories of reproductive endocrinologists (Society for Reproductive Endocrinology and Infertility), reproductive surgeons (American Society for Reproductive Medicine), and urologists (American Urological Association).

www.reprodsurgery.org

Society of Reproductive Surgeons, Birmingham, Alabama. Click on "Find a Reproductive Surgeon in Your Area" to search the database by state.

www.resolve.org

RESOLVE: The National Infertility Association, McLean, Virginia. The directory of services requires registration, which is free.

www.sart.org

Society for Assisted Reproductive Technology, Birmingham, Alabama. Click "Patient Benefits," then the "Find a Clinic" tab to search by state or ZIP code.

www.smru.org

Society for Male Reproduction and Urology, Birmingham, Alabama. Directory of members is searchable by state. Click on "For Patients," then "Find an SMRU Member in your area."

www.socrei.org

Society for Reproductive Endocrinology and Infertility. Click on the "Find Members" link for a database of obstetrician-gynecologists with advanced training in reproductive endocrinology and infertility, searchable by state.

www.theafa.org

American Fertility Association, New York, New York. See under "resources" for directories, by state, of physicians, therapists, and other professionals with fertility expertise, including providers of all types with particular expertise in LGBT issues.

www.urologyhealth.org

American Urological Association Foundation, Linthicum, Maryland. Click on "Find a Urologist."

### Finding Clinic Statistics

www.cdc.gov/art

Centers for Disease Control and Prevention's annual Assisted Reproductive Technology Report, with national summaries and clinic-by-clinic results going back to 1995, as well as a lesson on how to read the reports.

www.sart.org

Society for Assisted Reproductive Technology, Birmingham, Alabama. Includes a database of clinic statistics searchable by state or ZIP code.

### Finding Support

www.americanpregnancy.org/infertility/index.htm

American Pregnancy Association, Irving, Texas. Listing of support groups searchable by city and state or ZIP code (click on "Find Emotional Support"), and a section on working through the emotions of infertility.

www.fertileheart.com

Julia Indichova, Fertile Heart Studio, Woodstock, New York. Message boards and support groups (including phone support).

www.ihr.com/infertility/

Internet Health Resources. Links to an array of support groups.

www.inciid.org

The InterNational Council on Infertility Information Dissemination (INCIID; pronounced "inside"), Arlington, Virginia. Expert forums and peer chat groups on infertility, pregnancy loss, adoption, living child-free, and more.

www.infertility.bellaonline.com

BellaOnline: The Voice of Women. Click "Infertility Support" for a list of sites offering help, advice, and support.

www.nine-infertility.org

National Infertility Network Exchange (NINE), East Meadow, New York. Support groups and local chapters, and "the NINE line," which connects people with similar concerns via phone and Internet.

www.parenting.ivillage.com

iVillage's Pregnancy and Parenting section has a Trying to Conceive subsection with active message boards.

www.resolve.org

RESOLVE: The National Infertility Association, McLean, Virginia. Find local chapters and support groups, including online groups.

www.theafa.org

American Fertility Association, New York, New York. Online and in-person support groups and message boards. Toll-free support line: 888-917-3777.


### Finding More Information

We may not always agree with the opinions and advice on these sites, but they all offer much useful information when consulted in conjunction with our book.

www.americanpregnancy.org/infertility/index.htm

American Pregnancy Association, Irving, Texas. Information on male and female infertility; alternative treatments, including acupuncture and herbs; and reproductive technologies.

www.asrm.org/Patients/FactSheets/fact.html

American Society for Reproductive Medicine, Birmingham, Alabama. Patient information area on common fertility diagnoses.

www.easternharmonyclinic.com

Eastern Harmony Acupuncture and Herbal Clinic, founded by Dr. Randine Lewis, Houston, Texas. Information on acupuncture, herbs, and fertility and related women's health concerns, with links to medical journal articles.

www.fertilityplus.org/faq/infertility.html

Fertility Plus: "Information *for* TTC couples . . . written *by* TTC couples." Information on infertility and treatment, links to related newsgroups and other resources, and an extensive listing of acronyms and abbreviations to help you decipher both Internet slang and technical medical terms.

www.ihr.com/infertility/

Internet Health Resources. Information on infertility and treatment and related news items, plus information on infertility financing, legal issues, and social and psychological concerns. Section on infertility research programs, including clinical trials that provide treatment.

www.inciid.org

The InterNational Council on Infertility Information Dissemination (INCIID; pronounced "inside"), Arlington, Virginia. Wide variety of patient information, including a long glossary of acronyms to clue you in to both medical and Internet abbreviations and slang.

www.infertility.about.com

About.com. A wide array of information on fertility and coping with infertility.

www.infertility.bellaonline.com

BellaOnline: The Voice of Women. Wide-ranging articles and message boards on specific conditions related to infertility, alternative therapies, adoption, coping with infertility, and more.

www.nichd.nih.gov/health/topics/infertility_fertility.cfm

National Institute of Child Health and Human Development (NICHD), Rockville, Maryland. General information and links to ongoing clinical trials.

www.nine-infertility.org

National Infertility Network Exchange (NINE), East Meadow, New York. Informational meetings, fact sheets, and other resources for members.

www.nlm.nih.gov/medlineplus/infertility.html

Medline Plus. Authoritative information collected by the National Library of Medicine and the National Institutes of Health. Extensive links for the latest news on fertility, and information on diagnosis and symptoms, specific conditions, treatment, coping with infertility, legal issues, and relevant organizations. Links to ongoing clinical trials, research, and journal articles.

www.orientalhealthsolutions.com

Oriental Health Solutions, Durham, North Carolina. Information on fertility and related health concerns, acupuncture research, and treatment statistics.

www.parenting.ivillage.com

iVillage's Pregnancy and Parenting section has a Trying to Conceive subsection with a wide range of topics, including a column by Toni Weschler (author of *Taking Charge of Your Fertility*).

www.resolve.org

RESOLVE: The National Infertility Association, McLean, Virginia. Resource library, registration required.

www.sart.org

Society for Assisted Reproductive Technology, Birmingham, Alabama. Patient information about ART.

www.smru.org

Society for Male Reproduction and Urology, Birmingham, Alabama. Fact sheets about specific male reproductive disorders.

www.taoofwellness.com

Tao of Wellness Chinese medicine clinic run by Dr. Daoshing Ni, Santa Monica, California. Information on Chinese medicine in general and fertility in particular.

www.theafa.org

American Fertility Association, New York, New York. Information about trying to conceive, infertility prevention, and family building, including (but not limited to) some information and resources specifically geared toward same-sex couples.

www.urologyhealth.org

American Urological Association Foundation, Linthicum, Maryland. Click for more information under the "Patient Information" tab, then click "Adult Conditions" to find topics pertaining to male infertility.

www.yourtotalhealth.ivillage.com/fertility-issues

Your Total Health, by NBC and iVillage, has a Fertility Issues Center.

## Finding Products

www.bioorigyn.com

Pre-Seed. A list of where to buy Pre-Seed "fertility-friendly intimate moisturizer" locally — or order directly online.

www.blessedherbs.com

Blessed Herbs. For the monthlong herbal detox sold at YinOva and other herbal products.

www.ihr.com/infertility/

Internet Health Resources. Sources for fertility monitors, ovulation predictor kits, personal ovulation microscopes, fertility supplements, and more.

www.metagenics.com

Metagenics. For probiotics and other nutritional products.

www.quickspice.com

Quickspice. For rolls of hawthorn flakes (also known as "haw flakes"), if you can't get to a Chinatown shop.

## Finding the Authors

www.samidavid.com

Dr. Sami David, MD, PC, New York, New York, a reproductive endocrinologist and gynecologist specializing in the treatment of infertility with minimal pharmaceutical intervention.

www.yinovacenter.com

Jill Blakeway, The YinOva Center, New York, New York, specializing in complementary care for women and children. The Web site includes articles about alternative medicine and infertility.

# Acknowledgments

Special thanks to Jill Blakeway, my coauthor and dear friend, whose vision and encouragement inspired the creation of this book and much more. I would like to thank my staff of thirty years — Catherine, Barbara, Dorothy, and Rosanne — who have been devoted to my patients and to me every day. Also special thanks to Colleen Kapklein, who spent countless hours in the creation of this book; to our literary agent, Daniel Greenberg, who recognized the importance of this book for the general public; and to Tracy Behar at Little, Brown, who has brought the final draft to fruition. — S.D.

Thank you to everyone who has worked so hard on this book. In particular I am grateful to writer Colleen Kapklein for her patience, talent, and good humor, and to Dr. Sami David, a man who is rightly loved by thousands of patients for his caring, wise counsel. Thank you also to our patient and meticulous editor, Tracy Behar, and the many talented hands at Little, Brown who pitched in to bring this book to fruition: Barb Jatkola, Carolyn O'Keefe, Keith Hayes, Christina Rodriguez, and the many others working diligently behind the scenes. It truly takes a village. I'm indebted, too, to our kind editor at Virago, Rowan Cope; our fabulous agent, Daniel Greenberg; and the very capable Monika Verma.

I am grateful to my family for their love and support, especially my father, Gordon, who is always supportive and encouraging; my late mother, Ann, who worked hard to give me wings; my daughter, Emma, whose boldness and adventurous spirit make me proud; and my husband, Noah Rubinstein, a gifted acupuncturist and a solid source of practical advice and loving counsel.

The wonderful women of the YinOva Center in New York City have been a constant source of inspiration and advice. Marie Amato, Margaret Sikowitz, Liz Carlson, Beth White, Jane Titus, Sarah Rappaport, Melani Bolyai, Sharon Yeung, and Deborah Valentin are talented practitioners and wise, warm women who fill our office with love and humor. I thank them from the bottom of my heart.

I am indebted to many teachers of Chinese medicine, especially Z'ev Rosenburg, Alex Tiberi, Bob Damone, and Greg Bantick, who taught me to be rigorous in my practice of this beautiful medicine. The late Dr. Yitian Ni had a huge influence on my studies, and I have much appreciation for my beloved teachers Colleen Timmons and Carol Elliot, who modeled for me a way of practicing medicine with an open and loving heart and inspired me to try to be like them. I thank them all.

Several people read sections of this manuscript and gave insightful comments. They include acupuncturist and fertility specialist Caroline Radice, medical research expert Kell Julliard, and chiropractor Dr. Steven Margolin. Thanks also to Nicole Kruck, licensed massage therapist and all-around wise woman, for information about massage for fertility; Kerry Kane for getting the word out; and Greg Barton for working so hard on the illustrations.

Last but by no means least, thanks to my patients, current and past, who have inspired me with their courage. I have learned so much from them all. — J.B.

# Index